The Anthropology of AIDS

UNIVERSITY PRESS OF FLORIDA

Florida A&M University, Tallahassee
Florida Atlantic University, Boca Raton
Florida Gulf Coast University, Ft. Myers
Florida International University, Miami
Florida State University, Tallahassee
New College of Florida, Sarasota
University of Central Florida, Orlando
University of Florida, Gainesville
University of North Florida, Jacksonville
University of South Florida, Tampa
University of West Florida, Pensacola

The Anthropology of
AIDS

A Global Perspective

Patricia Whelehan

with contributions by Thomas Budd

University Press of Florida
Gainesville/Tallahassee/Tampa/Boca Raton
Pensacola/Orlando/Miami/Jacksonville/Ft. Myers/Sarasota

14   13   12   11   10   09   6   5   4   3   2   1

Library of Congress Cataloging-in-Publication Data
Whelehan, Patricia.
The anthropology of aids: a global perspective/Patricia Whelehan
with contributions by Thomas Budd.
p. cm.
Includes bibliographical references and index.
ISBN 978-0-8130-3292-4 (alk. paper)
1. Medical anthropology. 2. AIDS (Disease)—Epidemiology. 3. HIV
infections—Epidemiology. I. Budd, Thomas. II. Title.
GN296.W47 2009   306.4'619–dc22
2008044685

The University Press of Florida is the scholarly publishing agency for the
State University System of Florida, comprising Florida A&M University,
Florida Atlantic University, Florida Gulf Coast University, Florida In-
ternational University, Florida State University, New College of Florida,
University of Central Florida, University of Florida, University of North
Florida, University of South Florida, and University of West Florida.

University Press of Florida
15 Northwest 15th Street
Gainesville, FL 32611–2079
http://www.upf.com

John Francis Caravantes, October 23, 1957–January 5, 2003

John, you were my protector, a champion, a challenger, and the best "best boyfriend" any girl could have. You gave me a home and a place from which to conduct research, including one book, *An Anthropological Perspective on Prostitution,* several articles, and many discussions for ideas for this book, *The Anthropology of AIDS: A Global Perspective.*

Find my other soul mates, Andres and Doug, also lost to AIDS. It is up to us from your world to survive. It is up to me through this book to carry on your spirit and passion to educate, raise awareness, and, if at all possible, prevent just one new infection.

Contents

Illustrations

Figures

Tables

Abbreviations

ACTUP	AIDS Coalition to Unleash Power
ADA	Americans with Disabilities Act
ADAP	AIDS drug assistance programs
AIDS	Acquired Immune Deficiency Syndrome
AMA	American Medical Association
A/PI	Asian/Pacific Islanders
ART	Antiretroviral therapy(ies)
ARVs	Antiretrovirals
ATS	Alternative test site/anonymous test site
AZT076	Zidovudine 076
CALPEP	California Prostitute/Prevention Education Program
CBOs	Community-based organizations
CDC	Centers for Disease Control and Prevention
ELISA	Enzyme-Linked Immunosorbent Assay
FBOs	Faith-based organizations
FDA	Food and Drug Administration
FDC	Fixed Dosage Combination
FTMs/F2Ms	Female to males (transsexuals/transgendereds)
GRID	Gay-related immune deficiency
HAART	Highly Active Antiretroviral Therapy
HIV	Human immunodeficiency virus
HIV-	HIV negative
HIV+	HIV positive
HTLV	Human T-cell lymphotropic virus
IDU	Injection drug use
IDUs	Injection drug users
KAB	Knowledge, Attitudes, and Behavior model
KS	Kaposi's sarcoma
LAV	Lymphadenopathy-associated virus
MC	Male circumcision
MHC	Major histocompatibility complex
mRNA	Messenger RNA
MSM	Men who have sex with men

MSW	Men who have sex with women
MTF	Male to female (transmission of HIV)
MTFs/M2Fs	Male to females (transsexuals/transgendereds)
MTCT	Mother-to-child transmission
NIDA	National Institute of Drug Abuse
NIH	National Institutes of Health
NIMH	National Institute of Mental Health
N/SEPs	Needle/syringe exchange programs
NGOs	Nongovernmental organizations
NGU	Nongonococcal urethritis
OIs	Opportunistic infections
P-A	Penile-anal intercourse
PCP	Pneumocystis carinii pneumonia
PEP	Postexposure prophylaxis
PEPFAR	President's Emergency Plan for AIDS Relief
PhRMA	Pharmaceutical Research and Manufacturers of America
PI	Protease inhibitor
PLWH/As	Persons living with HIV/AIDS
PNAP	Partner Notification Assistance Program
P-V	Penile-vaginal intercourse
RT	Reverse transcriptase
SIV	Simian immunodeficiency virus
STDs/STIs	Sexually transmitted diseases/sexually transmitted infections
TAC	Treatment action campaign
TASO	The AIDS Service Organization (Uganda)
TB	Tuberculosis
TGs	Transgendereds
TSs	Transsexuals
TVs	Transvestites
WHO	World Health Organization
WSM	Women who have sex with men
WSW	Women who have sex with women

Preface and Acknowledgments

Since the recognition of HIV/AIDS more than twenty years ago, there have been volumes written on the topic. To date, however, there have been few textbooks written on the subject for liberal arts undergraduates. This book synthesizes data to present undergraduates with an overview of the epidemic from an anthropological perspective. This perspective integrates biocultural, gender, social, political, and economic factors in exploring HIV/AIDS epidemiologically, biomedically, and sexually, as well as how the epidemic impacts various groups and societies. This text can be supplemented with ethnographies, case studies, and edited sources about HIV/AIDS.

I would like to gratefully acknowledge institutions, groups, and individuals who made this book possible. First, I would like to thank SUNY–Potsdam, specifically the Anthropology Department, the dean of the School of Arts and Sciences, the provost, and the president for granting me a semester's sabbatical to write the first draft of this book. That time was invaluable. I also received a Research and Creative Endeavors grant from the Office of Research and Sponsored Programs at SUNY–Potsdam to defray some of the costs of manuscript preparation. The University Press of Florida, specifically editor John Byram, offered me a contract for the book early in its development. Thank you for your confidence in this project and for your insightful comments on drafts of the first chapters.

Appreciation goes to the fall 2002, 2003, 2004, and 2006 Anthropology of AIDS classes who read and commented on chapter drafts. Your dedication and commitment to the course and this project have helped considerably. I would like to recognize my "group of 7": Kathy Ladue, Susan Stebbins, Rachel Galgoul, David Barrett, Joyce Rice, Edward Hosley, and Linda Nelson, who once again provided invaluable criticisms of yet another book for me. Student research assistants and interns Amy Heimroth, Sarah Seeley, Mary Bailey, Amanda Pryce, Rebecca Polmateer, and Carol Michelfelder spent hours compiling and correcting the bibliography. I literally could not have completed this manuscript without your help. Sylvia Macey transformed chapters into presentable camera-ready copy form. Thank you all very much. Any errors of commission or omission rest solely with the author.

1

An Anthropological Perspective
on HIV/AIDS

CHAPTER HIGHLIGHTS INCLUDE

An overview of medical anthropology as a subfield of anthropology
and its place within anthropology
A discussion of the anthropological concepts, methodologies, and
theoretical orientations found in this book
An observation that an anthropological and medical anthropological
perspective can help us to understand and address the worldwide
AIDS epidemic

The HIV/AIDS Crisis

The bubonic plague (Black Death—Middle Ages (fourteenth century)
Smallpox—Late agrarian age (seventeenth century through the
twentieth century)
Tuberculosis—Industrial Revolution (nineteenth century through
the twenty-first century)
HIV/AIDS—Late twentieth and twenty-first centuries

These four diseases are some of the most virulent that humans have en-
countered. Before the virus's impact peaks, **HIV/AIDS** will take a greater
toll on the human species proportionately and in absolute numbers than
the bubonic plague, smallpox, and tuberculosis combined, according to
the United Nations and the Office of the Surgeon General (www.aarg.org
2001; Madhok et al. 1994; Office of the Surgeon General 2001). Smallpox has been eradicated, and the bubonic plague still occurs sporadically.
Tuberculosis (TB) continues to affect people in nonindustrialized societ-

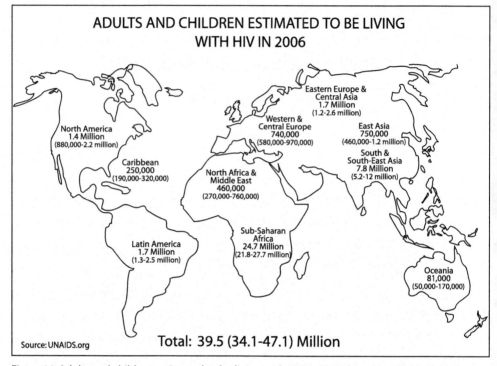

Figure 1.1. Adults and children estimated to be living with HIV in 2006, by region (Joint United Nations Programme on HIV/AIDS, May 2008, hereafter UNAIDS, 2008).

ies and compounds the seriousness of HIV/AIDS where both are found. Figures 1.1 through 1.3 indicate the spread of HIV around the world as of 2006 and the projected occurrence of HIV in key areas of the world as of 2010.

Human Immunodeficiency Virus (HIV) is the virus that causes **Acquired Immune Deficiency Syndrome (AIDS)**. AIDS, the end result of having HIV, is a collection of diseases and compromised immune states that almost always results in death if left untreated. Worldwide, AIDS kills more than 50 percent of the people infected with HIV. Global estimates since the beginning of the **epidemic** state that between 33 million and 57 million people have either HIV or AIDS (Merson and Dayton 2002: 13; UNAIDS 2007). Every day, 16,000 new infections occur (Sarche 2003:D5). Currently, HIV/AIDS is most widespread in sub-Saharan Africa and India.

If people are not personally aware of someone who has HIV or AIDS, it is easy to believe that this disease is someone else's problem. However,

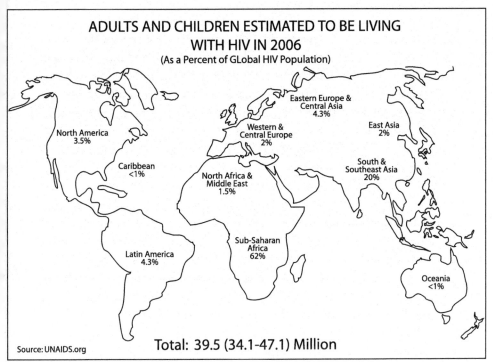

Figure 1.2. Adults and children estimated to be living with HIV in 2006, as a percentage of global HIV population (UNAIDS, 2008).

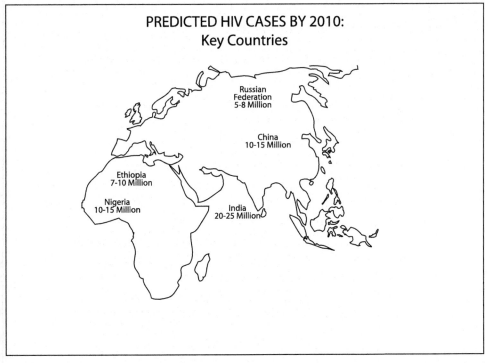

Figure 1.3. Predicted HIV cases by 2010: key countries (UNAIDS, 2008).

HIV/AIDS is a global concern. This disease affects the core of the societies where it is found, particularly in places such as sub-Saharan Africa and India, both of which have a large number of people infected as well as a significant percentage of these populations infected and affected by the disease (see chapter 2). The impact of the disease cuts across age, gender, sexual orientation and behavior, and sociocultural boundaries. It affects individuals and groups throughout the life cycle from conception through old age. The impact of HIV/AIDS crosses the sociopolitical, economic, religious and spiritual, and sexual domains of societies (Herdt et al. 1990). HIV/AIDS is an important topic of study because of how widespread and deadly it is, devastating societies and subcultures around the world. Given the global dispersal of the HIV/AIDS epidemic, it is a suitable topic for anthropologists to study. Anthropologists have specific skills that can help reduce infection, support HIV testing, and assist groups where AIDS occurs. These skills, discussed in this chapter, include in-depth knowledge of the values, beliefs, and symbols of a group as well as their behaviors; a relativistic perspective in which norms and practices are viewed within the context of the entire life of the group; and a comparative approach to data so that similarities and differences within and between groups can be assessed through time and space.

Anthropology, Medical Anthropology, and AIDS

This textbook addresses the HIV/AIDS epidemic from an anthropological perspective.

What is an anthropological perspective?
What is the relevance of anthropology and medical anthropology overall to the HIV/AIDS epidemic?

The answers to these questions form the core of this chapter.

Anthropology, the study of human behavior, formally began as a discipline in Europe and the United States in the eighteenth and nineteenth centuries (Kottak 2000). In both Europe and the United States, the discipline was largely academic and theoretical. In Europe, anthropology focused on understanding the behavior of colonized peoples in Africa, India, Southeast Asia, Melanesia, and Micronesia, to more effectively use resources in those areas. In the United States, anthropology's focus was chronicling and recording the "disappearing" native groups in the Americas.

Over the course of the past two hundred years, the nature, focus, interests, and research populations of anthropologists have shifted and expanded. With few, if any, totally traditional groups left that have not been influenced by industrialized contact and globalization, anthropologists have broadened their research base to include peasant societies, industrialized populations, and various subcultures in Euro-American and non-industrialized societies (Kottak 2000; Hahn 1995; Kleinman 2000).

Anthropology, as a discipline, includes five major fields:

ethnology or cultural anthropology, the study of living human groups;

biological anthropology, which includes the study of living primates, the human fossil record, and biological variations among groups;

linguistics, the study of languages within and between groups;

archaeology, the study of both historic and prehistoric populations from physical or material evidence and archival information; and

applied anthropology, the practical applications of an anthropological perspective to problems within and between cultures (Kottak 2000; Podolefsky and Brown 2002).

Since the early days of the AIDS epidemic in the 1980s, most anthropological involvement in the crisis has encompassed cultural and applied anthropology (www.aarg.org 2003). Medical anthropology is a subfield of cultural anthropology. However, some medical anthropologists are biological anthropologists who have interests in disease patterns.

Medical Anthropology

Medical anthropology dates to the nineteenth century. Anthropologists initially recorded the pharmacopoeia of indigenous groups, who the healers in the groups were, and their practices (Hahn 1995; Kleinman 2000; Northridge and Mack 2002). Currently, medical anthropologists also include the study of diseases within modern and ancient populations, conduct cross-cultural (that is, outside mainstream U.S. culture) growth and development studies, and specialize in certain diseases and illnesses cross-culturally or within populations (Kleinman 2000; Hahn 1995). They work in both academic and applied settings (Omohundro 2000; Joralemon 2006).

Medical anthropologists have been involved personally and professionally in HIV/AIDS efforts since the 1980s. The AIDS and Anthropology Research Group was formed in 1987 (www.aarg.org 1988), and a select group of anthropologists met in 1990 to organize and formalize their research and to provide support to each other (Herdt et al. 1990; Herrell 1991). Anthropologists who work with HIV/AIDS interventions are found in a variety of settings within and outside of academia. Their work includes data collection and education and prevention efforts in international and U.S. public health research. Medical anthropologists work in hospitals and clinics. They investigate U.S. and **cross-cultural** dimensions of sex, gender, sexual orientation, drug usage, and ecological factors that influence vulnerability to infection and the course of the disease in infected populations (American Anthropological Association 1997; www.aarg.org 2003).

Much of the medical anthropological work with HIV/AIDS is practice oriented and involves the subfield of applied anthropology. Applied anthropology does not disregard theory or academic involvement and research; rather, it seeks to use anthropological perspectives based on theory and research in practical situations and to solve problems. Many applied anthropologists also work in settings similar to medical anthropologists (Podolefsky and Brown 2002; Omohundro 2000; Joralemon 2006).

Applied medical anthropologists working in HIV/AIDS can be cultural liaisons between individuals and groups affected by the epidemic and local, regional, national, or international government agencies such as hospitals, clinics, and AIDS service organizations. These anthropologists may act as interpreters of cultural beliefs and practices of the groups being served by various agencies. Medical and applied anthropologists have experience with identifying and understanding the values and beliefs that underlie individual, group, and societal norms and behaviors. They know how to access local leaders and political power bases and how to interpret the unique culture to others (Podolefsky and Brown 2002; Vollmer 2000; Joralemon 2006). In a statement issued by the American Anthropological Association in 1997 at the "National Institutes of Health Consensus Development Conference," the association focused on anthropological involvement in HIV/AIDS since the 1980s and anthropology's unique ability to integrate and identify "contextual factors that predispose individuals and communities to HIV" (American Anthropological Association 1997).

Concepts

The roles of anthropology in addressing the AIDS epidemic are diverse. Since the 1980s, anthropologists have supported and encouraged an ethnographic, culture-specific, and culture-sensitive approach to HIV interventions that reflect community norms and values (Herrell 1991; American Anthropological Association 1997; Parker and Ehrhardt 2001; Parker, Barbarosa, and Aggleton, 2000). Applying an anthropological perspective to the study of HIV/AIDS involves having an understanding of anthropological concepts, methodology, and theory. Key anthropological concepts related to an examination of HIV/AIDS include

Culture—The learned, patterned beliefs, values, and symbols that are shared within a group.

Society—The learned, patterned, and shared organizational structures, behaviors, and rules found within a group.

Evolution—The study of how groups of organisms change and adapt to their environments over time.

Holism—A society's behaviors, beliefs, values, and customs as they relate to each other. The interdependency among the social, economic, political, material and expressive, and spiritual sectors of a society.

Cross-cultural comparison—The examination of cultures and societies holistically or by specific structures to understand the patterns of similarities and differences among groups.

Cultural relativism—The ability to understand cultures in terms of their own values, beliefs, norms, structures, and behaviors without imposing an external evaluation or judgment, that is, avoiding ethnocentrism (see below).

Ethnocentrism—The practice of using one's own worldview, values, beliefs, and norms to judge and evaluate another group's culture.

Emic and etic viewpoints—The examination of a culture either from the insider's point of view (emic) or from an external point of view such as that of the researcher, scientist, or anthropologist (etic) (Kottak 2000).

These concepts are best understood as operating along a continuum, and some, such as cultural relativism and ethnocentrism, become embroiled in discussions of universal or culture-specific human rights and generate their own debate within anthropology. The difficulties in maintaining cultural relativism and avoiding ethnocentrism, for example, will come to light in the chapters on HIV testing, sex, and drugs. However, incorporating all of these concepts in examining HIV/AIDS anthropologically illustrates what a variety of individuals and cultures share in the experience of HIV/AIDS, as well as the unique impact the virus has on diverse societies.

Methodology

The keystone of anthropological research is **participant-observation** (Omohundro 2000; Kottak 2000; Hahn 1995). The participant-observation approach to learning about a culture entails spending extended periods of time with the group or society that the anthropologist is studying. The anthropologist interacts with the members of the group while maintaining an observational stance. This approach involves observing and participating in the daily life and ritual aspects of the group that occur during the anthropologist's fieldwork, while remaining culturally relativistic. The anthropologist uses open-ended and structured interviews that can include questionnaires, interviews with **key informants** (those members of the culture who have specific or specialized knowledge of the group), and historical or archival materials when they are available. Anthropologists may also follow networks of people's interactions to locate new sources of data and to determine patterns among individuals and between groups. Use of networks can be particularly valuable for learning about sexual and drug-using behaviors (Singer 2005; Becklerleg et al. 2005; Clatts 1999; Needle et al. 1998). Participant-observation can incorporate the use of laptops, cameras, and tape recorders to record and obtain data.

Participant-observation provides what the anthropologist Robert Hahn refers to as **"thick data,"** which encompasses the nuances, details, comparisons, and changes in behavior and interactions that occur in a group (Hahn 1995). These "thick data" entail observations of behavior that lie beneath superficial interactions and what people say they do. These data allow the anthropologist to compare ideal behavior, which comprises the norms of the group and what people say they do, with real behavior, or what people actually do. Participant-observation provides texture, depth, and context to data that can be obtained quantitatively, such as the results of surveys, questionnaires, and structured, closed interviews. It provides observation of daily life over time, so that variations in norms and behaviors, rituals, and conflicts are experienced. Since human behavior does not always correspond to quantitative predictions, participant-observation provides anthropologists with a way to record society in action, not just measure the results of behavior. Participant-observation provides qualitative data that can be used as an organizational system of checks and balances for quantitative data (Carrier and Bolton 1991; American Anthropological Association 1997; Joralemon 2006).

As with any methodology, there is the potential in participant-observation for researcher bias and interpretational error. Anthropologists do not "go native." They rarely, if ever, become fully integrated members of the groups they study but instead maintain an observer role. The group granting access to the anthropologist does not usually accept the anthropologist as a fully integrated member of the group.

1.1

To clarify these ideas of real and ideal behavior and "thick data," think of these concepts in terms of what people are "supposed" to do compared to what they actually do. Marriage can be used to illustrate these differences in the United States. People getting married agree to "till death us do part": ideal behavior. However, 50 percent of our marriages end in divorce: real behavior.

By spending extended periods of time with the members of the group, anthropologists can check the validity of their initial observations as well as note discrepancies in people's behaviors and words. Lastly, anthropologists are trained to look at the assumptions and biases they may bring with them, to critically examine theoretical orientations that may influence their research, and to acknowledge potential sources of bias.

For example, I am a medical anthropologist, a certified sex educator and therapist, and a certified HIV test counselor in California and New York. I have been professionally and personally involved in HIV education and prevention efforts since 1984. I believe that it is professionally and ethically responsible to state my biases and perspectives at the outset.

Based on my research, applied work, and experience, I bring the following perspectives and biases to this book:

I take a cultural relativistic and culture-specific approach to issues concerning sexuality, gender, the concept of sexual orientation, women, and risks for infection.

I believe that intervention programs concerned with prevention, HIV testing, and treatments need to be culturally sensitive and appropriate to be effective.

I believe that grassroots, community, and peer-based efforts (emic) stand a greater chance of preventing infection, promoting HIV testing, and providing treatment to those with HIV than do those efforts imposed externally by outside agencies or groups (etic).

I believe that a culturally aware approach is necessary to acknowledge and respect local community norms and power structures among the targeted groups when developing and implementing prevention efforts.

I believe that ethnocentrism toward people at risk for HIV/AIDS in the United States and cross-culturally has impeded intervention efforts. Ethnocentrism has been expressed as **homophobia** (fear of homosexuals), **erotophobia** (fear of sexuality), sexism, and racism.

I believe that politics disguised as science and researchers who have not explored their own biases and assumptions have negatively impacted the course of the epidemic in the United States and cross-culturally (see Shilts 1987; Thomas 2001; Vernon 2001).

Anthropologists use both inductive and deductive approaches to research. An **inductive approach**, which continues to be the guiding force of current anthropological research, involves gathering data and searching for patterns within that data. From there, generalizations and descriptions of the patterns are made. The advantage of this approach is that analyses and generalizations remain close to the data and can be easily checked. An inductive approach provides descriptive data and can reduce researcher bias because the researcher is not necessarily imposing a theoretical model on the data. The major disadvantages of an inductive approach are that generalizations are limited to the data collected and it is time and labor intensive.

In contrast, a **deductive approach** often starts with theories. A deductive approach is the major one used in the natural sciences, as well as in psychology and sociology during much of the twentieth century. Theories are generalizations or statements that explain relationships between variables. Hypotheses are assumptions that provide the raw materials for testing the validity of theories. Evolutionary and Freudian theories are examples of the deductive approach. They provide broad explanations of how life forms change (evolution) and about human psycho-social development (Freud). Researchers start with a theoretical model and then test that theory with research on specific populations. A deductive approach provides quantitative data and works well with large populations and surveys. It tends to reflect ideal behavior and lends itself to statistical manipulation and analyses. Much of HIV/AIDS research, particularly that conducted in industrialized societies (which is derived from the basic sciences and biomedicine), is deductive and quantitative.

There are disadvantages to a deductive approach. Data may reflect what people say rather than what they do. There is a lack of cultural context for data. Importantly, biases may be introduced with a given theoretical orientation. For example, during the first decade of the AIDS epidemic in the United States, the frequent conceptualization of AIDS as a "gay disease"—and the initial label of it as **GRID**, or **Gay-Related Immune Deficiency**—limited awareness, knowledge, prevention, and treatment efforts (Shilts 1987; Vernon 2001). Women, infants and children, hemophiliacs, **injection drug users (IDUs)**, Latinos, African Americans, and members of other groups contracted HIV but were underrecognized and underdiagnosed because of the bias of AIDS as a "gay white boys'" disease (Shilts 1987; Schneider and Stoller eds. 1995; Roth and Fuller eds. 1998; Anderson 2001).

While excellent for conducting surveys with large groups and amassing quantitative data used in statistical analysis, a deductive approach is less effective than the qualitative inductive approach in providing the thick data discussed earlier (Hahn 1995; Herrell 1991). Thick data are important for prevention, intervention, and treatment efforts because they include the context and depth of human behavior and beliefs. Thick data provide information on attitudes, values, beliefs, and real behavior that can impact the efficacy of prevention, intervention, and treatment efforts (Hahn 1995).

A combined methodological approach is necessary when dealing with an epidemic as complicated as HIV/AIDS. Combining qualitative and quantitative, deductive and inductive methodologies provides

a comprehensive picture of the population under study;

a comparison of ideal and real behaviors that can provide the most accurate set of data;

"thick data" that provide in-depth cultural context and specificity, covering perceptions, beliefs, values, and attitudes (emic approach);

quantitative data on large groups that can be used as is and comparatively (etic approach);

a counter to the inherent weaknesses in either approach alone;

a large amount of survey data obtained relatively quickly and cheaply that complements the deeper data obtained from the more labor-intensive and costly qualitative data;

the data necessary to establish, implement, and evaluate prevention, intervention, and treatment programs in the present (synchronically) and over time (diachronically); and

the ability to develop program responses and interventions that are culturally sensitive and appropriate to the population to increase their efficacy.

Theoretical Orientations

Theories from several decades of medical and biological anthropological research are useful in understanding HIV and AIDS. An anthropological perspective on HIV/AIDS uses different theories to explain the global nature of the disease. These include a **systems/ecological approach** (Armelagos, Goodman, and Jacob, 1978, 1990), **critical medical anthropology** (Farmer 1992; Basu, Mate, and Farmer, 2000), and an understanding of our vulnerability to pathogens (Thomas 1984).

A systems/ecological approach posits a holistic interdependency among the individual, that person's culture, and the larger environment. This interdependency operates on a feedback mechanism in which changes in one of the parts affects changes in the other. The culture, through its system of rules and beliefs, mediates between the individual and the larger environment and aids in adapting the individual to the environment. Cultural artifacts, such as shelter, tools, and clothing, and means of food selection, preparation, and distribution are simple examples of this feedback mechanism. Resources available in the larger environment that the group defines and recognizes as useful, beneficial, or dangerous are incorporated by the individual into daily symbolic and material life.

George Armelagos, Mary Ryan, and Thomas Leatherman (1990) believe that an ecological model applies to understanding disease, including HIV/AIDS. In humans, cultural systems affect the disease process and diseases alter cultural adaptation. Ecological models of disease are holistic, incorporating the pathogen, the individual, and the group.

Relative to HIV/AIDS susceptibility, the larger environment can impact the types of **opportunistic infections (OIs)** that an HIV-infected individual may contract. Opportunistic infections are diseases usually found only in people with compromised immune systems. Fungal infections constitute one category of OIs. Some fungal infections are more common in subtropical regions or econiches than in northern areas of the world. Tuberculosis, the most common OI associated with AIDS, is found in sub-Saharan Africa, in South America, and in poverty-stricken urban areas of the United States. In these areas, substandard housing, crowded living conditions, and other immune-compromising behaviors such as injection drug use (IDU) and poor nutrition may also be factors. Cultural norms and values about marriage patterns such as the number of spouses allowed, the specific kinds of sexual behavior a culture accepts, and drug usage are other cultural factors that can affect an individual's susceptibility to infection.

A second theoretical model that complements the systems/ecology view is Lewis Thomas's theory of the integrity of the individual's "natural" biological defenses (Thomas 1984). Thomas, a biologist, believes that we are healthier than we think we are. The body's defenses such as the skin, **immune system**, and possibly one's genetic make-up are, or can be, "natural" barriers to disease (Thomas 1984).

This approach can be useful in explaining the variations in the spread of HIV within and between exposed individuals as well as among groups. For example, it is estimated that possibly 1 percent of Caucasian males in the United States (as well as a group of female prostitutes in Nairobi, Kenya, and Gambia, Africa) have a genetic protection against becoming infected with HIV despite multiple exposures to the virus (National Institute of

Allergy and Infectious Diseases 2002; Anon. 1998b; Fowke et al. 1996; Diaz et al. 2000). Their bodies may eradicate the virus before antibodies develop (Blower et al. 2002). This protective mechanism may also explain why some people are **nonprogressors** and **long-term survivors**. These individuals have been infected for more than fifteen or twenty years, yet either they do not progress to full-blown AIDS or they remain in good health if they receive a diagnosis of AIDS. The nonprogressors and those who appear to be immune to infection are of scientific interest. Studying their biochemistry may help researchers to develop a vaccine to prevent HIV infection (Blower et al. 2002). Research on specific genetic markers, gender, ethnic, or lifestyle differences continues to attempt to determine why some people either do not get infected or, if infected, remain healthy.

The third major theoretical perspective used in this text is from critical medical anthropology (Farmer 1992; Basu, Mate, and Farmer, 2000; Herdt 2001). Based on his research in Haiti as both an anthropologist and a physician, Paul Farmer explains vulnerability to infection, and the course of the disease once infected, as a function of larger political, social, and economic practices within and between cultures (Farmer 1992). As will be discussed in later chapters, Farmer and colleagues (2000) believe that gender inequality and poverty contribute significantly to the risk of HIV infection.

The "global village" dimension of HIV/AIDS encompasses most of the world's population and societies where malnutrition and other health problems exist, such as malaria, tuberculosis, or infant diarrhea. These societies are subject to industrialized societies' international economic, political, and social policies, as well as indigenous social and sexual practices. The combination of culture change and indigenous practices influences who becomes infected, how they are treated once infected, and the spread of the virus (Farmer 1992; Basu et al. 2000).

Concepts of health, illness, disease, and healing within a cultural context are considered within both a medical and a critical medical anthropological perspective on HIV/AIDS. According to the **World Health Organization** (WHO), "Health is a state of complete physical, mental, and social well-being, and not merely the absence of disease or infirmity" (1946/1948). Health is a state of relative equilibrium in which the physical (biological), sociopsychological, emotional, and spiritual aspects of an individual integrate to allow an individual to function according to the norms of that person's culture (WHO 1946/1948; Weil 2004). This definition of health is holistic, reflecting a systems/ecological model (WHO 1946/1948; Armelagos, Goodman, and Jacob, 1978). The term *disease* generally refers to the pathogens and physical manifestations, including psychiatric, that disrupt that equilibrium to the extent that the individual cannot function in his or her respective society for a culturally defined period. In contrast, *illness* refers to the socioeconomic, political, and psychological side effects of the disease for both the individual and the group (Vernon 2001). These side effects can include the inability to work and bring in resources, maintain social and kinship relations and obligations, and other culturally defined impaired functions that affect both the individual and the group. In many indigenous societies, such as the Navajo in the United States and the Yanomamo in South America, when an individual is sick, the group is in danger until the individual can be restored to health (Perrone et al. 1989; Vernon 2001).

In twentieth- and twenty-first-century biomedical practice, the use of antibiotics, public health measures such as potable drinking water, safe disposal of wastes, and immunizations have resulted in the ability to cure a number of bacterial infections or prevent some viral infections such as polio. These developments lead many people in the United States to believe in the efficacy of cures, that is, the removal of the disease-causing agent and restoration of health (Perrone et al. 1989; Sargeant and Bretell 1996). The success rate of curing numerous diseases also created a shift away from the concept of healing in the United States until very recently (Weil 2004; Perrone et al. 1989; Sargeant and Bretell 1996). Andrew Weil, a physician and anthropologist, suggests that healing involves accepting the illness and restoring balance and harmony to both the individual and the group (2004).

Healing is a common practice among Native American groups and support groups in the United States. Among Navajos, for example, who use both biomedical and traditional practices, people will visit the tribal clinic and have a "sing" to restore their spirit and achieve harmony with themselves and nature (Perrone et al. 1989; Vernon 2001). Twelve-step programs such as Alcoholics Anonymous recognize that there is not a cure for alcoholism but that the person can live a full and rewarding life without being cured of the disease of alcoholism. Healing may exist with or without a cure. For example, a person with a terminal illness—which AIDS is for most people who have it worldwide—may be able to come to peace with the disease (HIV infection and AIDS) without being cured, that is, rid of the virus. These five concepts (health, disease, illness, healing, and curing) will be incorporated throughout the text.

Anthropology and medical anthropology have definite roles to play in resolving the AIDS epidemic. At the beginning of the twenty-first century, HIV/AIDS is a global pandemic disease. Currently, there is neither a vaccine nor a cure. Largely because of cost and accessibility, the drugs used to slow the progression of the disease are available to only a small percentage of the world's population who are infected. Even within industrialized societies that have access to **Highly Active Antiretroviral Therapy (HAART)** and biomedical care, there are problems with availability of and access to the drugs, serious side effects, and adherence to the drug regimen (*HIVPlus* 2002a, 2002b; Anderson 2001; Wormser and Horowitz 1996).

As a global phenomenon, HIV/AIDS is described as a disease and topic of study that fits well with an anthropological perspective. The physical, biological, sociocultural, political, and economic aspects of HIV/AIDS filter through each society's values, beliefs, and institutions in relation to health, illness, disease, sexuality, men and women, life and death. Because anthropologists have a history of qualitative as well as quantitative research, they have the ability to discern the symbols and constructs underlying people's behaviors and to work in intercultural health settings (Carrier and Bolton 1991).

HIV/AIDS affects human groups across the life cycle. The anthropological perspectives of holism, relativism, and comparison are helpful in understanding the cultural complexities of this disease. Medical anthropology, a subfield of cultural anthropology, has a century-old history of examining not only patterns of disease among human populations but also how responses to disease reflect the sociocultural systems in which they occur.

The applied, critical medical anthropological perspectives integrate theoretical, methodological, and practical approaches to understand how this disease and illness affects different populations, and the perspectives also offer means of preventing and responding to the epidemic. Of the world's AIDS cases, 80 percent occur in sub-Saharan Africa alone (UNAIDS 2002, 2004; Anon. 2000a; Daley 1999). Without a cure or vaccine, culturally sensitive intervention methods are an important means of reducing infection. Medical anthropology offers an integrated approach in response to the specific impact that HIV/AIDS has on various groups. Using an emic perspective, anthropologists take active roles in prevention and treatment efforts by examining the effects that larger socioeconomic and political factors have on risk and vulnerability among individuals and groups at the local, national, and international levels (Parker and Ehrhardt 2001; Parker 2001).

This book discusses the phenomenon of HIV/AIDS globally, across the life cycle, and cross-culturally. It includes chapters on **epidemiology** (the study of the patterns of disease), the biomedical aspects of the epidemic, women and AIDS, and HIV testing, as well as the socioeconomic, political, and sexual components of HIV/AIDS. This book discusses specific groups and societies to illustrate the impact that HIV/AIDS has had on them. These include areas of sub-Saharan Africa, Latin America, Southeast Asia, and subcultures in the United States. There are discussions of the ethical issues involved in HIV testing, the availability and access to HAART, and sexual and gender factors. The book concludes with suggestions about how to respond to the epidemic anthropologically in the twenty-first century.

The next chapter examines the history and epidemiology of HIV/AIDS globally. It discusses various origin theories and controversies found in AIDS research and introduces some of the ethical dilemmas involved in the AIDS epidemic.

1.2

Discussions of HIV/AIDS are rife with ethical considerations. Various ethical situations appear throughout this text. Louise de la Gorgendière, an anthropologist who conducts research on women's risk of HIV infection in Zaire, cautions anthropologists about the ethical issues surrounding HIV/AIDS investigations. She states: "In the interest of promoting equality and participation, as anthropologists and HIV/AIDS researchers, we must ensure that we do not play into the hands of the local hierarchy disempowering and excluding local people. . . . We must ensure that people in developing countries are treated with respect, and most importantly, that the research 'will do no harm'" (2005: 176).

SUMMARY

HIV/AIDS is a devastating global problem.

An interdisciplinary approach to understanding HIV/AIDS is necessary because of the complexity of the disease and illness.

HIV/AIDS affects individuals, groups, and societies throughout the life cycle.

A medical anthropological perspective brings unique methodological and theoretical approaches to examining HIV/AIDS.

Thought Questions

What kinds of ethical problems do researchers' biases present for responding to the AIDS epidemic?

Why is using only one methodological or theoretical approach (reductionism) insufficient to explain, prevent, or treat HIV/AIDS?

Resources

Books

Farmer, Paul. *AIDS and Accusation: Haiti and the Geography of Blame.* Comparative Studies of Health Systems and Medical Care 33. Berkeley: University of California Press, 1992.

Kottak, Conrad. *Cultural Anthropology.* New York: McGraw-Hill, 2000.

Shilts, Randy. *And the Band Played On: Politics, People, and the AIDS Epidemic.* New York: St. Martin's Press, 1997.

Web Sites

AAA (American Anthropological Association): http://www.aaanet.org.

AARG (AIDS and Anthropology Research Group): http://www.puffin.creighton.edu/ aarg.

CDC (Centers for Disease Control and Prevention): http://www.cdc.gov/hiv/stats/ htm#cumaids.

UNAIDS (Joint United Nations Programme on HIV/AIDS): http://www.unaids.org/ hivaidsinfo/statistics.

USAID (United States Agency for International Development): http://www.USAID. gov/pop_health/aids/TechAreas/prevention/ index.html.

WHO (World Health Organization): http://www.who/int/en.

2

The Changing Face of AIDS

A Historical and Epidemiological Overview

CHAPTER HIGHLIGHTS INCLUDE

Basic epidemiological concepts and definitions

Global HIV/AIDS statistics as of 2006

Discussions of the changing patterns of infectivity and affectivity in the United States and cross-culturally

The modes of transmission of HIV infection

Discussions of the controversies and theories surrounding the origins of AIDS and the role of HIV in AIDS

An introduction to some of the ethical epidemiological and intervention issues

---

> Our struggle is—as it has been for so long—a struggle for survival as a people. We are not being alarmist(s) when we raise the potential of another demographic collapse due to AIDS and the disappearance of entire indigenous cultures. An epidemic which primarily affects those individuals in their most fecund years can destroy a tribe's future.
>
> Ron Rowell, executive director, National Native American AIDS Prevention Center (Vernon 2001)

This statement reflects the kind of devastating effect that HIV/AIDS has on communities. HIV/AIDS wreaks havoc socially, economically, and politically as people become infected and die. This chapter presents the devastating toll exacted by HIV/AIDS on individuals and groups by examining how the disease manifests itself in the United States and cross-culturally. Variables such as age, gender, ethnicity, and geographic location are part of the distribution of HIV/AIDS globally. (HIV/AIDS statistics change rapidly. For current information, please contact the Web sites listed at the end of this chapter or your local AIDS task force.)

I examine these variables by looking at epidemiological and histori-cal data and by discussing origin theories about HIV/AIDS. Using spe-cific groups and societies to illustrate concepts, this chapter explores the "**changing face of AIDS**," that is, who is infected and affected by this dis-ease (Watkins 2002) and controversies surrounding when and how HIV/AIDS developed. This chapter also introduces some of the ethical issues about and biases toward HIV found among some social science research-ers, physicians, biological scientists, and laypeople that affected our initial understanding of and response to HIV/AIDS.

Epidemiology Overview

Epidemiology is the study of the patterns of disease. Knowing the patterns of who, where, when, and how many people are infected is important. It is also important to know the causative factor(s) of a disease, as well as the demographic characteristics (such as age, gender, **ethnicity** [identity and affiliation with a group], and socioeconomic conditions) that may influ-ence one's susceptibility to disease. In any examination of the patterns of how HIV/AIDS affects individuals, groups, and societies, it is important to adopt a culturally relativistic perspective. This disease has impacted various groups differently, having more to do with larger and global so-cioeconomic and political factors than with membership in a particular sexual, ethnic, or other population (Singer, Huertas, and Scott, 2000).

With this information, effective intervention programs can be devel-oped. Intervention efforts in the AIDS epidemic include prevention, test-ing for **antibodies** or antigens to the virus (with **HIV tests**), and treatment for those who are infected. In general, these programs include prevention efforts such as vaccine development or education. Testing for the presence of the pathogen and treatment of the disease and illness occur in conjunc-tion with prevention efforts.

Educational and risk-reduction efforts exist in the United States and cross-culturally to prevent sexual and injection drug use (IDU) transmis-sion of HIV as well as **mother-to-child transmission (MTCT)**. As part of prevention and treatment, HIV counseling and testing are available. Preventively, if someone tests **HIV negative (HIV-)**, educational efforts can help to maintain one's HIV- status. If someone tests **HIV positive (HIV+)**, education can occur to prevent transmission to sex and needle-sharing partners or to the fetus and child before and after birth. If someone does test HIV+, education about treatment options and information about maintaining one's health can also be provided (see chapter 3).

Prevention of mother-to-child transmission (MTCT) involves education, prenatal HIV testing, and provision of **antiretroviral** therapy (**ARV/ HAART**) to those pregnant women who are HIV+. Treatment interventions for pregnant women in the United States have made MTCT "statistically insignificant" over the past few years. For women in nonindustrialized societies, however, access to treatment is riddled with political and economic complications (Global Health Council 2005; De la Gorgendière 2005; see chapters 7 and 8). Treatment involves education about the disease and drugs to improve the immune system and reduce the risk of contracting opportunistic infections (OIs). As discussed in chapter 1, these are the diseases that people with compromised immune systems often get. Information about the patterns of HIV infection can influence decisions regarding allocation of intervention resources.

Incidence rate and **prevalence** and epidemic, **endemic**, and **pandemic** aspects of disease are key concepts in epidemiology. Related concepts include **acute**, **chronic**, and **terminal** illnesses. Incidence rates refer to the number of new cases of a disease in a given period. For example, globally, there are about 16,000 new HIV infections daily (Sarche 2003:D5) (see figures 2.1–2.3).

The incidence of HIV in the United States ranges from about 40,000 to 42,000 new cases a year, a figure that has remained relatively stable for at least the most recent decade of the epidemic (Sarche 2003:D5). What has changed since the first diagnosed case of AIDS in the United States in 1981 is "the face of AIDS." The face of AIDS refers to the profile or common pattern of who is infected relative to incidence. This "face" in the United States has shifted from largely middle-class, Anglo **Men Who Have Sex With Men (MSM)** who are in their twenties and thirties, to Latinas and African American women and adolescents (Robinson et al. 2002; CDC 2001a). About 50 percent of these new infections occur among "people of color" (Sarche 2003; CDC 2001a) (see table 2.1).

Prevalence refers to how widespread a disease is in a population. Prevalence connotes a degree of stability and persistence of a disease within a group. For example, estimates indicate that in South Africa, 20 percent of the adult population is HIV+; in Botswana, about 38 percent of the adult population is HIV+; and in Swaziland, almost 40 percent of the adult population is HIV+ (UNAIDS 2002, 2004; *HIVPlus* 2002b; *AIDS Treat-*

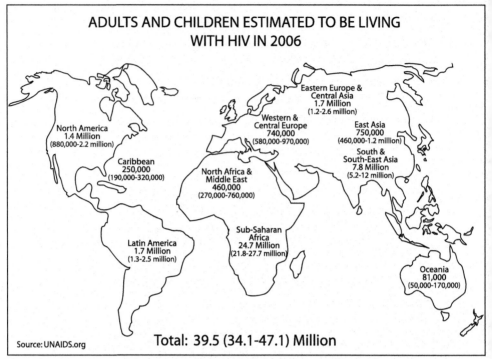

Figure 2.1a. Adults and children estimated to be living with HIV in 2006 (UNAIDS, 2008).

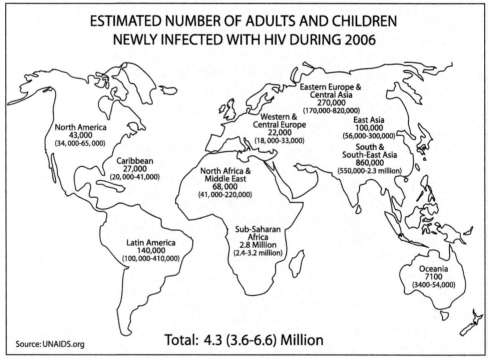

Figure 2.1b. Adults and children estimated to be newly infected with HIV during 2006 (UNAIDS, 2008).

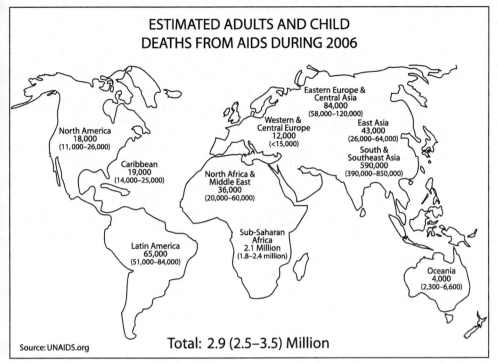

Figure 2.1c. Estimated number of deaths of adults and children from AIDS during 2006 (UNAIDS, 2008).

Table 2.1. AIDS cases by race/ethnicity

Race or ethnicity	Estimated number of AIDS cases	Cumulative estimated number of AIDS cases[a]
White, not Hispanic	11,780	385,537
Black, not Hispanic	20,187	397,548
Hispanic	7,676	155,179
Asian/Pacific Islander	483	7,659
American Indian/ Alaska Native	182	3,238

Source: Centers for Disease Control and Prevention (CDC Fact Sheets, October 2008, hereafter CDC, 2008)

a. Includes persons with a diagnosis of AIDS from the beginning of the epidemic through 2005.

HIV/AIDS AROUND THE WORLD

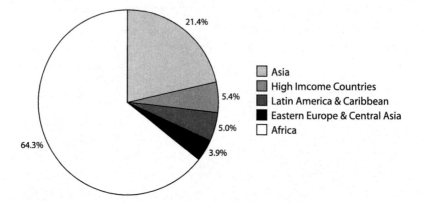

Figure 2.2a. HIV/AIDS around the world (CDC, 2008).

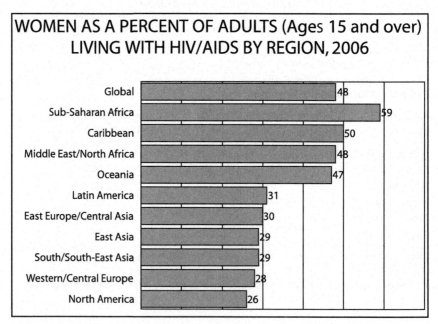

Figure 2.2b. Women as a percentage of adults (ages 15 and over) living with HIV/AIDS, by region, in 2006 (UNAIDS, 2008).

ESTIMATED NEW AIDS CASES, AIDS DEATHS, AND PEOPLE LIVING IN UNITED STATES WITH AIDS 1985–2006

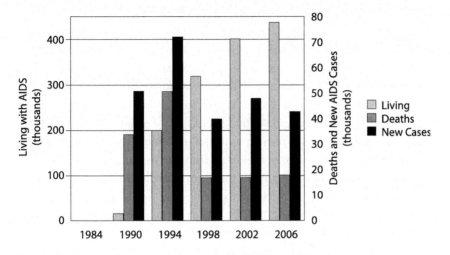

Figure 2.3. Estimated new AIDS cases, AIDS deaths, and people living with AIDS in the United States, 1985–2006 (Henry J. Kaiser Family Foundation, HIV/AIDS Policy Fact Sheet/The HIV/AIDS Epidemic in the United States, July 2007).

ment Now 2003: issues 40, 41; UNAIDS 2006). In the United States, 1 in 125 people overall and 1 in 500 college students are estimated to be HIV+ (CDC 1999).

The terms *epidemic, endemic,* and *pandemic* all refer to the ways in which a disease appears and spreads through a population. Epidemics are diseases that often appear relatively suddenly and spread through a group quickly. The number of new cases of a disease (incidence) can help to define an epidemic. The flu is an example of an epidemic. A disease becomes endemic when it is relatively stable and prevalent within a population. Obesity in the United States is endemic. A pandemic disease is global.

HIV/AIDS is an epidemic, endemic, and pandemic disease. Based on recorded accounts and diagnosed cases, HIV/AIDS appeared relatively suddenly in the United States in 1981 (epidemic), and it remains in the general population at about 1 in 125 people infected (endemic). Globally, it is found on every inhabited continent and in more than 165 countries, making it pandemic (Stine 1997; UNAIDS 2002; CDC 2001b). Since 1981, an estimated 57.9 million people worldwide either have been infected with

HIV or have AIDS. More than 90 percent of those infections occur in non-industrialized societies, largely because of poverty and politics (Merson and Dayton 2002: 13; see chapter 8). Throughout this book, I will use the term *epidemic* when referring to HIV/AIDS within a specific population or society and *pandemic* when referring to it globally.

The terms *acute, chronic,* and *terminal* relate to epidemiological concepts and apply to configurations of disease and illness. Acute, chronic, and terminal refer to the course of and potential outcome of a disease in an individual. Acute diseases usually have a sudden onset in an individual and a relatively quick progression. Measles and colds are examples of acute diseases. Chronic diseases usually develop more gradually. Generally incurable, chronic diseases remain with the individual but may be manageable over time. Chronic diseases may impact the individual's long- and short-term functioning. Diabetes, autoimmune diseases such as lupus or thyroid disorders, and arthritis are examples of chronic diseases. Terminal diseases that result in death may be either acute or chronic. Some heart disease and several cancers are terminal.

HIV/AIDS has the characteristics of being acute, chronic, and terminal. In the United States, about 50 percent of the people with HIV develop flulike symptoms shortly after infection. This passes fairly quickly (acute) (Cohen, Sande, and Volberding, 1999). With the availability of HAART in industrialized countries since 1996, many researchers and physicians hope that people who can tolerate the rigorous drug regimen may be able to cope with HIV as a chronic but manageable disease (*HIVPlus* 2001, 2002b). For most people in the world who have HIV/AIDS, it is a death sentence. Only about 17 to 20 percent of the world's population with HIV/AIDS receives treatment for it (*AIDS Treatment Now* 2003: issue 44; UNAIDS 2006; http://www.aids2004.org). Again, this discrepancy in treatment worldwide is primarily due to global and regional political and economic factors (see chapter 8).

The average length of time in the United States that elapses between the initial AIDS diagnosis and death without taking HAART is about four years. In sub-Saharan Africa, where HAART is largely unavailable, longevity is less (Spira et al. 2000; CDC 2000). Nutritional status, other health problems, **cofactors** such as **sexually transmitted infections (STIs)**, and access to antiretroviral drugs determine longevity in the nonindustrialized world (Keersmaekers and Meheus 1998; Patton 1994; Thomas 2001; Fletcher et al. 1999; Ferry 1995; Daley 1999).

In discussions of the course of HIV/AIDS since 1981, the terms *patterns* and *waves* have been used. Patterns describe the progression of HIV/AIDS cross-culturally, and waves apply to discussing it in the United States. Patterns and waves roughly correspond with the decades of the epidemic. Initially, HIV/AIDS incidence was described as found in **Pattern I, II, or III** areas of the world.

Patterns I, II, and III follow the international reporting of AIDS. AIDS was first reported in Pattern I sites, which include North America and Western Europe, with an incidence largely among men who have sex with men (MSM). Pattern II sites include sub-Saharan Africa, parts of Latin America such as Brazil, and parts of the Caribbean. Pattern II areas of infection largely involve heterosexual transmission of the virus, particularly **male-to-female transmission (MTF)**. Pattern III sites initially included Southeast Asia, Japan, China, and the South Pacific. HIV was believed to have been introduced to these regions by infected people from Pattern I and II areas (Stine 1997; Merson and Dayton 2002). The widespread nature of the pandemic since the late 1990s has made the delineation into Pattern I, II, and III areas of the world less meaningful.

The waves of the AIDS epidemic apply to the United States. As of 2003, three waves have been identified in the United States. The first wave occurred in the 1980s, primarily among young, Anglo MSM who identified as gay. Many of these men were middle class. The second wave occurred from the late 1980s through the 1990s. With better surveillance procedures and tracking methods available, and with a revised definition of AIDS by the CDC in 1993, people from other groups were more accurately included in the statistics. These included women, adolescents, injection drug users (IDUs), and ethnic minorities, specifically African Americans and Latinos (CDC 2001a; Anon. 1998a; Brookmeyer 2002; Loue 1999). The third wave began in the late 1990s and continues to the present. Wave three is characterized by a resurgence of AIDS in 18–24-year-old MSM (Clay 2002; CDC 2003a; Yee 2003a; *Infectious Disease News* 2004).

In early 2003, the incidence of AIDS in the United States increased overall for the first time since the mid-1990s (Anon. 2003a; Yee 2003a). There continue to be high incidence rates in the United States among African American MSM, women in general, and African American, Latina, and Native American women specifically (Herek and Glunt 1995; Vernon 2001; Loue 1999; CDC 2001a, 2003a). For example, 83 percent of the women with AIDS in the United States are African American or Latina

(CDC 2001a, 2003a). Worldwide, almost half the people with HIV/AIDS are women (Gayle 2003).

Applying Epidemiology to HIV/AIDS

There are several key points involved in understanding the application of these epidemiological concepts and statistics to the AIDS crisis. First, even though a disease exists in a population, not everyone exposed to it will become infected (Thomas 1984; Abel 2002). In addition, several variables influence one's vulnerability to disease and infection. These include factors of age, sex, socioeconomic status, ethnicity, overall states of health and nutrition, and the presence of cofactors such as STIs. Cofactors increase one's susceptibility to a disease, although they do not actually cause the disease. They affect risk, the course of the disease, and its outcome. For example, an STI such as genital herpes depresses one's immune system, and the lesions can allow HIV to more easily pass through membranes. The graphs, maps, and charts that follow depict the breakdown of HIV/AIDS in the United States and cross-culturally according to these factors.

Those people who contract a disease such as HIV/AIDS do not necessarily experience the disease similarly. The variables and cofactors referred to bear on the course and outcome of the disease and illness. Societal beliefs, norms, values, and behaviors influence not only susceptibility to the disease but also recognition that a disease exists, and the appropriate response to it. Having HIV/AIDS is stigmatized. Societal responses to the **stigma** affect both the risk for infection and prevention and treatment efforts (Herdt 2001; Sontag 1995; Wang and Ross 2002; Green and Sobo 2000; Singer 2003b, 2005; Brown, MacIntyre, and Trujillo 2003). As a stigmatized disease, HIV/AIDS is also underreported.

Global and regional incidence and prevalence rates as well as demographic data help to present an overall picture of disease. But with HIV/AIDS, incidence and prevalence rates are underestimates of the scope and impact of the disease. HIV/AIDS is underreported even in industrialized societies, including the United States (*HIVPlus* 2002b; Yee 2003b). Daniel Klein and colleagues (2003) found that in a clinic on the West Coast that treats a large number of people with HIV, 30–40 percent of the clients were not diagnosed with HIV until after they had received an AIDS diagnosis.

Cross-culturally, HIV/AIDS is underdiagnosed and misdiagnosed in a number of nonindustrialized societies (*HIVPlus* 2002a; d'Adesky 2002a, 2002b, 2002c). In addressing the basic epidemiological aspects of HIV/ AIDS, deeply entrenched sociocultural values and structures factor into risk. These include ethnocentrism, erotophobia, and homophobia.

Ethnocentrism, the practice of judging another society by one's own beliefs and practices and imposing one's values on another group, impedes intervention efforts. According to Tim Vollmer, a medical anthropologist, indigenous sexual, marital, social, and intergenerational relationships need to be considered and respected as valid. Attempts to impose Euro-American beliefs about these practices have resulted in failed prevention efforts and inaccurate epidemiological data (Vollmer 2000). Ethnocentrism extends to viewing women in the United States and elsewhere as **"vectors of transmission"** or **"reservoirs of infection"** (Stine 1997; Patton 1994). These views ignore basic epidemiological data and modes of transmission. Men are more likely to transmit HIV to women than women are to men. In any penetrative sexual encounter—anal, vaginal, or oral— the inserter is at less risk for infection than the receiver is (UNAIDS 2002; Schneider and Stoller 1995; Roth and Fuller 1998).

In addition, the vocabulary used to identify risky behaviors can be problematic and do reflect an ethnocentric and Eurocentric perspective. For example, applying the term *gay* to men who have sex with men may have little meaning cross-culturally or within ethnic groups in the United States. In nonindustrialized societies in Southeast Asia and in Latin American societies such as urban Brazil as well as among ethnic Latinos and African American men in the United States, men may engage in same-gender sexual behavior but not identify as gay. The extent to which men adopt a gay identity may depend on peer-group acceptance or the degree of assimilation into the larger culture for Latinos in the United States (Aggleton et al. 1994; Parker and Aggleton 1999; Clay 2002; Tielman 1991; Diaz 1998). Men can have sex with men under a variety of circumstances and not consider themselves to be "gay" or "homosexual." For example, in Mexico as well as Brazil, men who are the inserter in sex with other men retain their identity as male and as heterosexual or "straight" (Parker and Aggleton 1999; Carrier 2001; Diaz 1998; Doll et al. 1991; Garcia et al. 1991).

Erotophobia and homophobia also influence obtaining and interpreting accurate epidemiological data. Erotophobia is the fear of sex, particularly sexual behavior or identities that occur outside culturally defined norms and values. Homophobia is the fear, distrust, and dislike of people known or perceived to engage in same-sex sexual and romantic love relationships (Bolin and Whelehan 1999). If these concepts become part of the belief system and are then acted upon by an individual or group, they can impact accurate data collection, interpretation, and presentation. In the United States in 2003, researchers applying for HIV/AIDS grants with the **National Institutes of Health (NIH)** and **National Institute of Mental Health (NIMH)** found that the use of words such as *homosexual* and *anal intercourse* could classify their research as "controversial." These researchers were cautioned by federal health officials that conducting "controversial" sexuality research could jeopardize their chances of funding (Sherman 2003; Goode 2003). Randy Shilts, a journalist for the *San Francisco Chronicle* who died of AIDS, and Patricia Thomas, a medical journalist, discuss how the federal government (and, by extension, the **Centers for Disease Control and Prevention [CDC]**, which is part of, and thus funded by, the federal government) hindered scientific investigation into HIV/AIDS because of biases concerning sexuality and orientation (Shilts 1987; Thomas 2001).

2.1

In response to the NIH/NIMH statement, many social scientists (including anthropologists) and other researchers signed petitions and wrote responses to this position. They expressed outrage and concern about the politicization and moralization of scientific endeavors in connection with HIV prevention (Kaiser 2003; Kaiser Daily HIV/AIDS Report 2004).

Other factors introduced here that complicate epidemiological research and program implementation include politics, economic policies, and specific sexual behaviors. These complications exist both in the United States and cross-culturally. For example, until very recently, the stigma associated with having AIDS in China meant that people with HIV/AIDS could be prosecuted and jailed (Beyrer 1998; Becker 2003; Stanmeyer 2003; Lau and Tsui 2002; Wu et al. 1999). This situation in China impeded educational efforts and caused people to delay or avoid testing or seeking appropriate medical treatment. This resulted in massive underreporting of the incidence and prevalence rates and modes of transmission of HIV in China until about 2000 (Stanmeyer 2003; Becker 2003; Wu et al. 1999, 2002).

By 2003, China's approach to HIV/AIDS had become more open, which made establishing an identity as gay or as an MSM easier (Stanmeyer 2003). Health-care workers are encouraged to become more knowledge-able about HIV/AIDS and to accept HIV-infected patients. The period of intense sex negativism in China largely occurred between the eighteenth and twentieth centuries. Reasons for this include culture change, contact with Europeans and the impact of their views about sexuality, and the Cultural Revolution of the Communists in the 1930s. Chairman Mao's negativity about sexuality in part was a reaction to his perception of the "West" as "decadent" (Ruan 1991). The recent emergence of a more positive view toward sexuality is closer to traditional Chinese views as expressed in the original Taoist philosophy than it is to the policies of the Cultural Revolution (Ruan 1991; Becker 2003). A 2003 news report of the publicized marriage of an HIV+ heterosexual couple in the Chinese province of Sichuan is one example of an increasingly open approach to HIV/AIDS in China (Liu 2003).

Since societal norms and beliefs can affect data collection, HIV/AIDS statistics are estimates, at best. The CDC is the epidemiological source for HIV/AIDS statistics in the United States. It publishes national HIV/AIDS incidence and prevalence rates semiannually. Because these statistics are published semiannually, they are somewhat dated when released. These data, however, do have a degree of validity in that epidemiological data illustrate shifts and continuities in incidence and prevalence rates and demographics over time.

Despite the problems with accurately accruing HIV/AIDS data both in the United States and cross-culturally, epidemiological data provide valuable information about patterns of disease that are used to develop intervention programs ranging from education to testing to treatment. In other words, epidemiological data provide a baseline. These data are used to allocate funding for interventions and to conduct follow-up studies and program evaluations.

Figures 2.4–2.7 and tables 2.2 and 2.3 illustrate known, reported cases of HIV/AIDS in the United States and elsewhere through 2006 (CDC 2002; UNAIDS 2004; Kaiser Family Foundation 2006). These illustrations include data on age, gender, ethnicity, geographical location, and mode of

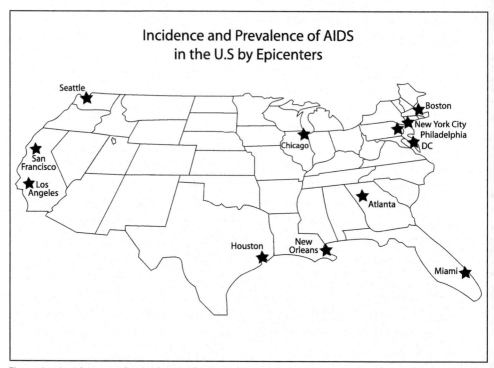

Figure 2.4. Incidence and prevalence of AIDS in the United States, by epicenters (Silvia Macey, 2008).

In 2005, the estimated number of diagnoses of persons living with AIDS in the United States and dependent areas was 433,760. This included 418,084 adults and adolescents and 3,787 children under the age of thirteen.

In 2005, the estimated number of new diagnoses of AIDS in adults and children in the United States was 45,669. Adult and adolescent AIDS cases totaled 45,611. There were 58 AIDS cases estimated in children under the age of thirteen.

The cumulative estimated number of diagnoses of AIDS in adults and children in the United States is 988,376. Since the beginning of the U.S. epidemic, an estimated 182,822 adult and adolescent women have been diagnosed with AIDS. The number of new AIDS diagnoses among women of color rose by an estimated 17 percent between 2001 and 2005, to 80 percent.

Figure 2.5. Persons living with AIDS in the United States (CDC, 2008).

RACE/ETHNICITY OF U.S. WOMEN WITH HIV/AIDS DIAGNOSED DURING 2005

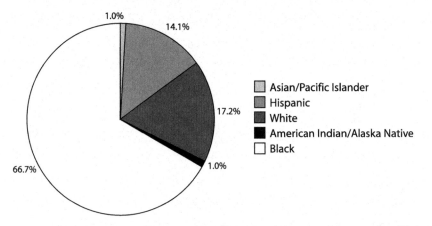

Figure 2.6. Race/ethnicity of U.S. women with HIV/AIDS diagnosed during 2005 (CDC, 2008).

U.S. PEOPLE LIVING WITH AIDS, 2006

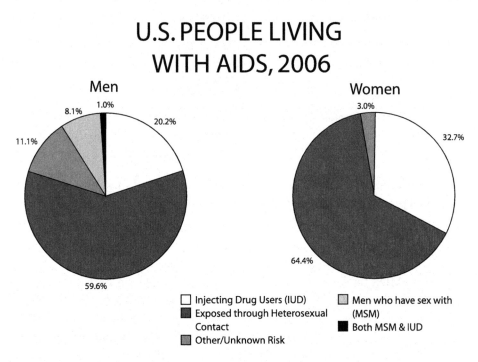

Figure 2.7. U.S. people living with AIDS in 2006 (CDC, 2008).

Table 2.2. Top ten U.S. states/territories in number of AIDS cases, 2005

Number of AIDS cases	State/territory
6,299	New York
4,960	Florida
4,088	California
3,113	Texas
2,333	Georgia
1,922	Illinois
1,595	Maryland
1,510	Pennsylvania
1,278	New Jersey
961	Louisiana

Cumulative number of AIDS cases[a]	State/territory
172,377	New York
139,019	California
100,809	Florida
67,227	Texas
48,431	New Jersey
32,595	Illinois
31,977	Pennsylvania
30,405	Georgia
29,116	Maryland
29,092	Puerto Rico

Source: Henry J. Kaiser Family Foundation, HIV/AIDS Policy Fact Sheet/
The HIV/AIDS Epidemic in the United States, July 2007.
a. From the beginning of the epidemic through 2005.

transmission (that is, how the virus was contracted). U.S. statistics include the **epicenters** of the epidemic. Epicenters are those cities with high incidence and prevalence rates of AIDS.

Age

HIV/AIDS tends to be a disease of younger people in both the United States and cross-culturally. Currently, 50 percent of the new infections in the United States are in people under twenty-five years old (Anon. 1998a; Farmer, Walton, and Furin 2000; CDC 2001b). Worldwide, including the United States, most people diagnosed with AIDS are in their thirties and forties, followed by the numbers of people in their late teens and twenties.

Table 2.3. AIDS cases in the United States by age, 2005

Age[a]	Estimated number of AIDS cases	Cumulative estimated number of AIDS cases[b]
Under 13	68	9,112
13–14	86	1,065
15–19	447	5,289
20–24	1,836	34,795
25–29	3,407	114,141
30–34	5,122	193,926
35–39	7,246	208,505
40–44	8,210	165,697
45–49	6,418	102,732
50–54	3,935	56,950
55–59	2,064	30,424
60–64	967	16,493
65 or older	801	14,503

Source: Centers for Disease Control and Prevention (CBC).

a. Age of a person in the United States at the time of diagnosis of AIDS.

b. From the beginning of the epidemic through 2005.

Pediatric AIDS, defined as AIDS in children from birth to twelve years old, is considered separately by the CDC and the World Health Organization (WHO) (CDC 2001b; CDC/HHS 1999; WHO 2004a; National Institutes of Health 2002).

Because HIV is a disease of primarily younger people, the consequences of having a large segment of a culture's young adult population sick and dying can have profound effects on the survival of the group (Basu, Gupta, and Krishna 1997; Im-em et al. 2002). Late adolescence through mid-adulthood is the time in most societies when reproduction occurs, ensuring the continuation of the group. This phase of the life cycle involves socializing the young into the ways of the group. If there are not sufficient numbers of adults to do this, cultural continuity is interrupted and the ways of the group can be lost. In most parts of the world, the extended kin group—composed of parents, grandparents, cousins, aunts, and uncles—jointly raise the young. In parts of sub-Saharan Africa, enough members of these kin groups have died of AIDS to leave children both homeless and parentless. There were an estimated 1.5 million AIDS orphans in Africa at the end of the twentieth century (Anon. 2000a). In some situations, schools become home and teachers fulfill parenting roles (Anon. 2000a).

Late adolescence through mid-adulthood is also the time when individuals tend to contribute most of their labor to the group. Loss of labor and resources because of AIDS illness and death by this segment of the population puts an additional strain on the group's survival (Basu , Gupta, and Krishna 1997). This situation is beginning in parts of Thailand and India and is common in sub-Saharan Africa (Bond et al. 1996; Pitayanon et al. 1997; Anon. 2000a; Basu, Gupta, and Krishna 1997; Schoofs 1999). The impact of HIV/AIDS in these societies weakens the socioeconomic base and at its most extreme threatens group survival (see chapters 7 and 8).

Although younger people are at the greatest risk, older people are not immune to contracting HIV/AIDS. For example, 14 percent of the people in the United States with AIDS are over fifty (G. Anderson 1996; Edwards 2005). There is increasing concern about AIDS among older adults in Thailand because of the Thais' acceptance of sex across the life cycle (Imem et al. 2002).

Gender

Gender is an important demographic variable in the AIDS epidemic (see figure 2.8). As primarily a sexually transmitted infection, HIV is transmitted through unprotected penile-vaginal (p-v) intercourse in 80 percent of cases worldwide (UNAIDS 2002). Globally, 50 percent of the people with HIV/AIDS are women (UNAIDS 2002; Gayle 2003). In sub-Saharan Africa, approximately 1.2 to 1.5 women are infected for every man who is HIV+ (UNAIDS 2002). In the United States, the male-female ratio of AIDS has shifted since 1981 from 11:1 to 3:1 (CDC 2001a; Edwards 2005).

Women, in general, and African American, Latina, and Native American women in the United States are disproportionately affected by and infected with HIV/AIDS (Robinson et al. 2002; Vernon 2001; CDC 2001a). The biological, economic, social, and political reasons for this disparity are discussed in chapters 7 and 8.

A sexist, ethnocentric, and homophobic view of HIV/AIDS during the first decade of the epidemic contributed to understating the numbers of women infected and affected by the virus in the United States and cross-culturally (J. Anderson 1996, 2001; Vernon 2001; Loue 1995, 1999). The initial focus on HIV/AIDS as GRID among middle-class, Anglo, self-identified gay men reinforced biases that researchers, epidemiologists, and physicians held about the reality and risks of HIV and AIDS for women in the United States. This bias carried over to women and AIDS cross-culturally (Corea 1992; Loue 1999; Vernon 2001; Schneider and Stoller 1995). In reality, women were infected and affected by HIV from the beginning of the epidemic, and they have a much different experience with it than do men (Schneider and Stoller 1995; Anderson 2001; Gomez 1995; Campbell 1999; O'Leary and Jemmott 1996; chapter 7).

Ethnicity

Ethnicity is a third variable in HIV/AIDS epidemiology (see figure 2.9). Ethnicity is the identification an individual has with a particular socially or culturally defined group or groups (Barth 1998). People who share an ethnic identity may speak a similar language, hold a common worldview, have a recognized set of values and beliefs (including religious ones), and have a relatively homogeneous gene pool (Barth 1998). In a highly stratified and heterogeneous society such as the United States, there are clear ethnic differences related to the risk for infection and the incidence and prevalence of HIV (CDC 2001a, 2001b). For example, African Americans and Latinos comprise about 15 percent and 12 percent of the U.S. popula-

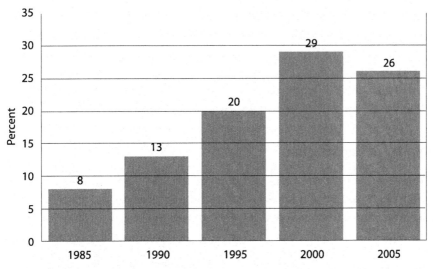

Figure 2.8. Women as a proportion of new AIDS diagnoses, 1985–2005 (CDC, 2008).

ETHNICITIES OF U.S. PEOPLE LIVING WITH AIDS, 2006

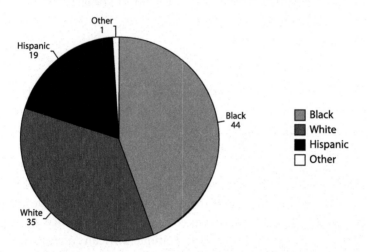

Figure 2.9. Ethnicities of U.S. people living with AIDS in 2006 (CDC, 2008).

tion respectively, but they comprise a disproportionate number of AIDS cases. As of 2001, 49 percent of new adult AIDS cases occurred among African Americans (CDC 2001a). AIDS is the leading cause of death among African American females twenty-five to thirty-four years old, as well as among African American males thirty-five to forty-four years old. Of the women with AIDS in the United States, 83 percent are African American or Latina (CDC 2001a; http://www.aids2004.org; see figures 2.8 and 2.9). Most of these people are also poor (Vernon 2001). These ethnic differences also elicit different responses from the larger society toward those who are HIV+ or have AIDS (see chapters 8, 9, and 10).

Modes of Transmission

The means of transmitting and contracting HIV (that is, the modes of transmission) became known during the first wave of the epidemic and have remained unchanged to the present (see figure 2.10). While HIV can be isolated from any body fluid or tissue, there are sufficient concentrations of the virus to be infectious only in certain body fluids: blood and all of its components, semen, vaginal secretions, and breast milk. Pregnant

TRANSMISSION CATEGORIES AND RACE/ETHNICITY OF WOMEN LIVING WITH HIV/AIDS, 2005

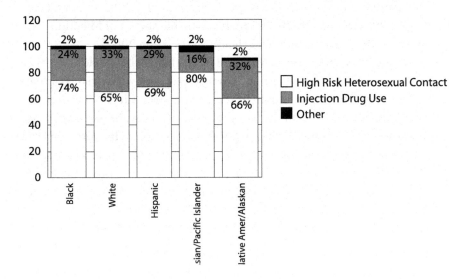

Figure 2.10. Transmission categories and race/ethnicity of women living with HIV/AIDS in 2005 (CDC, 2008).

women can also transmit HIV to their offspring during pregnancy and birth. Therefore, only those behaviors that expose individuals to these infected fluids can transmit the virus. HIV is not airborne. It is not a casual-contact infection.

Those behaviors that can put someone at risk for infection include unprotected penetrative sex, sharing needles, transfusions with HIV+ blood or its products, pregnancy and birth, and breast-feeding. Having unprotected penetrative intercourse involves vaginal, anal, and (to a significantly lesser extent) oral sex, either **fellatio** (oral sex on a man) or **cunnilingus** (oral sex on a woman), without the use of either latex or polyurethane barriers such as condoms and vaginal dams. Sharing sex toys such as dildos that come in contact with infected blood, semen, or vaginal fluid is also risky. Cuts or other breaks in the skin that can come in contact with infected blood, semen, or vaginal fluids during sex can also transmit HIV (see chapter 5).

Sharing needles or drug paraphernalia (works) of any type that are "dirty" (that is, contain fresh or dried blood or blood products that are

HIV-infected) can transmit the virus. Needle usage occurs in a variety of circumstances. These include medical procedures such as blood draws or injection of medicine such as insulin in diabetics or vitamins, a practice that is common in Mexico. Needles are used in IDU and in tattooing and body piercing. Sharing razors is a possible source of infection as well (Body 2003a; American Social Health Association 2003).

Pregnant women can transmit HIV to their babies before or during birth or during breast-feeding. During pregnancy, the risk is greatest if there are microscopic tears in the placenta (Preidt 2005). The risk of transmission depends on the woman's overall HIV status such as her **viral load** (how much virus she has in her system) and **T-cell** count (a measure of her immune system), as well as birthing practices. The risk of transmitting HIV during breast-feeding depends on these and other factors. Additional factors include whether the infant has mouth sores and whether the woman's nipples are cracked, as well as the mother's general state of health (White 1999) (see chapter 7).

Cofactors

Cofactors are varied and culture-specific. For example, the presence of another sexually transmitted infection (STI)—particularly one that can create genital ulcers, sores, or lesions, such as syphilis or herpes simplex virus—can increase the chances of infection (Choi et al. 2000; Keersmaekers and Meheus 1998; Musher and Baughn 1999). Sexual practices such as using substances to dry and constrict the vagina in parts of Islamic Africa and Southeast Asia are another cofactor that can increase the risk of infection (Brown, Ayowa and Brown 1993; Wolffers and Bevers 1997; Feldman 2003a).

The role of male circumcision in HIV transmission is controversial (Bailey, Neema, and Othieno 1999; www.aarg.org 2003; Aggleton 2007). In the United States, most of the first wave of HIV among MSM occurred among circumcised males and in Europe among uncircumcised males (Bailey and Halperin 2000; Bailey, Plummer, and Moses 2001; Cold and Taylor 1999). In Africa, there are differences in the incidence of HIV between populations that practice male circumcision and those that do not. Data indicate that in areas of West Africa where male circumcision is customary, there are lower rates of HIV (WHO 2007). These countries are also largely Islamic, a belief system that has fairly strict beliefs and behaviors about sexuality and drug usage that could reduce the risk as well (Gray 2003). In East Africa and parts of Southeast Asia where male circumcision occurs less often, rates of HIV are higher (Halperin and Bailey 1999). However, other variables such as the presence of STIs and overall states of health may be confounding factors in risk (Bailey, Neema, and Othieno 1999; Bailey and Halperin 2000) (see chapter 5). Poverty that leads people to engage in risky sexual or needle-using behavior is another cofactor (Farmer 1992; Basu, Mate, and Farmer 2000). Individual societies' economic and social practices influence the risk for HIV. Thus, most cofactors involved in the risk for HIV infection are culturally created.

Political and Economic Cofactors

Cuba has one of the lowest incidences of HIV/AIDS in the world (UN-AIDS 2002). The treatment of Cubans with HIV/AIDS has stirred international controversy over the limits of cultural relativism, civil rights, human rights, and the care of people with HIV/AIDS (Scheper-Hughes 1994; Manlowe 1997). Cuba is not a democracy. It is a communist state where the needs of the individual are subsumed to the needs of the group. There is voluntary HIV testing in Cuba; however, until 1993, anyone who tested positive in Cuba or who was diagnosed with AIDS was quarantined (separated from the larger community). Under quarantine, the individual received housing, food, medical care, and visits from family and friends for the duration of the illness (Scheper-Hughes 1994; Manlowe 1997; Parameswaran 2004; see chapter 4).

2.2

Iran is another country with a relatively low prevalence of HIV/AIDS. Known as a conservative Islamic country, Iran also has a progressive needle exchange program for its prison population; contraceptives (including condoms) available for both prisoners and the general population; and an effective rural health-care outreach program (Allam 2006; Larsen 2003).

The issue of quarantining people with HIV/AIDS is not restricted to Cuba. During the first decade of the epidemic, quarantines and generalized mandatory testing were suggested by various groups and individuals in the United States (Bayer 2000; McGuire 2000). For a brief period, Illinois required premarital HIV testing. That law was abandoned when premarital HIV testing proved cost-ineffective and did not detect many cases of HIV (Bayer 2000; McGuire 2000). New York conducts mandatory testing on newborns, and there is debate over whether or not pregnant women in the United States should receive voluntary or mandatory testing (Zierler and Krieger 2000; Bayer 2000; McGuire 2000). Currently, the federal government strongly supports abstinence-only sex and HIV education programs in public schools. These kinds of political decisions affect the demographics of risk and the epidemiological data.

Economics are a major cofactor in HIV risk. Currently, most people with HIV/AIDS worldwide are poor. Poverty, as discussed in chapter 8, impacts people's health throughout the life cycle, influences the kind of medical care they receive, and contributes to HIV risk-taking (Farmer 1992; Farmer, Walton, and Furin 2000; Basu, Mate and Farmer 2000). Economics determine what kinds of prevention, testing, and treatment programs exist, for whom, and under what circumstances. The cost of HAART/ARVs, for example, ranges from US$12,000 to $15,000 per year. Certain individual drugs such as T-20 that are given to people for whom other drug regimens have failed may cost that much alone. The inability to provide drugs to the more than 33 million people with HIV worldwide is one of the most pressing concerns of the pandemic (Waterston 1997; Koenig et al. 2004; Harder 2005; Desclaux et al. 2003). Economics present local, national, and global challenges to HIV prevention.

From an etic perspective, some of the more confounding epidemiological cofactors in HIV infection are sociosexual practices. These include various kinship, marital, and sexual behaviors found among subcultures in the United States and cross- culturally. In AIDS-dense societies such as Kenya, Uganda, Tanzania, Botswana, and South Africa, **polygyny** (having more than one wife), the **levirate** (marrying one's deceased husband's brother), ritual sexual cleansings, and genital surgeries as part of initiation ceremonies are common practices (Malungo 1999, 2001; Orubuloye, Caldwell, and Caldwell 1994; Feldman 2003a). These practices contribute to social and economic functioning and stability within the groups where they occur. They also can directly or indirectly act as a mode of transmission for HIV. Balancing societal behaviors and risk for HIV necessitates an emic or insider approach, cultural relativism and sensitivity, and respect for a culture's worldview (see chapter 5).

Table 2.4. AIDS timeline

1981: CDC reports cases of rare pneumonia in MSM

1982: Media and health-care workers increasingly refer to illness as GRID; CDC develops acronym AIDS; first AIDS case reported in Africa; GMHC formed in New York City

1983: First AIDS Candlelight Memorial Service held

1984: Luc Montagnier in Paris the first person to isolate HIV; Robert Gallo simultaneously working on isolating HIV in the United States

1985: HIV antibody test developed; Rock Hudson dies from AIDS complications; Ryan White barred from attending school; first international AIDS conference/International AIDS Day, December 1

1986: AIDS reported worldwide; AZT, first antiretroviral, developed; first panel of the Names Project/AIDS Quilt made

1987: TASO formed in Uganda; the Names Project (the AIDS Quilt) first displayed in Washington, D.C.

1988: More women than men in sub-Saharan Africa reported with HIV/AIDS; ACTUP stages its first demonstration against slow approval of antiretrovirals

1989: A foreigner with AIDS barred from entering the United States

1990: ADA declares AIDS a protected category; pop artist Keith Haring dies of AIDS

1991: Magic Johnson announces that he is HIV+; Freddy Mercury, lead singer of rock group Queen, dies of AIDS

1992: Arthur Ashe, tennis champion, announces he has AIDS

1993: CDC changes its definition of AIDS; female condom available in the United States; Rudolf Nureyev, classical ballet dancer, dies of AIDS

1994: AIDS becomes the leading cause of death for people between the ages of 25 and 44 in the United States; first oral HIV test approved by the FDA

1995: Rap artist Eazy-E dies of AIDS

1996: HAART becomes available in the United States; at-home HIV antibody tests become available; Brazil makes ARVs available to its citizens, first nonindustrialized society to do so

1998: Treatment failures and side effects reported for HAART

2001: 20 years since the first reported case of AIDS

2003: United Nations announces "3×5" plan; PEPFAR initiated

2005: International AIDS organizations announce efforts to make generic ARVs available to people in nonindustrialized societies; 700,000 people treated with ARVs in these societies

2006: 25 years since the first reported case of AIDS

2007: WHO and UNAIDS recommend "provider-initiated" HIV testing

Source: Henry J. Kaiser Family Foundation, HIV/AIDS Policy Fact Sheet/The HIV/AIDS Epidemic in the United States, July 2007.

Origins of HIV/AIDS

One approach to understanding the incidence and prevalence of HIV/ AIDS globally and within specific groups is to determine the origins and nature of the virus (Shilts 1987; Garrett 1994) (see table 2.4). Although most researchers believe that HIV/AIDS originated in Africa, the theories that have been proposed to explain the origin and dispersal of HIV and its role in causing AIDS are varied and controversial. Unfortunately, some of them are also racist and sexist. They include the theory that AIDS was spread in Africa through bestiality and through "wanton" sexual behavior (Patton 1994).

Other theories take on conspiracy connotations. Conspiracy theories state that HIV/AIDS is a genocidal plot against African societies, African Americans, gays, or other stigmatized groups (Rambaut et al. 2001; Dickson 2000). There were suggestions that a form of oral polio vaccine (OPV) given to people in Central Africa during the 1950s was contaminated with HIV from infected chimpanzee tissue (Dickson 2000; Hahn et al. 2000). This controversy raised disturbing questions about how research is conducted and the quality of drugs given to people in nonindustrialized societies. Recent research indicates that HIV-contaminated OPV was not given to Congolese and other Central African peoples (Dickson 2000; Rambaut et al. 2001; Hutchinson 2001). The vaccine used was not made from chimpanzees: "The structure of the HIV-1 phylogenes (the most common form of HIV worldwide) is the result of epidemiological processes acting within the human populations alone" (Rambaut et al. 2001: 1047; Dickson 2000).

Historically, HIV/AIDS may have been in Africa as early as 1940, and definitely by the late 1970s (Cohen, Sande, and Volberding 1999). In 1978, a Scandinavian physician working in Africa became the first European believed to be infected with HIV. How she became infected remains unknown (Shilts 1987; Cohen Sande, and Volberding 1999).

Currently, the most widely accepted theories to explain the origin of AIDS have appeared in the journal *Science* since 2000 (Hahn et al. 2000; Bailes et al. 2003; Keele et al. 2006). These theories posit a **zoonotic**, or "species jumper," transmission of HIV to humans (Hahn et al. 2000; Hutchinson 2001; Beil 1999; Bailes et al. 2003; Lovgren 2003).

On the basis of genetic analysis, researchers believe that simian immunodeficiency virus (SIV) crossed over from monkeys to chimpanzees relatively recently (Bailes et al. 2003; Hahn et al. 2000; Hutchinson 2001).

Monkeys and some apes contract simian AIDS. Simian AIDS is not fatal to these animals, and it is not transmissible to humans.

Chimpanzees hunt two different kinds of monkey species for food. These monkey species carry a form of SIV (SIVcpz) that eventually recombined (changed its genetic structure) in chimpanzees and was spread to humans as HIV-1, the more common form of the virus (Lovgren 2003; Bailes et al. 2003; Keele et al. 2006). Humans do not contract simian AIDS. HIV evolved and mutated from SIV. Chimpanzees are hunted by humans for food and as trophies. Ironically, the mode of transmission from monkeys to chimpanzees and from chimpanzees to humans is the same: hunting.

Hunting practices provide numerous opportunities for blood exchange. It is a bloody endeavor. With predators and prey, there is a high probability that the blood of both will be exchanged during the kill and as a result of processing and/or eating the meat. Safari big game hunting was popular in Africa from the 1920s through the 1950s. Wealthy Europeans and Americans would travel to Africa to hunt game, largely for trophies. Decapitation and amputation of the animals' heads and hands exposed guides to blood and injury.

During this period of big game hunting and later, when monkey and chimpanzee meat also served as a source of protein for indigenous groups and became a delicacy for wealthy foreigners, the simian AIDS virus mutated, eventually evolving into HIV-1. Mutation of pathogens over time is common; it has occurred with other diseases such as syphilis (Garrett 1994). The virus, through mutations, was thus able to "jump" to humans initially during hunting, butchering, and preparing the meat (Hahn et al. 2000; Keele et al. 2006).

Changes in socioeconomic, sexual, and demographic patterns also contributed to the spread of HIV during this period. We have become a "global village" with relatively quick and easy international travel and contact (Garrett 1994). Economic conditions that create a desire for "exotic" meat and a need for alternative protein sources for some malnourished populations contributed to the spread of HIV among humans (Hahn et al. 2000). To date, these are the scientifically accepted theories for the origins of HIV among humans (Hutchinson 2001; Keele et al. 2006).

There are other controversial theories concerning HIV/AIDS. One of the most controversial theories concerns the role HIV plays in causing AIDS (Goodman 1995; Adams 1989). Whereas most scientists believe that HIV causes AIDS, Peter Duesberg, a biologist at the University of California–Berkeley, presents a different explanation for AIDS (1996). In the late 1980s, Duesberg proposed that HIV does not cause AIDS. He does not deny that AIDS exists, but he states that HIV is not the precipitating virus (Duesberg 1996; Adams 1989). Duesberg believes that lifestyle factors including IDU, recreational drug use such as "poppers" (amyl nitrate), and sexually transmitted infections (STIs) such as syphilis are the causative agents for AIDS. Each of these agents or a combination of them can weaken the immune system, leaving one susceptible to OIs, resulting in death (Duesberg 1996; Goodman 1995).

Duesberg initially proposed his theory before much was known about the mutability and replication abilities of the virus, its different strains, and the immediate and insidious effect HIV has on the immune system. He believes that HIV does not meet the criteria of Robert Koch's postulates. Koch's postulates are a set of four principles that must be met to accept that a virus is the causative agent for a disease. Since HIV antibody tests do not test for the virus itself, and people can be immune-compromised for reasons other than being infected with HIV, Duesberg believes that if HIV exists, it is a cofactor but not the cause of AIDS (Duesberg 1996; Adams 1989; Goodman 1995; see chapter 3).

The **AIDS Coalition to Unleash Power (ACTUP)** is an AIDS activist group. Early in the epidemic, ACTUP accepted that HIV caused AIDS and supported the use of antiretroviral drugs. ACTUP was a critical force in changing how clinical trials for new drugs to slow the progression of AIDS were conducted and in challenging major pharmaceutical companies about the prices for early antiretroviral drugs (Thomas 2001; Shilts 1987; Stoller 1998).

However, by the 1990s, ACTUP had changed its views in support of Duesberg (ACTUP 2003). The reasons for this change are rooted in politics and the lack of either a cure or a vaccine for HIV/AIDS. ACTUP now believes that HAART and other antiretroviral drugs destroy the immune system, not HIV (ACTUP 2003). The organization also believes that the lack of a cure or vaccine is due in part to homophobia in the United States.

HAART is a highly toxic drug regime. People with HIV/AIDS will be on HAART indefinitely until either a cure or a vaccine becomes available. For ACTUP, HAART has become a symbol of homophobia, insensitivity to the gay community, and the power that the U.S. pharmaceutical industry has over drug costs and drug distribution (ACTUP 2003). ACTUP's philosophical changes illustrate both the connection between theory and behavior and the impact that Duesberg's work has had in various communities. His position has had far-reaching consequences and generated international debate.

Although most people in the biomedical community, basic and social science researchers, and epidemiologists renounce Duesberg's theory, the controversy generated by him and others about HIV has had international implications. President Thabo Mvuyelwa Mbeki of South Africa announced prior to the beginning of the Thirteenth International AIDS Conference in Durban, South Africa, in 2000 that he doubted that HIV caused AIDS and that he accepted Duesberg's explanation for AIDS. President Mbeki called for an international panel, including both supporters and opponents of Duesberg's ideas (Cherry 2000a, 2000b; Anon. 2000a; Commentary 2000). President Mbeki believes that poverty and malnutrition, not HIV, cause AIDS (Cherry 2000a, 2000b; Basu et al. 2000). About 20 percent of South Africa's population is HIV+. The average per capita health care expenditure in parts of sub-Saharan Africa is US$14 per year (Basu, Mate, and Farmer 2000). While most scientists and others involved in HIV research, prevention, treatment, and program development recognize the effects of poverty on overall health, and its role as a cofactor in HIV infection, the overwhelming position by these communities is that HIV causes AIDS (Commentary 2000; Basu et al. 2000). In response to international criticism and lack of support for his position, Mbeki later withdrew from the debate over the cause of AIDS (Anon. 2000a; Cherry 2000b).

In 2000, an international panel of AIDS researchers, physicians, and activists issued a multipoint statement challenging Duesberg (Commentary 2000). This statement includes the following points:

- HIV-1 and HIV-2 are closely related to SIV that infects chimpanzees and sooty mangabey monkeys respectively.
- HIV-1 and HIV-2 "species jumped" to humans and are now spread from human to human. HIV-1 is the more common of the two viruses.
- HIV meets Koch's criteria for viral diseases. These include the following. First, people with AIDS are infected with HIV. If untreated, people with HIV develop AIDS within five to ten years. HIV can be detected by the presence of antibodies to it, through gene sequences, or by virus isolation. Next, people who receive HIV+ blood develop AIDS, whereas those who do not receive HIV+ blood do not develop AIDS. Most HIV+ children contract

HIV from their mothers either in utero, during childbirth, or while breast-feeding. Furthermore, the higher the viral load in the mother, the greater the risk to the fetus/child. Under laboratory conditions, HIV infects white cells in people with AIDS. Lastly, HAART blocks HIV in the lab and in people.

Given what is currently known about viral load, viral replication, and mutability, the scientific community maintains that HIV causes AIDS (Stine 1997; Thomas 2001; Cohen, Sande, and Volberding 1999). The scientific community's response to Mbeki was rapid and equally vitriolic. The community's detailed response can be read at http://www.tac.org.za/.

2.3

Harper's, a respected magazine, set off a maelstrom of criticism in the scientific community when it published an article by Celia Farber in its March 2006 issue. Farber, a reporter, basically challenged the scientific community's position on HIV as the cause of AIDS, reinvoking Duesberg's arguments and the toxicity of the AIDS drugs as the primary destroyers of the immune system (2006).

There are many reasons why racist, sexist, and conspiracy-based origin theories as well as competing theories for AIDS causation exist and gain acceptance. The reasons are complex. As Cindy Patton states, Africa still is seen by outsiders as the "dark" continent. Racist theories about African sexuality, particularly about African women, persist (Patton 1994; Orubuloye et al. 1994). When a disaster occurs, having an "other" to blame for it is much easier than examining one's own behavior as a contributing factor. Many people in the United States and cross-culturally believe that HIV/ AIDS is a punishment, a moral transgression, or "God's revenge." Blaming others for a virus reinforces sexist and racist origin theories (Patton 1994; Vernon 2001; Bockting and Kirk 2001).

Conspiracy theories can also develop from racism and sexism. Racism and sexism are widespread cross-culturally and in the United States. Euro-American politicians and researchers have not always behaved responsibly and humanely toward disenfranchised people in their own and other societies. Two examples illustrate this point. The Tuskegee experiments in the United States allowed African American men with syphilis to be left untreated so that researchers could "learn" about the disease's progression. International testing of oral contraceptives without informed consent in nonindustrialized countries during the 1950s created distrust of U.S. medical and political systems (Loue 1999; Vernon 2001; Mayer and Pizer 2000).

Origin theories pose several problems. First, they are hard to prove and, once accepted, to disprove. The interpretation and acceptance of origin theories by the larger society can affect people in their daily lives. For example, the belief that HIV/AIDS was introduced by the oral polio vaccine (OPV) resulted in parents in some communities not inoculating their children, for fear of HIV transmission (Dickson 2000). Second, many origin theories for HIV/AIDS reinforced stigma and blame, were ethnocentric and racist, and attributed the virus and its spread to an "other," an outsider, reinforcing existing stereotypes (Sontag 1995; Patton 1994; Wolffers and Josie 1999).

We are now in the third decade of the epidemic, with estimates of up to 57 million people having been infected with HIV or having AIDS worldwide since 1981. There is no "limit" predicted on the incidence or prevalence of HIV/AIDS that will be seen in the future (UNAIDS 2002a, 2002b, 2004; Merson and Dayton 2002: 13). Some researchers suggest that focusing on prevention and treatment would be more useful at this time than determining origins of the virus (Farmer, Walton, and Furin 2000).

Ethics

This overview of the epidemiology, history, and origins of AIDS leads to an introduction of the ethics involved in AIDS intervention. Controversy seems to exist with whatever facet of HIV one explores—biomedical, epidemiological, sociocultural, or politico-economic (Fletcher et al. 1999; Bennett 1999; Bennett and Erin 1999). The controversies extend to ethics and AIDS. Ethnocentrism, erotophobia, homophobia, and sexism have all been involved in reporting incidence and prevalence rates, the labeling of the disease in its early years, and deciding how to establish profiles of behaviorally at-risk individuals and groups (Loue 1999). As discussed earlier, unexamined assumptions and biases about "morality," sexuality, women, subcultures, and drugs have influenced early and current investigations into the incidence and prevalence of HIV (Vollmer 2000).

Ethical discussions impact funding research and access to and distribution of resources for prevention, testing, and treatment, as well as affect drug and vaccine development and trials. There are debates over applied and research aspects of HIV, as well as over informed consent and who develops and implements programs (Kendall 1996; LeVine 2000; Heitman and Ross 1999; Thomas 2001). Historically and currently, there are ethical arguments about the use of human subjects in medical research, particularly in using groups in nonindustrialized societies to test drugs and in giving people expired or less-effective drugs that are no longer used in industrialized countries (De la Gorgendière 2005; Bond 1997). The ethical debates about drugs include whether to deny people access to HAART because of international patent laws (Kendall 1996; Loue 1999).

With the development and availability of HAART in 1996, and the administration of **AZT076** to pregnant women to reduce perinatal transmission since 1994 in the United States, the ethical controversies about drug access and administration have become divisive and pervasive (Bennett 1999; Bennett and Erin 1999). The different approaches to prevention and treatment between industrialized and nonindustrialized societies have widened since the availability of these two drug regimens. With HAART, people live longer and experience improved health. Since most people with HIV/AIDS worldwide do not have access to HAART, they face debilitating illness and death.

Disenfranchised groups within and outside the United States such as African Americans and people in sub-Saharan Africa and parts of Southeast Asia are suspicious of industrialized countries' and governments' motives for testing and distributing medical resources (Vernon 2001; Loue 1999; Thomas 2001; Patton 1994; Fletcher et al. 1999; Blankenship 1997). Because these suspicions are grounded on actual abuses, participants at the Helsinki Conference issued clear international guidelines concerning ethical issues and procedures when conducting medical research, testing, and treatment across borders (Kendall 1996; LeVine 2000).

Economic, political, and social policies advanced by industrialized societies toward nonindustrialized ones have created distrust, fear, and anger. These feelings can result in conspiracy theories, backlash reactions, and compromises in people's health when HIV is involved.

HIV/AIDS is a relatively new disease. The cultural response to it is as complex as the virus itself. Responding to the epidemic requires a continuous, interdisciplinary, and international response that is culturally sensitive and cognizant of the intricacies involved in this illness.

2.4

Two unresolved, ongoing ethical controversies surrounding HIV prevention and treatment in nonindustrialized societies involve the use of Nevirapine, an ARV, to prevent **mother-to-child transmission (MTCT)** and
the testing of Tenofovir, another ARV, as a preventive drug. Nevirapine
can effectively reduce MTCT, is cheaper and more easily administered
than some of the other drugs used for this purpose, and has fewer negative side effects than other drugs. For these reasons, it is seen by many as
the drug of choice to give to pregnant women in nonindustrialized societies. However, administering Nevirapine for this reason can also lead to
later drug resistance for the woman.

Tenofovir is seen as a possible HIV preventive drug for sexually active
people. However, in clinical trials begun in Southeast Asia, local and international activist groups protested the lack of safety measures for the
research population, sex workers. The trial was halted. Ethical controversies surround every aspect of HIV intervention, from prevention to HIV
testing and treatment. These two topics are addressed in more detail in
chapters 5 and 7, respectively.

SUMMARY

HIV/AIDS is pandemic. As of 2008, there is neither a cure nor a vaccine
   available.

HIV/AIDS is decimating nonindustrialized societies, particularly in sub-
   Saharan Africa.

Risks for infection include individual behavior, societal norms and values about sexuality and drugs, and larger politico- economic policies
   that affect health.

Cofactors in HIV infection include nutrition, other STIs, overall state of
   health, and economic stability.

The origins of AIDS are controversial. Current explanations involve an
   evolved species-jumping (zoonotic) transmission from chimpanzees
   to humans.

Ethical issues surround most aspects of AIDS intervention both in the
   United States and cross-culturally.

Thought Questions

Why are origin theories of AIDS so controversial? What ethical questions do these theories present?

Why is a culturally sensitive and specific approach needed to develop and provide HIV intervention efforts?

Resources

Articles

Aggleton, Peter. "'Just a Snip?' A Social History of Male Circumcision." Reproductive Health Matters 15, no. 29 (2007): 15–21.

Books

Garrett, Laurie. The Coming Plague. New York: Harper Collins Canada, 1994.
Office of the Surgeon General. The Surgeon General's Call to Action to Promote Sexual Health and Responsible Sexual Behavior. Rockville, Md.: Office of the Surgeon General, 2001.
Shilts, Randy. And the Band Played On: Politics, People, and the AIDS Epidemic. New York: St. Martin's Press, 1987.
Sontag, Susan. Illness as Metaphor and AIDS and Its Metaphors. London: Peter Smith Publishers, 1995.
Thomas, Patricia. Big Shot: Passion, Politics and the Struggle for an AIDS Vaccine. New York: Public Affairs Press, 2001.
Vernon, Irene S. Killing Us Quietly. Lincoln: University of Nebraska Press, 2001.
Wolffers, Ivan, and Mascha Bevers. Sex Work, Mobility and AIDS in Kuala Lumpur, Malaysia. Amsterdam, Netherlands: Caram-Asia and the Free University of Amsterdam, 1997.

Videos

Bilheimer, Robert. A Closer Walk. Santa Monica, Calif.: Direct Cinema Limited, 2003.
D'Entremont, D. Breaking the Silence (South Africa). Glenwood Springs, Colo.: Media for Development International, 1996.
Pike, R. (ed.). AIDS in Africa. Ontario Center, Montreal, and Ottawa: Canadian Film Board (National Film Board [NFB]), 1990.
Reid, F. The Faces of AIDS: Human Experience in Africa. A Family Health International AIDS/TECH/AIDSCA Production (Arlington, Va.: USAID). Glenwood Springs, Colo.: Media for Development Intl., 1992.
Roodt, Darrell James. Yesterday. New York and Los Angeles: HBO Films, 2004.

Web Sites

AEGIS (AIDS Education Global Information System): http://www.aegis.com.

CDC: http://www.cdc.gov.

UNAIDS: http://www.unaids.org/en/.

World Health Organization, 2007. "WHO and UNAIDS Announce Recommendations from Expert Consultation on Male Circumcision for HIV Prevention." http://www.who.int/hiv/medicacentre/news68/en/index.html, accessed April 2, 2007.

3

The Biomedical Aspects of HIV/AIDS

Thomas Budd

CHAPTER HIGHLIGHTS INCLUDE

An overview of viruses

A description of HIV

HIV infection and detection of the virus

A description of the biochemical process that occurs with seroconversion and the development of AIDS

Reverse transcription and HIV progression

A discussion of the efficacy and challenges of taking HAART in the United States and cross-culturally

A discussion of the challenges involved in vaccine development

> Over the course of our evolution, "genetic changes in humans may have left us more susceptible to infection by human immunodeficiency virus type 1 (HIV-1)."
>
> Kaiser, Malik, and Emerman: abstract 1756

Knowledge of the circumstances and consequences of HIV infection can be understood through an overview of the basics of cell biology. Most social and cultural considerations cannot be discussed without understanding the biology of the virus and the resulting medical consequences. With several excellent texts, Internet sites, and a huge body of literature (both scientific and lay) available, this chapter will focus on the basic biological factors needed for an understanding of the anthropological aspects of the AIDS pandemic. Most of this chapter will be an explanation of two diagrams. The first is referred to as the course of AIDS and the second, the HIV cycle.

The Course of AIDS Begins with the Viruses

Viruses are not infectious organisms, even though we classify them using the same nomenclature conventions as organisms. They are normal cell products. Virtually every living cell, from bacteria to human, has the ability to produce viruses if appropriately stimulated to do so, as part of its normal genetic makeup. Often, that stimulation is the uptake of the virus by the host cell, but many cells have long-term viral-making potential—that is, the virus has become a normal, permanent genetic component of the host cell, called a **provirus**. Examples include herpes simplex (which causes cold sores) and Epstein-Barr virus (which causes mononucleosis). These viruses stay in our bodies for life. Unfortunately, many viruses have evolved in a way that disrupts the delicate homeostasis of the mammalian organism. When this situation occurs in an organism, we call this condition a disease or pathology, regardless of whether it is influenza, the common cold, or HIV (see figure 3.1).

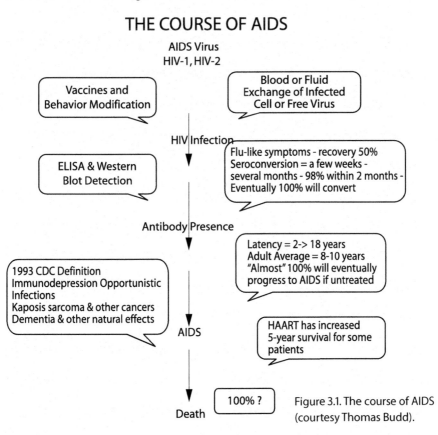

Figure 3.1. The course of AIDS (courtesy Thomas Budd).

Human Immunodeficiency Virus (HIV) Components

Envelope

The outermost layer of the virus is called the **envelope**. It is composed of a biological membrane that is derived from the infected (host) cell's surface membrane. This membrane is referred to as the cytoplasmic or plasma membrane when that cell buds off creating the new **virons** (viral particles) (see figure 3.2).

Envelope Proteins: gp120 and gp41

The *gp* stands for glycoprotein, a molecule made up of both protein and carbohydrate parts. The number stands for the molecular mass of the glycoprotein in scientific units called kilodaltons; thus, the larger the number, the larger the protein. The proteins that occur in the envelope of the viron have to be placed in the host cell's membrane and positioned at the site of the budding process (see figure 3.2).

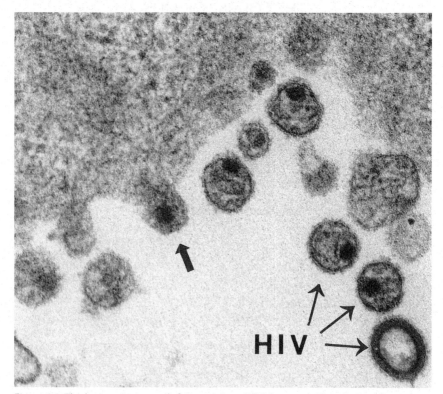

Figure 3.2. The human immunodeficiency virus (HIV) (courtesy Thomas Budd).

Matrix Layer

Just beneath the viral envelope lies a layer of matrix proteins. These proteins bind to each other to form a structural layer that provides some durability. Many nonenveloped viruses use this protein layer as the main coat or capsid of the viron (figure 3.3).

Core Particle

The core particle is found inside the matrix layer. This particle is made up of "core" protein molecules that bind together to give the particle a tapered, cylindrical, cigar-butt shape. Within this core protein layer are two copies of the RNA viral genome with a molecule of an enzyme called **reverse transcriptase (RT)**. This enzyme is attached to each RNA copy. Reverse transcriptase is an enzyme used by **retroviruses** to transcribe genetic information from RNA to DNA. The RNA is in a highly condensed shape because it is bound with several copies of a protein called p7.

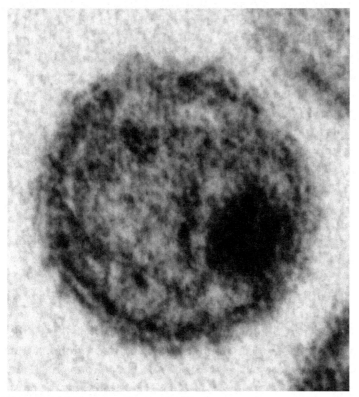

Figure 3.3. HIV (courtesy Thomas Budd).

There is also a molecule of an enzyme called **integrase** inside the core particle, along with a few other viral proteins (Alcamo 2003; Fan et al. 2004; Bartlett 2006; Hutchinson 2001).

Does HIV Really Cause AIDS?

As discussed in chapter 2, there are still some who are not convinced that HIV is the cause of the current AIDS pandemic. They argue that medical experts have not satisfied Koch's postulates and that there are some case reports of persons with clinically defined AIDS who show no evidence of HIV infection (see chapter 2 for a discussion of Koch's postulates and HIV).

There are some reported cases of acquired immune deficiencies without evidence of HIV infection. However, these reports do not prove that HIV does not cause AIDS. There have been many cases of adults acquiring a wide variety of immune-based deficiencies, some of which may cause clinical symptoms similar to AIDS. Theoretically, this situation is analogous to adult-onset diabetes, which may be attributed to genetic predisposition, to environmental effects of obesity, to age-related mutation burden, or to autoimmune diseases. The current AIDS pandemic repeatedly illustrates the link between HIV and AIDS. Today, with the present level of sophisticated molecular techniques, we have identified every HIV gene and understand most of each gene's contribution to the pathogenicity of AIDS. This understanding is alarming because we have not been able to develop either a cure or a vaccine for HIV/AIDS, and that presents a definitive biological puzzle.

HIV Variations

Unfortunately, HIV is not a single, stable virus but instead a large family of viruses. There are two major forms: HIV-1 and HIV-2. HIV-2 is a relatively minor contributor to the AIDS pandemic. It is mostly endemic in northwestern Africa but has also occurred in other parts of the world. HIV-1 has caused most of the AIDS cases worldwide (Keele et al. 2006; Hutchinson 2001). There are three groups of HIV-1, designated "M" (the "main" group), "O" (the "outlier" group), and "N" (a "new" group). Most AIDS cases in the world are caused by viruses in the M group. There are several subgroups of HIV-1 group M (labeled A–H, with B being the most prevalent in North America and Western Europe, for example). Each subgroup has hundreds, perhaps thousands of genetic variants (Alcamo 2003; Fan et al. 2004). This is because the virus mutates (evolves) very rapidly, more rapidly than any other virus studied to date. If an individual were to be infected with one viral variant, within one year, there could be dozens of other genetically different virons within the infected host. This rapid mutation ability presents us with several serious problems. For example, how does one develop a vaccine, a process that takes years, against a target that changes genetically in weeks? What if the virus evolves to become more easily transmitted?

When HIV was first discovered in the United States, it was thought to belong to a family of viruses called **human T-cell lymphotrophic viruses (HTLV)**. These viruses were implicated in the causation of some leukemias, and the AIDS-associated isolate was called HTLV-III. French scientists at the Pasteur Institute in Paris who were also studying HIV called their isolate **lymphadenopathy-associated virus (LAV)** (Shilts 1987; Hutchinson 2001). When scientists understood the genetic makeup in more detail, the virus was assigned to its own classification group and named HIV (Shilts 1987; Hutchinson 2001).

HIV Infection

HIV is transmitted through sex (anal, vaginal, and oral, in order of efficiency of transmission), through nonsterile syringes and/or needles (anytime one penetrates one's skin with any needle that has penetrated someone else's skin, one is at risk of infection), and through MTCT. MTCT has been shown to be significantly minimized by antiviral drugs (see chapter 7).

These modes of transmission are how many people conceptualize HIV transmission. There is, however, another component that is an important part of understanding HIV transmission. Theoretically, a person can be infected with a free virus particle. Free virus particles consist of the virus itself, not encapsulated into a cell. (The free virus might be found in laboratory settings, for example.) The free viron is extremely fragile and is inactivated by sunlight, soap, rubbing alcohol, diluted bleach, or drying. After thirty minutes, culturing the virus from a smear of free virus on a dried surface becomes nearly impossible. Thus, it would be almost impossible to be infected with free virus.

However, if cells are infected, they can transmit the virus. Cells can remain viable much longer than the free virus. This probably accounts for why the infection is spread not by casual contact but by contact with secretions containing infected cells. This difference might seem trivial, but it is not. Most HIV is transmitted through infected cells, a factor that is of paramount importance in how we test vaccines and how we design antiviral drugs.

Because the virus is found within a cell, it can move across cell wall barriers. For example, HIV can pass through the placental barrier as well as the blood brain barrier. These barriers are made up of endothelial cells, which form the capillaries at these boundaries and are easily infected by HIV. These boundaries filter what passes into the brain and across the placenta. Neurons are also easily infected by HIV, which can lead to AIDS-related dementia. We cannot actually "kill" HIV (since it is not an organism), but it can be inactivated by antiretrovirals.

Since almost all infections are probably due to the transfer of infected cells that contain the viral genome from an infected person to the new host, the lymphocytes and other white blood cells that are a normal component of semen and vaginal secretions make them good hosts for HIV. Because most HIV is encapsulated in cells, urogenital infections such as sexually transmitted infections (STIs) significantly increase the probability of transmission of HIV. Such infections cause cells of the immune system to accumulate in the genital system to fight the infection. If these cells are infected with HIV, it increases their probability to carry the HIV to the new host. Once a person is infected, the immune system usually recognizes the presence of the virus, responding by making special serum proteins called antibodies and by activating special cells to kill HIV-infected cells.

Immunology

The immune system is made up of a fascinating collection of cells that keep the human body under constant surveillance for foreign invaders (see figure 3.4). The immune system comprises white blood cells, primary and secondary immune tissues, and a second circulatory system in the body. The major cell components of this system are called T-lymphocytes or T-cells (the "T" stands for thymus, and these cells are processed in the thymus gland before being released into the body); B-cells (in humans these originate in the *b*one marrow, thus *B*-cell); and macrophages. The other white blood cells function as accessory cells that help the T-cells, B-cells, and macrophages (Alcamo 2003).

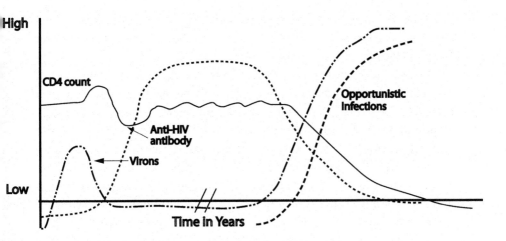

Figure 3.4. Time course to AIDS (courtesy Thomas Budd).

Most simply, macrophages are cells that migrate throughout the body's tissues and detect foreign material. They leave the blood vascular system at the capillary beds (which are composed of endothelial cells that line the entire vascular system for blood and lymph). Macrophages enter tissues and are then drained into the lymph vascular system. This system leads to what are called secondary lymphatic tissues, mostly lymph nodes and fol- licles, and eventually re-enters the blood stream. When the macrophages arrive back at secondary lymphatic tissues such as lymph nodes, they present any foreign material found in the tissues to specific T-cells. These T-cells (called helper T-cells or CD4 cells) then direct B-cells to make and secrete special proteins called antibodies that will specifically bind to the HIV components, leading to the destruction of the virus. Other T-cells (called cytotoxic or killer T-cells) are activated to attack and kill any cells that are producing new HIV (Alcamo 2003; Hutchinson 2001).

Although helper T-cells are a high-affinity target of most HIV (owing to the high binding affinity between the HIV envelope gp120 and the T- cell's CD4 surface protein and a co-receptor called CXCR4), some HIV are able to target macrophages because of the occurrence of another specific co-receptor, called CCR5, on the macrophage cell surface. Thus, mac- rophages also take up the HIV provirus early in the infection. This is most troublesome because the normal role of macrophages is to keep all of the bodies' tissues (cells) under immune surveillance through direct cell-to- cell contact. This, of course, lends itself to the possibility for transfer of the viral genome or, at the very least, close-up transfer of budded virons.

Regardless of the method, we now know that there is a very long list of cell types that can become host cells for HIV (Hutchinson 2001; McBride and Bradford 2004).

The viral production (load) will fluctuate throughout the latency period between infection and AIDS but overall will usually be held at relatively low levels. At some point, the viral load begins to increase, with a corresponding decrease in CD4 cell count and eventually a decrease in the amount of anti-HIV antibodies, thus the onset of immunodeficiency.

There are two main theories pertaining to this phenomenon. The first theory states that the virus takes up residence in CD4 cells (the provirus) and enters a quiescent phase. The viral genes are thought to be activated in individual cells at a relatively low but steady frequency and thus cause a low-level, continuous production of free virons that can progressively infect many other cells, leading to the later acquisition of AIDS. We can call this theory the "quiescent" theory.

The other theory contends that the immune system is very efficient at killing off the infected CD4 cells, many or most of which are producing the virus. We have already noted that this viral production causes the viral envelope components to be displayed on the surface of infected cells, subjecting the cells to efficient immune destruction. The immune system attempts to replace these destroyed cells at such a rate that it depletes the lifetime supply of these cells during the latency period. We can call this the "burn out" theory, which is consonant with a major theory of biological aging. The CD4 cell is the immune cell that directs the production of antibodies against foreign material. If this population of cells is eventually depleted, the level of anti-HIV antibodies will also decrease. Which of these theories is correct? There is evidence that both models are valid: there is a rapid turnover of helper T-cells, and there is also a large reservoir of infected cells (containing the provirus) that persist long term throughout the body (Hutchinson 2001; Bartlett 2006; Alcamo 2003).

Unfortunately, HIV is able to take up residence in many different cell types, not just helper T-cells. This list includes most other white blood cells (especially macrophages), endothelial cells (which line the inner surface of the entire vascular system and also form capillaries), neurons and glial cells, epithelial cells, and fibroblasts. Almost any cell is potentially capable of harboring HIV. This is because cells may transmit HIV or its genome via cell-to-cell contact. There is no need for the free virus particle. Mammalian cells are very capable of taking nucleic acids (such as DNA or RNA) from solution. Also, when **histocompatible** cells (cells that are not foreign to one another—for example, from within the same organism) come into physical contact with each other, there are often transient membrane fusion events that can allow the transfer of cellular material, including HIV components. These phenomena are known to exist even in primitive bacterial cells. As a result, even if our antibodies can bind to and neutralize free HIV, the provirus form still persists since antibodies cannot penetrate into the interior of infected cells (Hutchinson 2001; Alcamo 2003).

The production of antibodies by the immune system is how we determine whether one is infected by HIV. One's **sero-status** goes from being **seronegative** for anti-HIV antibodies (that is, no HIV-specific antibodies in the serum) to **seropositive** for anti-HIV antibodies. Thus, one **seroconverts** from negative to positive for these proteins that bind very specifically to HIV components. This usually happens within the first two to three months following the receipt of HIV into the body. About half of infected persons experience a flulike illness that is rarely realized as being linked to HIV infection. The other half of infected persons have no indication that there is something new in their bodies. Some persons take a longer time to respond immunologically to HIV, which is referred to as delayed seroconversion. Delayed seroconversion can sometimes take months. These people's blood would test negative for HIV despite their being infected. This small number of persons is why the donated blood supply is not perfectly safe. Despite vigilant screening efforts, some HIV-infected blood still makes its way into the blood supply (see chapter 6).

ELISA (Enzyme-Linked Immunosorbent Assay)

The **Enzyme-Linked Immunosorbent Assay** (**ELISA**) is a test designed to detect anti-HIV antibodies in blood samples. Because it is very inexpensive, we also use this assay to test people. If one has antibodies against HIV in one's serum, it is somewhat reasonable to assume that one is infected with HIV. Remember that HIV is closely related to other retroviruses such as the HTLV family of viruses. If one is infected with an HTLV, the antibodies made against these viruses might "cross-react" with HIV virus components. Thus, there are actually two assays used to determine HIV infection. The ELISA is the first test. This assay was designed to give more false positive results than false negative results, the theory being that we should reject more noninfected blood than accept infected blood. If the first ELISA is negative, people can reasonably assume that they are

HIV negative. Because of this test bias, if people test positive on the first ELISA, they should not assume that they are positive for HIV. If the first test is positive, the ELISA is repeated a second time. If the first ELISA was positive and the second ELISA was negative, this first result was most probably a false positive reading. If people receive two positive ELISA results, it is highly improbable that they would have two false positive readings in a row. This means that they are infected with a retrovirus, but it is not necessarily HIV; it could be an infection with a cross-reactive HTLV. Nor, if people are infected with an HTLV, does this necessarily mean that they will develop leukemia, because HTLV infection is only one of several steps that can lead to the development of leukemia (Bartlett 2006).

To discern between these related viruses, a second test, called a **Western Blot**, is performed. The Western Blot is a test that determines not only whether testers have anti-HIV antibodies but also which components of HIV the antibodies will specifically bind to. The assay first separates the HIV components and then measures which of them are bound by serum antibodies. This then differentiates whether people are infected with HIV or a related virus. If the Western Blot is negative, even with two positive ELISAs, people are not considered to be infected with HIV. If the Western Blot is positive, then the tester is considered to be HIV positive (Bartlett 2006). This testing scenario is important for everyone to know. There are numerous reports of persons erroneously thinking they were infected when they received positive ELISA results but negative Western Blot results. Having an HIV test is a serious decision. The intricacies of testing are discussed in chapter 4.

3.1

Since the Western Blot test is the confirmatory HIV test, why isn't it administered first instead of the ELISA? The answer rests with demographics (see chapter 2) and finances. The ELISA is sensitive to viral presence, relatively inexpensive, and easy to administer, making it a good initial screening test. The Western Blot test, while much more specific than the ELISA, is a more expensive and complicated test. Therefore, the initial HIV screening test is the highly sensitive but not specific ELISA.

Progression to AIDS

What happens between infection with HIV and progression to AIDS? As defined and discussed in chapters 1 and 2, an AIDS diagnosis is a classification of symptoms. The consequence of infection is quite variable from individual to individual. Because of this, the definition of AIDS was expanded in 1993 (see chapter 2). However, there is an average latency period between infection and the acquisition of the symptomatic form, AIDS, of eight to ten years in adults (without drug therapy). Infants infected with HIV usually develop AIDS sooner because their immune systems are not fully developed.

The progression of the HIV infection is now tracked predominantly by measuring the viral load, which represents the number of HIV virons in the blood circulation system. This increases early in the infection and then usually decreases to varying low levels for several years in response to the immune response. Then, an average of eight to ten years later, the viral count increases and the number of helper T-cells decreases, with a concomitant increase in opportunistic infections; this is classified as a case of AIDS. This lowered resistance to infection is predominantly due to a decrease in antibody production. The opportunistic infections are often life-threatening (Hutchinson 2001; Fan et al. 2004; Alcamo 2003).

It is interesting to note that some individuals have been infected with HIV for much longer than the average latency period without developing the symptoms of AIDS. We refer to these people as long-term survivors or nonprogressors. Everyone else who becomes infected with HIV will very probably progress to AIDS and without successful treatment will most likely die.

Once the immune response against HIV is compromised, there is an increase in opportunistic infections (OIs). We all have what is referred to as a normal flora of microbes that live in and on our bodies: stomach, intestines, lungs, throat, mouth, and skin. They are everywhere and include bacteria, fungi (molds), and protozoa. Our primary and immune defenses normally hold these organisms in check. When our immune defenses are compromised, these microbes have the opportunity to grow out of control and can cause opportunistic infections. Which OIs manifest would depend on whether the microbes were present in one's normal flora.

There may be other consequences of immune deficiency than opportunistic infections. Neurons are easily infected with HIV. When they display HIV components on their surface membranes, they are subjected to destruction by cytotoxic T-cells, just as were the CD4 cells. That is, they are killed while attempting to produce and release HIV. If enough neurons are killed, this may result in AIDS-related dementia. This phenomenon may occur in the absence of other classic opportunistic infections. The immunodeficiency may also allow some cancers to establish more readily than normal, especially **Kaposi's sarcoma** and malignant lymphoma. There is no longer one definition of classical AIDS. This is due in part to the variability in the genetics of the human immune system (see chapters 1 and 2) (Hutchinson 2001).

The vigor and durability of the immune system is determined by a cluster of genes called the **major histocompatibility (gene) complex (MHC)**. In humans, this cluster of genes is found on chromosome number 6. The term *major histocompatibility (gene) complex* implies that there are minor histocompatibility gene complexes. There are, but the MHC genes collectively determine the vigor of the immune system (Hutchinson 2001; Alcamo 2003). We always theorize that there are individuals who have a natural immunity to a malady. That is why you are reading this chapter; your ancestors survived smallpox and other lethal diseases. In the realm of AIDS, we refer to these persons as long-term nonprogressors. There is a group of infected persons who have been HIV positive for more than eighteen years and have not progressed to the symptomatic stage of AIDS. How is their MHC different from the normal progressors? This remains to be determined.

3.2

A recent article in the journal *Science* posits that during the course of primate evolution, sometime after humans separated from other primates, we lost a gene common to chimpanzees. Loss of that gene eventually made us more susceptible to HIV-1 (Kaiser, Malik, and Emerman 2007: 1756–1758).

Despite the length of the latency period, most people infected with HIV will progress to AIDS. We will explain soon how some drugs (that is, chemotherapy) may postpone this. Currently, we are seeing a significant decrease in mortality because of this therapy. Those persons who either do not have access to this therapy or have drug-resistant HIV die of the consequences of immunodeficiency.

Cellular Production of HIV

Let us now examine in more detail the cycle of HIV production by cells using the diagram in figure 3.5. HIV genes are not made of DNA. HIV, like the HTLV family, is referred to as a retrovirus because the HIV genes are in the form of RNA. Most genes in our biological world are in a form called DNA. In the normal course of biology, DNA (genes) does basically one thing: its gene sequences are transcribed into RNA. The RNA is used (translated) to make proteins. Proteins do the work of cells, making up cell structures and causing the synthesis of cell structures. This overall process has been called the central dogma or primary metabolism (see figure 3.6).

DNA also undergoes replication (indicated by "Rep." in figure 3.6), so that when cells divide, each daughter cell receives a copy of the cell's ge-

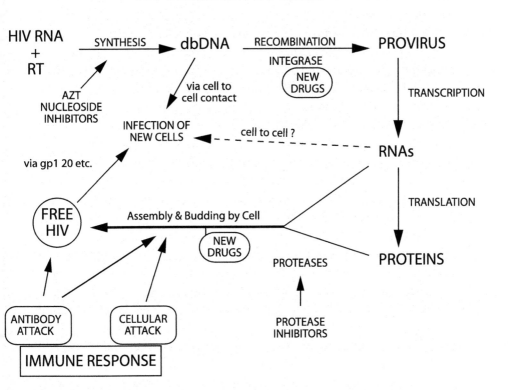

Figure 3.5. HIV infection of cells (courtesy Thomas Budd).

TRANSCRIPTION PROCESS

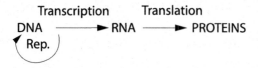

Figure 3.6. Transcription process (courtesy Thomas Budd).

nome. This replication of the DNA is done by a group of enzymes called DNA-dependent DNA polymerases (they use DNA as a template to make an exact copy of DNA). To do the reverse of transcription—that is, to turn RNA into DNA—we need an RNA-dependent DNA polymerase enzyme, and that is what the reverse transcriptase enzyme is. It uses the RNA gene sequence as the template to make a DNA copy of the gene sequence. This process also involves some enzyme activity called RNAse to accomplish this task. This activity is needed to form double-stranded DNA, the form that host cell genes are made of. After this process, the HIV genes are in the same chemical form as normal cellular genes (Hutchinson 2001).

Remember that reverse transcriptase is associated with the HIV RNA in the viron core particle. Thus, our process begins with the virus's entry into a cell. This is facilitated by receptor proteins on the surface of the virus that bind specifically with cell surface proteins. An example of this is the binding specificity between the viral envelope protein called gp120 and the protein called CD4, which occurs almost exclusively on the surface of helper T-cells. This binding also involves another co-receptor protein on the cell surface, referred to as a chemokine receptor. Thus, most HIV has a preference for infecting the helper T-cells. When these proteins become bound to each other, they change shape, causing the viral envelope membrane and the cell membrane to fuse. This allows the viral core particle (containing the viral RNA and reverse transcriptase [RT]) to enter the cell interior. The normal cellular machinery for protein degradation and turnover (all proteins and protein structures in cells are constantly being degraded and resynthesized) disassembles the core particle. This releases the two RNA copies of the viral genome to be converted into the form of the double-stranded DNA, the same form as normal cellular genes. There are three genes that are found in all retroviruses: they are called env, pol, and gag (Hutchinson 2001; Alcamo 2003; Fan et al. 2004).

The RT enzyme is very error prone when making the DNA form of the HIV genes. The cells' regular DNA polymerases have a proofreading mechanism to ensure accuracy in synthesizing the DNA, but RT lacks this proofreading activity. With no proofreading as a check on RT replication, HIV mutates and evolves very rapidly. This also makes RT a good target for antiviral drugs and explains why we have a large selection of RT inhibitor drugs in our treatment arsenal.

Forming the Provirus

HIV contains an enzyme called integrase that, when released from the core particle, works with other normal cell proteins to integrate the DNA viral genome among the other cell genes in the nucleus. This normal cellular process is called genetic recombination. Many cellular genes can be moved (that is, cut out and inserted) to different locations on the chromosomes and even to different chromosomes. The HIV DNA is transported into the cell nucleus, where the cellular DNA is cut open and the HIV DNA is inserted by connecting each end of the HIV DNA to the terminus on each side of the cut. The viral genome thus becomes, for all metabolic purposes, a normal component of the host cell genome. We refer to this arrangement as a provirus. If the infected host cell divides, the viral genes are replicated along with the cell's normal genome (Hutchinson 2001).

As you might imagine, this is a very intricate and complicated process; thus, it is also a good target for inhibiting HIV. Indeed, integrase inhibitor drugs are under development. Great care is needed, however, because the normal cellular process of cutting and splicing genes (recombination) might also be disrupted or misregulated.

Expression of the HIV Genes

As noted above, genes do basically two things: they are used as templates to make more copies of the genes, and they are transcribed and translated into proteins. Proteins do the work of cells (and viruses—for example, enzymes), and they make up some structures of cells (and virons—for example, matrix and core proteins). When activated, the proviral DNA is used to make two kinds of particular forms of RNA (called messenger or mRNA). One kind of mRNA will be arranged as the RNA genome in the core particles for new virons. The other kind of mRNA will be translated into proteins that will be either packaged into new virons (such as matrix or core proteins) or used to control the cellular process of making some viral components. This latter function is very important in making new virons and is a focal point of antiviral drug design. A key viral protein in this process is called **protease**; it is responsible for cleaving some of the proteins translated from the mRNA into their final form before being used to make a new viron. Without this posttranslational maturation process, assembling new virons would be impossible. Thus, we have several new drugs called **protease inhibitors** that are designed to disrupt this protein's maturation process (Hutchinson 2001; Alcamo 2003; Fan et al. 2004).

All of the HIV components must be trafficked to a location near the cell surface membrane, assembled into new viron structures, and released by a complex process called budding. This trafficking and budding process is another ideal target for drug design. Usually, the more complex a process is, the easier the occurrence of errors becomes.

When new virus particles are released, they can then infect other cells with compatible surface receptors. The new virons are also susceptible to being bound and neutralized by antibodies. Likewise, when the cells are assembling the viral envelope proteins on their surface just prior to the budding process, anti-HIV antibodies can bind to these and mark the cells for destruction by the cytotoxic T-cells (and some other immune processes). This is what ultimately causes a decline in the number of helper T-cells (CD4+) observed with the onset of AIDS.

Something very unfortunate can happen during this whole process of going from RNA to DNA and back to RNA. There is the possibility of cell-to-cell transfer of the viral genome. We will see later that there is also an opportunity for cells to absorb genetic material that is free in serum solution (for example, when an infected cell is killed and destroyed, releasing its contents, including HIV genomic material, into serum solution). These phenomena are most likely what causes the many different types of cells beyond helper T-cells to become infected.

HAART—Highly Active Antiretroviral Therapy

HAART therapy is usually the combination of two RT inhibitors along with a protease inhibitor (see figure 3.5), thus disrupting viral production at two different points in this very complex process. There are currently several different RT-inhibiting drugs and protease inhibitors approved for use in the United States. More are in development. There is also one approved drug designed to inhibit the fusion of HIV with the host cell membrane. The selection of which drugs to include in the HAART regime is a difficult process; it requires a detailed history of previous drug administration to the patient. With HIV able to mutate so rapidly, drug resistance develops relatively easily; and since many of the drugs act in similar ways, resistance to one drug often provides resistance to other similar drugs. The efficacy of HAART is usually monitored by measuring the serum viral load. If successful, the viral load can decrease to undetectable levels, usually resulting in improved health in those with AIDS symptoms and a prolonging of the latency period in asymptomatic patients (Hutchinson 2001; McBride and Bradford 2004).

Unfortunately, HAART does not work for every patient. The reasons for this vary. The main reasons include viral resistance to the selected drugs (often because of previous use of the same or similar drug), mutation of the virus itself, or lack of adherence to a strict schedule needed for taking the drugs. Not only are there many pills to be taken each day (sometimes including drugs against OIs), but the drugs also usually have unpleasant side effects. Physicians will adjust the selection of drugs while monitoring viral load, hoping for efficacy. Patients need to adhere to the drug regimen for the rest of their lives.

3.3

Since adherence is so vital to effective drug treatment, measures of adherence are important. In a study of adherence among HIV-infected people living in Belgium, social scientists Ralph Bolton and John Vincke measured adherence from three perspectives: the people infected, their significant others, and their medical team. Variations regarding adherence among the three groups led the authors to conclude that the medical team's objective measures of viral load, T-cell counts, and lack of OIs were the best indicators of adherence (Vincke and Bolton 2002).

It is very important to continue the development of new HAART drugs. The drug pipeline needs to equal or exceed the rate of drug resistance development as HIV continues to evolve. HAART is our only current means to combat HIV infection, beyond education and behavior modification for preventing infection. Developing these new drugs is very expensive, costing millions of dollars for each. The cost of the drugs themselves as well as developing them are major obstacles in providing worldwide access to them. This has created an anthropological quandary, as it directly affects the global dynamics of HIV evolution.

The Cultural Dimensions of HAART/ARVs and Vaccines

Ideally, there would be both a cure for HIV/AIDS and a preventive vaccine. More than halfway through the first decade of the twenty-first century, and more than twenty-five years after the first diagnosed case of AIDS, there is neither. As stated in previous chapters, controversy and ethical issues accompany any discussion of HIV/AIDS. This applies to treatment and vaccines as well, with topics often conceptualized as biological and medical. These next two sections on treatment and vaccine development introduce some of these issues and discuss options and progress in these areas.

Abundant data in both the United States and cross-culturally indicate the success that HAART/ARVs have in improving the health of those people who take it (at least for several years) HAART/ARVs have side effects ranging from the redistribution of fat in the body to nausea, vomiting, and diarrhea, to potentially life-threatening cardiac complications (Bartlett 2006; Hutchinson 2001; Desclaux et al. 2003; Gillett et al. 2005; Pankhurst 2006).

We also know that people in nonindustrialized societies who have access to the drugs take them and adhere to the treatment regimen (Desclaux et al. 2003; Pankhurst 2006; Mills et al. 2006). However, only about 17 percent of the people worldwide who need the drugs get them. Most of those people live in the United States or other industrialized societies (Edwards 2005; Global Health Council 2005; *Newsweek* 2006). The reasons for lack of more-widespread access to and availability of ARVs are merely introduced here; they are critically discussed in chapter 8.

The primary reasons for lack of access to and availability of HAART/ARVs are political and economic (Koenig et al. 2004). These drugs are expensive and require both some level of societal infrastructure that can disseminate them and a social support system that can reinforce their usage. Cuba and Brazil have had high success rates in providing ARVs to their HIV-infected populations (Parameswaran 2004; Okie 2006). Senegal and Ethiopia have also had success in making ARVs available to at least some of their populations.

An interdisciplinary research team led by anthropologist Alice Desclaux was part of a pilot project to bring HAART/ARVs to Senegal. Her team believed that economic and infrastructure problems should not prevent people from receiving treatment. In her study, anyone with HIV who was a resident of Senegal was eligible for treatment; people paid according to their ability, with the poorest having fully subsidized treatment. This project also oversaw a coordinated medical team to implement the program and monitor patient progress (Desclaux et al. 2003).

Another study, conducted by anthropologist Alula Pankhurst, examined people's response to HIV/AIDS in twenty Ethiopian villages (2006). In Ethiopia, "HIV/AIDS has become the most important health problem and a threat to the social and economic threat to the fabric of the nation" (Pankhurst 2006: 1). Although their responses differed along some aspects of the situation (such as who was more at risk, the poor or the rich), the participants in the study agreed on the importance of HIV testing and the economic devastation the epidemic was wreaking on their villages. They wanted HAART but also recognized that being open about one's HIV status was difficult.

Access to and availability of HAART/ARVs involves an interdisciplinary approach. Within nonindustrialized societies, this includes use of traditional healers and practices. Using local healers who often have positions of authority and respect within a community can increase the use of drug therapy and lessen the stigma surrounding HIV/AIDS (Vollmer 2000; Traditional Medicine and HIV/AIDS Workshop 2006; Thornton 2002). Use of complementary medicine and alternative treatments occurs in the United States as well. James Gillett and colleagues found that HIV-infected people used acupuncture and meditation as well as other therapies to address the side effects of HAART (Gillett et al. 2005).

Vaccines

There are now over sixty vaccines in clinical trials being monitored by the **Food and Drug Administration (FDA)** (Lahey 2004). Most of these focus on either envelope or core particle proteins, while others are nucleic acid (gene) based, and some use other live viruses to deliver genetically modified HIV components (antigens). All of these are designed to elicit the production of anti-HIV antibodies and activate cytotoxic T-cells capable of attacking HIV infected cells. Do not expect a successful preventative or therapeutic vaccine for HIV/AIDS in the near future, though, given the general definition of a vaccine! Vaccines are designed to cause the production of specific antibodies and/or a cellular attack on the foreign material, in this case the free virus or virus-infected cells.

Developing a vaccine to protect us against this virus is a challenge. Once infected with HIV, we actually become hyperimmunized against it.

3.4

In 1984, Margaret Heckler, Secretary of Health and Human Services under President Ronald Reagan, promised a vaccine within ten years (Shilts 1987). Twenty-two years later, despite millions of dollars spent on vaccine research, vaccine trials completed or in process worldwide, and the establishment of several vaccine development agencies, we are not much further along in having a preventive vaccine available. There are concerns about poorly administered funds and studies, ethical issues, and erosion of public support and confidence in an effective vaccine. Timothy P. Lahey, a physician and researcher, reflects on a comment made by scientists in the journal *Science* regarding HIV vaccines: "One price for repetitive failure could be crucial erosion of confidence by the public and politicians in our capability of developing an effective AIDS vaccine collectively" (Lahey 2004: 1).

Because the immune system is unable to rid the body of the virus, it is like having a constant "booster" shot. We make lots of antibodies against every component of the virus. Our immune system kills off millions of infected cells each day, yet the virus persists within the body. This is not unusual; as noted, there are lots of viruses that can persist in our bodies for our lifetime. So why should we expect a vaccine that promotes the formation of anti-HIV antibodies to prevent infection or to help shed the infection from the body? There is some evidence that many of the vaccines currently in clinical trial do not work (that is, they do not prevent infection). There have been no effective preventive vaccines to date (Lahey 2004; Bartlett 2006).

The development and provision of a preventive HIV vaccine is a global effort. Given that more than 70 percent of HIV/AIDS occurs in sub-Saharan Africa alone, devising vaccine trials that are culturally sensitive and maintain ethical standards cross-culturally can pose a challenge. There are concerns about participants' ability to provide informed consent, their understanding of the nature of clinical trials, and the likelihood that they may develop a false sense of security about their HIV risk by participating in a trial (McGrath et al. 2001). For informed consent to be obtained, research teams need to have an understanding of the participants' culture and be prepared to engage in pre-vaccine-trial education before implementing the study (McGrath et al. 2001).

In addition, since there is not a reliable animal model for this disease, vaccine prospects diminish even further. Our current best model is the chimpanzee, which is our closest primate relative; however, not very many of them are available for vaccine testing. In addition, the chimpanzee does not seem to give the same clinical result with HIV infection as do humans. Nor do humans give the same clinical result as chimpanzees when infected with SIV (simian immunodeficiency virus). Why should we expect a vaccine developed in chimpanzees to work effectively in humans? None of the early vaccines tested in chimpanzees protected them from infection.

To progress in vaccine development, we need to get beyond the mindset of the traditional vaccine that causes antibodies and cytotic cell pro-

---

3.5

There are also controversies about the use of animal models for medical research that benefits humans. Jane Goodall, a noted primatologist, has spoken out about using sootey mangabeys as HIV research subjects. HIV-2 is seen as having mutated and species-jumped from sootey mangabeys. These monkeys have been on the endangered species list. As such, there is concern about using them in medical research (Kaiser Daily HIV/AIDS Report 2006b). A compromise is needed between animal rights activists and scientists relative to HIV vaccine development.

---

duction. There is a more promising way to combat HIV, but we do not quite have the technology yet. We need to be able to selectively mutate every copy of the HIV genome (provirus) in every infected cell. We are a generation or two away from having that level of technological precision. Although we can selectively mutate genes in simple bacteria, our cells are quite a different matter.

SUMMARY

HIV is in the family of retroviruses.
HIV is difficult to contract, but once a person is HIV infected, there is a progressive deterioration of the immune system until a person develops AIDS, the end point of HIV infection and disease.

Because of the structure of HIV, its progression to AIDS can be interrupted at several points.

HAART disrupts the viral replication process, but its effectiveness is
dependent on several factors.

A successful preventive vaccine for HIV will require years of ongoing
research and testing.

Thought Questions

Since HIV is not contracted casually, why is there such a fear-based
response to it?

What are some of the factors involved in successfully treating people
with HIV?

What aspects of the HIV replication process make it so difficult to develop either a vaccine or a cure?

Resources

Articles

Kaiser, Shari M., Harmit S. Malik, and Michael Emerman. "Restriction of an Extinct
Retrovirus by the Human TRIM5{lga} Antiviral Protein." *Science* 316, no. 5832 (June
22, 2007): 1756–58.

Thornton, Robert. "Traditional Healers, Medical Doctors and HIV/AIDS in Gauteng
and Mpumalanga Provinces, South Africa." Report to the Margaret Sanger Institute
and Medical Care Development International Center, October 16, 2002.

Books

Alcamo, I. Edward. *AIDS: The Biological Basis.* 3rd ed. Boston: Jones and Bartlett,
2003.

Fan, Hung Y., Ross F. Conner, and Luis P. Villarreal. *AIDS–Science and Society.* 4th ed.
Boston: Jones and Bartlett, 2004.

Thomas, Patricia. *Big Shot: Passion, Politics and the Struggle for an AIDS Vaccine.* New
York: Public Affairs Press, 2001.

Web Sites

AEGIS (AIDS Education Global Information System): http://www.aegis.org.

AmFAR (American Foundation for AIDS Research): http://www.amfar.org.

Body, The: http://www.thebody.com/index.shtml.

Johns Hopkins School of Medicine: http://www.hopkins-aids.edu/.

NAPWA (National Association of People with AIDS): http:// www.napwa.org.

4

HIV Testing

CHAPTER HIGHLIGHTS INCLUDE

A definition of HIV testing and a discussion of the types of HIV tests that
  are available
A discussion of HIV pre- and posttest counseling procedures in the
  United States
A discussion of what HIV test results mean
A discussion of the controversies surrounding voluntary versus manda-
  tory testing in the United States and cross-culturally
A discussion of the culture-specific and ethical issues involved in test-
  ing in the United States and cross-culturally

> Early awareness of HIV+ status can get people into drug therapy earlier.
>
> Stryker and Coates (1997)

HIV Tests

HIV antibody testing became available in North America and Western
Europe in 1985. The HIV test detects antibodies to the virus, not the virus
itself. It is *not* an AIDS test. Although there are tests to determine viral
load and other AIDS markers, there is *no* AIDS test per se (see chapter
3). AIDS is the diagnosis received at an advanced stage of HIV infection
and immune suppression. An HIV positive antibody test is necessary for
a diagnosis of AIDS, but it is not the same as having AIDS.

HIV testing within the U.S. and cross-culturally is controversial. Issues
involve culture-specific decisions about who gets tested as well as where
and what kind of testing occurs (Kaiser Family Foundation 2005). A decision to have an HIV test is also determined, in part, by what resources are
available for those who test positive. Factors involved with testing include

considerations about what legal, social, economic, and political repercussions occur for people who have an HIV test, particularly for those who test HIV positive (HIV+) (Hammar 2004).

There is much debate about the dissemination of HIV test results. This includes interpretation of the results, who has access to them, and what is done with them (Synergy Project 2003; Bayer 2000; Powers 1991). There are ongoing arguments concerning **mandatory HIV testing** versus voluntary testing for different individuals and groups, such as pregnant women (Geller and Kass 1991; Mayer and Pizer 2000), and whether testing should occur at **alternative/anonymous test sites** or **confidential test sites**. The definitions of *confidential, voluntary,* and *informed consent* in and of themselves are culture-specific, as are the interpretation of results and access to them (Strauss and Falkin 2001; Mitchell, Kaufman, and Pathways 2002; Bennett 1999; Bennett and Erin 1999). This chapter addresses these controversies and explores the basics of HIV testing.

While there are several means to detect HIV, the standard test worldwide to determine someone's **sero-status**—that is, whether an individual is HIV+ (HIV positive) or HIV- (HIV negative)—is through an HIV antibody test (Bartlett 2002, 2006). The standard HIV antibody test is a blood test. A small amount of blood is drawn and then analyzed for the presence of antibodies to the virus. There are also tests that use cheek cells (buccal membranes) to detect antibodies, and there are urine tests, which are very expensive (Bartlett 2002, 2006; CDC 2002). Most HIV tests performed in the United States and other industrialized societies take place in clinics, at **alternative or anonymous test sites (ATS)**, in doctors' offices, or, less commonly, at home (Bartlett 2002, 2006). In nonindustrialized societies such as India, Thailand, and much of sub-Saharan Africa, tests usually occur either in clinics or in hospitals (Coodvadia 2000; Jiraphongsa et al. 2002; Machekano et al. 2000; Bakari et al. 2000; Balmer et al. 2000; Kaiser Daily HIV/AIDS Report 2005, 2006d).

The term *sero-status* refers to whether or not there are antibodies to HIV detectable in a person's blood. The time between exposure to HIV and seroconversion, when there are detectable antibodies to HIV, is called the "**window period**" (PAEG 2002). Getting tested during the window period will yield inaccurate test results. Most likely, a person who is infected and has an HIV test during the window period will have a false negative test result (Bartlett 2002; PAEG 2002). A false negative result means that the person actually is HIV+.

Generally, with standard HIV tests, it takes at least thirty days after infection for an individual to develop sufficient antibodies to the virus to be detectable, that is, to seroconvert. In the United States, most people seroconvert within thirty days; about 95 percent of infected people seroconvert within three months of infection; and about 98 percent of infected people seroconvert within six months of infection (CDC 2003a; Bartlett 2002, 2006).

A person can test HIV+, HIV-, or **HIV indeterminate**. An indeterminate result rarely occurs and indicates unclear test results (Bartlett 2002). An HIV- (negative) test result indicates either that the individual is not infected with the virus or that the person has been exposed to HIV but there has not been sufficient time for antibodies to develop. Therefore, it is important to observe the window periods when obtaining an HIV antibody test. An HIV- test result does not mean that the person is immune to contracting HIV in the future. To maintain HIV negative status, people are encouraged to follow safer sex practices and safer needle usage (see chapters 5 and 6 respectively for an explanation of these terms).

Testing HIV+ (positive) requires three tests on a sample of blood before the results are confirmed as HIV+. The first blood test performed is an ELISA. If the first ELISA tests positive, a second ELISA is performed to eliminate false positives (Stine 1997; Bartlett 2002, 2006; MMWR 2003: 329–332). If the second ELISA is negative, the first, positive ELISA is discarded and the person is considered HIV-. If the second ELISA is positive, however, a third test is performed on the same sample of blood. This test is called a confirmatory Western Blot test. It specifically tests for antibodies for HIV to eliminate false negatives (Bartlett 2002). (See chapter 3 for a detailed description of ELISAs.)

The Western Blot test can have three results: negative, indeterminate, or positive. A negative result indicates that the person is HIV-. The previous ELISAS may have yielded false positives or may have detected other kinds of activity in the person's blood, but not HIV. This could be due to other kinds of viral activity. An indeterminate Western Blot means that there are not sufficient antibodies to HIV present in the blood. Usually, an indeterminate HIV test result indicates that the person has not met his or her individual window period for seroconversion and insufficient antibodies were found. Often, a person with an indeterminate HIV test is advised to be retested when the next window period has passed (Bartlett 2002, 2006). If both ELISAs and the Western Blot tests are positive, then the individual is said to have seroconverted and is HIV+ (Bartlett 2002, 2006; Stine 1997). An HIV+ antibody test does *not* mean that the person has AIDS, however. AIDS is the end point of HIV infection and has other diagnostic criteria (see chapter 3).

Since 2002, a **Rapid Immuno-Assay Test**, the **OraQuick®** HIV Rapid Test, or OraQuick®, has been available in both the United States and other parts of the world (U.S. Department of Health and Human Services 2003; Bakari et al. 2000). In the United States, this test was initially given to health-care workers who had been exposed to blood through needle-stick, surgical, or other invasive medical procedures that can expose them to a patient's blood. OraQuick® is sometimes given to women who have been raped (Bartlett 2002). These forms of exposure may place someone at risk for HIV infection.

There are pilot studies to determine whether OraQuick® can be used in other situations. Glide Church in San Francisco, California, is administering OraQuick® to the homeless and other indigent people in its neighborhood (Galgoul 2003, personal communication, July 12). This HIV test requires a finger prick of blood, and results are obtained within twenty minutes. It provides a baseline sero-status marker for most people. If the person tests positive with OraQuick®, he or she needs a confirmatory Western Blot test (U.S. Department of Health and Human Services 2003). As of 2006, problems with false positive results from OraQuick® administered in Los Angeles and San Francisco, California, in late 2005, have been resolved. This rapid test is now recommended as an alternative for special groups in the United States and elsewhere (Kaiser Daily HIV/AIDS Report 2006c).

There are several advantages of the Rapid Immuno-Assay test. First, it provides baseline results quickly, whereas standard HIV antibody tests usually take two weeks to get results. Second, it is a reassuring way to respond to blood exposure in health-care settings. With this test and a negative result, the person has the option of receiving **postexposure prophylaxis (PEP)** to reduce the chances of HIV transmission (see chapter 6). Third, OraQuick® can be administered outside of traditional health-care settings. Finally, it is an easy way to screen pregnant women or newborns for HIV antibodies (CDC 2003a).

Cross-culturally, OraQuick® can quickly serve as a screening method without expensive laboratory equipment, refrigeration, the need for a trained phlebotomist (someone who draws blood), or the need to return for results. Testing and results can occur in the same visit, saving time and money and reducing suspicion from family and community about why a person is traveling twice to the health-care facility (Bakari et al. 2000). Again, if the person tests HIV+, a confirmatory Western Blot test is necessary.

At-home HIV tests became available in the mid-1990s in the United States. The Home Access Express Test can be obtained on-line, through television ads, by mail, from some pharmacies, or by calling 1-800-HIV-TEST. The cost of an at-home test ranges between $35 and $50 per test (Bartlett 2002, 2006). However, at-home HIV tests may be more expensive than going to an HIV alternative/anonymous test site (ATS), as these often base their fees on a sliding scale. ATSs are generally found in states that have epicenters of HIV/AIDS.

Initially, at-home tests were marketed as valuable for individuals who lived far from HIV test sites, who did not want to use standard testing facilities such as clinics or doctors' offices, or who were concerned about confidentiality. They were also recommended for the "**worried well**," those people who were concerned about their HIV status but engaged in low-risk behaviors. At-home tests were seen as assuaging their fears without relying on and burdening publicly funded testing resources (Stryker and Coates 1997: 261–262). These tests involve a finger prick of blood that is then mailed to a lab. Results generally are accurate and are available within a week either by mail or by phone. However, people who take at-home HIV tests may not receive **pretest counseling**, and they receive **posttest counseling** by phone, regardless of the results (Bartlett 2002).

Receiving both HIV pretest counseling and posttest counseling is important for several reasons. Pretest counseling provides information about what the test entails and what the results indicate. It assesses the individual's window period for seroconversion. It allows the individual the opportunity to ask questions and receive information about safer sex, prevention, and potential responses to test results. Face-to-face posttest counseling provides a complete explanation of test results, can suggest ways to maintain a HIV- status, and offers resources for a person who tests HIV+. In-person pre- and posttest counseling also provides the opportunity to address any psychological issues that arise for the person taking the test (Hammar 2004). The September 2006 CDC decision to "streamline" or eliminate pre- and posttest counseling runs the risk of missing an important educational opportunity (MMWR 2006b).

HIV Test Counseling

Since 2003, the CDC has been updating recommendations about HIV testing (CDC 2003a, 2005b; Kaiser Family Foundation 2005). With a rise in incidence among heterosexuals, women, and men who have sex with men (MSM), and a decrease in the effectiveness of HAART since 1999, the CDC now recommends general screening for HIV as part of routine health care for adults 13–64 years old. This includes screening pregnant women, newborns whose mothers may not have received a prenatal HIV test, and **opt-out** consent practices, by which a person can decline testing. Previous recommendations included screening people living in epicenters of the epidemic or who engaged in "high-risk" behaviors (CDC 2003a; Kaiser Daily HIV/AIDS Report 2006g).

4.1

Although the CDC, WHO, and UNAIDS in 2007 all recommended routine HIV testing in part to reduce the stigma associated with HIV/AIDS and testing, the reality is that stigma continues to exist both in the United States and cross-culturally around this issue (Bray-Preston et al. 2007; O'Leary et al. 2007: 210). This is particularly true for sexual and ethnic minorities and women, and it can be found in both health-care settings and people's residential living areas (Bucher et al. 2007; Chase 2006; UNFPA 2007a). Unless these issues are addressed, promotion and implementation of universal HIV testing will be problematic here and elsewhere. In addition, researchers such as David R. Holtgrave who have done cost-benefit analyses of routine HIV testing say that continuing to fund high-prevalence areas for testing may be more effective than dispersing funds across the board (Holtgrave 2007). Funding for routine testing is another facet of this complex and controversial recommendation.

In the United States, HIV testing occurs at either confidential or anonymous test sites. A confidential test site includes doctors' offices, health clinics, and student health centers on college campuses that offer HIV testing. Confidential test sites maintain identifying demographic data such as name, address, age, gender, ethnicity, and mode(s) of transmission. The person's test results become part of his or her medical record.

Anonymous test sites do not keep any identifying information such as their clients' names or addresses. The person being tested receives a number before being tested and must submit that number to obtain his or her results.

With the exception of at-home tests, HIV test results legally must be given to the individual in person, not over the phone or by mail. Legally, people having an HIV test must receive HIV pretest and posttest counseling for both HIV+ and HIV- test results (Bartlett 2002; Stine 1997; New York State Department of Education 1990). However, current recommendations by the CDC endorse much-abbreviated pre- and posttest counseling sessions in order to screen everyone (CDC 2005b; Kaiser Family Foundation 2005).

Pre- and posttest HIV counseling involves a minimum of two conversations between the counselor and the client/patient. The content of the counseling is the same whether it occurs at a confidential or an anonymous test site. During pretest counseling, the person is asked about specific sexual and needle-using behavior that could transmit HIV. The window period is assessed, and the person is asked about prior HIV tests. This is important because three months exist between window periods. Getting tested more frequently than that probably will not provide accurate results. The person should also be asked whether testing is being done voluntarily, what he or she expects the results to be, and how he or she would respond to an HIV+ test result.

4.2

States and countries have varying criteria as to who is a HIV test counselor, their training, and background qualifications. In New York State, where I am a test counselor, the criteria changed since I was certified in 1994 and 2000. Currently, the training and background credentials for certification are based on where the counselor works and the population served. Outside the United States, counselors generally are health-care workers working in clinics or hospitals. In 2005, the Lesotho government in sub-Saharan Africa recommended universal testing done as a door-to-door effort (Kaiser Daily HIV/AIDS Report 2005).

In states with **mandatory name reporting** for people with HIV+ test results, the person should be informed during pretest counseling at confidential test sites that HIV+—but *not* HIV- —test results will be reported to the state department of health and then to the CDC. The person's name, address, age, gender, ethnicity, and mode of transmission will be reported to the state department of health; only general demographic data about the person's sex, gender, age, and mode of transmission go to the CDC. If the state also has **mandatory contact tracing** of the HIV+ person's sex- and needle-sharing partners, that information should also be discussed during pretest counseling at a confidential test site. A list of states that require mandatory name reporting can be found in the HIV/AIDS Policy Fact Sheet released by the Henry J. Kaiser Family Foundation in 2005 (available at http://www.kff.org).

Mandatory contact tracing is a fairly common public health practice for other communicable sexually transmitted infections/diseases, such as syphilis. Mandatory contact tracing involves letting the person's sexual and needle-sharing partners know that they may have been exposed to HIV. The name of the contact is not disclosed, nor is the possible mode of transmission. Contact tracing and the reporting of names occur only at confidential test sites, not at anonymous test sites.

If, after completing pretest counseling and having any questions about the test answered, the person wants to have an HIV test, he or she signs and dates a consent form. The individual has his or her blood drawn and returns in two weeks for results. Some test sites provide the individual with a pamphlet that explains HIV testing (see figure 4.1)

Posttest counseling involves some similarities and variations, according to whether the person tests at an anonymous or a confidential test site. At both sites, the person receives his of her test results and an explanation of what they mean (see figure 4.2 and figure 4.3).

If the person tests HIV-, there should be a discussion about how to remain HIV-. Testing HIV- does *not* protect the person from contracting HIV in the future. It means that on the day that the person's blood was drawn, there were no antibodies to the virus present. HIV- test results are not reported to either the state department of health or the CDC at either confidential or anonymous test sites.

Anonymous and confidential test sites in the United States differ when giving HIV+ test results. There is no personal identifying information on record at an anonymous test site. The person receives his or her results by turning in the number received during the pretest counseling session.

WHY

SHOULD

I

WORRY

ABOUT

HIV?

Knowing Your Status

Could Save Your Life!

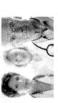

I HATE TESTS! WHAT DOES THIS ONE INVOLVE?

An HIV test looks for antibodies to the virus in your body. Your health care provider has different tests that they use. Here are the more common ones:

Blood test – This test is just like any other blood test you take at the doctors. A small amount of blood is taken to the lab and the antibody test is run.

Oral test – No needles are involved. The health provider takes a cotton swab and runs it against your cheek to collect the cells necessary for the test.

Rapid test – This test involves a needle prick or an oral swab. Initial test results come back within 20 minutes.

Home based test – If you do not feel anonymous enough, you may purchase a home testing kit. With this, you prick your finger, draw blood, and send the kit to the lab which runs the test and gives you the results over the phone. It takes about a week for these results to come back. The Food and Drug Administration has approved an HIV home testing kit and it can be obtained through their website (www.fda.gov).

Most HIV tests done at public health care centers are free, but there will be a charge at your family physician or by using the HIV home testing kit. Also cost is dependant on the type of test you want to take.

WHERE CAN I GO FOR THE TEST?

The tests are given at most doctors' offices, hospitals, family planning clinics, county health departments, drug treatment facilities, and even s ome university health care centers. Call your local health department for the testing center nearest you.

SHOULD I RELY ON THE FIRST TESTS RESULTS?

If you first test results were negative, but you think you have been exposed, you may be in what experts call the "window period." The window period is a time when you have been exposed to HIV, but do not have sufficient number of antibodies to be detected. The window period can be as early as 3 weeks after exposure to 6 months.

HOW DO I ENCOURAGE MY PARTNER TO BE TESTED?

It is always a good idea for you and your partner to be tested so you both know your status. By both being tested, you are not only protecting yourself but your partner also.

1. Have an open discussion early in your relationship about the need for testing. This ensures that both of you are aware of the possible risks of infection
2. Have the discussion away from your friends and relatives in a quiet location.
3. Plan what you will say. Make it simple, but direct.
4. Go together. There is strength in companionship.

To learn more about HIV and other sexually transmitted disease, contact your local health department, your family physician, or call:

CDC NATIONAL STD AND AIDS HOTLINE
(800) 227-8922 OR (800) 344-7432
(24 HOURS A DAY)

CDC NATIONAL HIV TESTING RESOURCE
WWW.HIVTEST.ORG

AMERICAN SOCIAL HEALTH ORGANIZATION
www.ashastd.org/stdfaqs/index.html

*INFORMATION PROVIDED BY American Social Health Association.
Other sources include AVERT and The Body.

Figure 4.1. "Why Should I Worry about HIV?" pamphlet (courtesy Linda Martindale).

continued

WHY SHOULD I WORRY: THE NEED FOR HIV TESTING*

HIV (Human Immunodeficiency Virus) can infect anyone, of any age, race, ethnicity, or sexual orientation. While people with the virus can look and feel healthy for years, they can still infect others, and HIV can damage their immune systems, even when they feel well. The only way to know if you have the virus is to take an HIV test. While the test will not protect you from HIV, the process of taking it can provide you with information and the motivation to make healthy choices.

WHAT IS HIV?

HIV is a retrovirus that leads to a depletion of immune cells and eventually a diagnosis of AIDS.

WHAT IS AIDS?

AIDS (Acquired Immune-deficiency Syndrome) is the latter stages of HIV infection characterized by a positive HIV antibody test, and/or low or absent T-cells, and one or more Opportunistic Infections. It can lead to death.

I CAN'T GET HIV OR AIDS! I'M NOT GAY!

HIV and AIDS is not a "gay" disease. While first considered a disease that was based in the homosexual community, it is now found in a number of communities, including college students. This is a disease caused by a virus and transmitted by specific sexual and needle sharing behaviors.

HAVE YOU EVER?*

had unprotected sex (anal, vaginal)?
    Yes   No
had unprotected sex (oral)?
    Yes   No
shared needles or works for drugs, tattoos, body piercings, steroids, hormones?
    Yes   No
had a Sexually Transmitted Infection (STI)?
    Yes   No

If your sexual partner can answer "yes" to any of the questions above, especially to anal or vaginal sex, then you should think about getting tested for HIV. Unprotected anal or vaginal sex puts you more at risk than oral sex. A test would be wise even if you answer "no" to all four questions.

WHY SHOULD I BE TESTED?

For many, HIV will not be a concern in your lifetime. For others, HIV will develop and you may not even know you have it, as it is not a visible condition.

* As a college student, the need for testing lies in not only your personal health, but that of any sexual partners you may have. Whether you realize it or not, people you have had unprotected anal or vaginal sex with could have exposed you to the risk of HIV. Getting tested in a relationship can help you make decisions about safer sex and birth control.

* Another reason is that you may decide you want to have a child. By becoming pregnant without knowing your status, you are exposing yourself and your child to potentially dangerous health risks.

* If you have shared a needle with anyone, you run the risk of contracting the HIV virus from the needle or equipment.

* To alert your health provider to special needs that may develop and to get you any necessary medication or additional treatments that may be needed.

WHAT IF SOMEONE FINDS OUT THAT I WAS TESTED?

Your HIV test results can be confidential or anonymous. In an anonymous HIV test, you are assigned a number which identifies your test. When you contact your health provider for your results, you would give him/her the identification number and s/he would then give you the results. No one will know unless you feel the need to inform others of your results in an anonymous test. In the confidential test, your name appears on the test results and the administering health provider gives you the results.

It is wise though to alert your sexual and needle using partners, and your doctors (including dentists) to your status so they are aware of your condition.

WHAT DOES A NEGATIVE RESULT MEAN?

A negative result means two things.
1. There is no sign that you have HIV at the time of the test.
   There is still a chance you could get the virus in the future.
2. You have HIV but the virus hasn't shown up yet. You may still develop the antibodies and infect others.

WHAT DOES A POSITIVE TEST RESULT MEAN?

A positive result means that you have the HIV antibodies in your system. You can pass the virus on to others. It does not mean you have AIDS but that the virus is there that causes the disease. You can become immuno-compromised and you should seek medical care for continued monitoring.

Figure 4.1.—continued

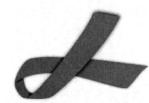

Being

HIV

Negative

continued

Now you need to take steps so you won't be faced with the possibility of becoming HIV infected. So, here are some suggestions:
* use a latex, lubricated, non-spermicidal condom during anal and vaginal sexual intercourse.
* use a dental dam during oral sex.
* talk with your partner about how to practice safer sex and needle usage.
* be tested if risky sex or needle-usage happens.

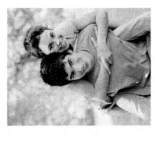

WHAT ABOUT MY PARTNER?

Remember, in many instances people are unaware of the HIV status. You can't see the disease because the symptoms do not become obvious until you develop full-blown AIDS. The only way to be sure that your partner is HIV negative is for him or her to be tested too!

The main thing you need to do is to talk to your partner about the HIV risk you both face. It may be difficult but this type of openness will save you from the fear in the future. Be proactive and find out! Be honest yourself. After all, it is ultimately your health and life!

HIV AND OTHER SEXUALLY TRANSMITTED DISEASES

While you have tested negative for HIV, you need to be aware that if you are exposed to other sexually transmitted diseases, you have a stronger chance of developing HIV in the future. Be aware that the sores or rashes caused by an STD leave you more vulnerable to HIV.

WHERE CAN I GET MORE INFORMATION?

To learn more about HIV and other sexually transmitted disease, contact your local health department, your family physician, or call:

CDC NATIONAL STD & AIDS HOTLINE
(800) 227-8922 OR (800) 344-7432
(24 HOURS A DAY)

CDC NATIONAL HIV TESTING RESOURCE
WWW.HIVTEST.ORG

AMERICAN SOCIAL HEALTH ORGANIZATION
www.ashastd.org/stdfaqs/index.html

*INFORMATION PROVIDED BY American Social Health Association.

Information provided by the American Social Health Association (ASHA), the Centers for Disease Control and Prevention, AVERT.org, and The Body.

Figure 4.2. "Being HIV Negative" pamphlet (courtesy Linda Martindale).

WHAT IS HIV?

HIV stands for human immuno-deficiency virus. Your immune system keeps you healthy through CD4 cells that fight diseases to which you are exposed. If you are HIV-positive, your immune system will start to fail as the CD4 cells are destroyed. You will no longer be able to fight infections or diseases.

HIV can lead to AIDS (Acquired Immune Deficiency Syndrome). When you are HIV+ and your CD4 cells fall to a count of less than 200 and/or you have an Opportunistic Infection (OI), you have developed full-blow AIDS. There are ways of keeping yourself healthy and slowing down the onset of AIDS, but you need to know your status and for you this you need to be tested!

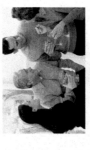

WHY SHOULD I WORRY: THE NEED FOR HIV TESTING*

HIV (Human Immunodeficiency Virus) can infect anyone, of any age, race, ethnicity, or sexual orientation. While people with the virus can look and feel healthy for years, they can still infect others, and HIV can damage their immune systems, even when they feel well. The only way to know if you have the virus is to take an HIV test. While the test will not protect you from HIV, the process of taking it can provide you with information to make safer choices.

WHY SHOULD I BE TESTED? I'M CAREFUL!

Have you . . .

... had unprotected anal or vaginal sex (no condom)?
... shared a needle, syringe, or other drug paraphernalia?
... had sex with more than one partner?
... had sex with a partner who has had sex with others or shared drug paraphernalia?
... had a sexually transmitted disease?
... had a blood transfusion before 1985.
... been raped or didn't know your partner?
... questioned your possible exposure?

Are you . . .

... a man or woman who has had unprotected anal sex with another man?
... a health care provider who may have been exposed to someone else's blood through a needlestick injury or other medical procedure.

If you can answer yes to any of these questions, then it could be good to be tested to be sure that you haven't been exposed to HIV.

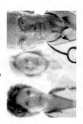

WHERE CAN I GO FOR THE TEST?

The tests are given at most doctors' offices, hospitals, family planning clinics, county health departments, drug treatment facilities, and even some university health care centers. Call your local health department for the testing center nearest you.

I HATE TESTS! WHAT DOES THIS ONE INVOLVE?

An HIV test looks for antibodies to the virus in your body. Your health care provider will help you determine which test suits your needs. Common ones include:

Blood test – You have these at the doctors during physicals. They will take a sample of your blood and run an antibody test on it.

Oral test – This one involves no needles. A cotton swab is wiped inside your cheek to collect cells for the test.

Rapid test – The test involves a needle prick or oral swab. Initial test results come back within 20 minutes.

Home based test – For anonymity, a home testing kit may be purchased. You prick your own finger and draw the blood. The test is sent to a lab and results come to you by calling a telephone number in about a week.

AND THE TEST RESULTS ARE . . . NEGATIVE!

Congratulations on being HIV negative. These results are only accurate as of the day the test was taken. You should consult with your health provider to see about whether you should be retested if you engage in risky sex or needle usage after your test was done. There is usually a three month "window" period wheer the virus can be dorminat. They will probably recommend that you be retested after the three month window period.

SO WHAT DO I DO NOW?

Figure 4.2—continued

Being

HIV

Positive

Make an appointment with a health care provider to discuss treatment options. If your personal care provider feels the need, s/he will send you to an HIV specialist. The important thing is to get help in evaluating your options and choosing the right treatment for you.

Ask your doctor about:
* HIV treatments and their risks;
* other diseases you may be vulnerable to;
* lifestyle modifications for healthy living;
* how to prevent yourself from infecting others.

WHAT IS THE TREATMENT AND HOW LONG WILL IT LAST?

Your health care providers will have guidelines which will help them determine the best course for your treatment. They may want to wait until your CD4 cells reach a certain level. In most instances when you are put on a drug regimen, it will be HAART (Highly Active Antiretroviral Therapy), i.e., the cocktail. You and your health care provider should consider the following:
* the results from various tests to measure how much virus there is in your body and the number of T-cells you have;
* the number of pills and when they are to be taken;
* the HIV drugs' interaction with your other medications;
* whether you are pregnant.

HIV treatment will continue for the rest of your life.

WHAT ELSE DO I DO?

It is important to contact sex and needle-sharing partners and encourage them to be tested. Either you can do that yourself, or a counselor can contact them and protect your identity.

Also learn ways to keep yourself healthy.
* Consistently practice safer sex!
* Take all medications you are given!
* Reduce the risk of exposure to other STDs!
* Eat healthy and exercise!
* Get enough sleep!
* Practice stress reduction techniques and think about joining a support group for people with HIV.

WHERE CAN I GET MORE INFORMATION?

To learn more about HIV and other sexually transmitted disease, contact your local health department, your family physician, or call:

CDC NATIONAL STD & AIDS HOTLINE
(800) 227-8922 OR (800) 344-7432
(24 HOURS A DAY)

CDC NATIONAL HIV TESTING RESOURCE
WWW.HIVTEST.ORG

AMERICAN SOCIAL HEALTH ORGANIZATION
www.ashastd.org/stdfaqs/index.html

*INFORMATION PROVIDED BY American Social Health Association.

Information provided by the American Social Health Association (ASHA), the Centers for Disease Control and Prevention, AVERT.org, and The Body.

Figure 4.3. "Being HIV Positive" pamphlet (courtesy Linda Martindale).

continued

WHAT IS HIV?

HIV stands for human immuno-deficiency virus. Your immune system keeps you healthy through CD4 cells that fight diseases to which you are exposed. If you are *HIV- positive*, your immune system will start to fail as the CD4 cells are destroyed. You will no longer be able to fight infections or diseases.

HIV can lead to AIDS (Acquired Immune Deficiency Syndrome). When you are HIV+ and your CD4 cells fall to a count of less than 200 *and/or you have an Opportunistic Infection (OI)*, you have developed full-blow AIDS. There are ways of keeping yourself healthy and slowing down the onset of AIDS, but you need to know your status and for you this you need to be tested!

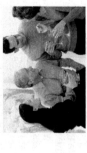

WHY SHOULD I WORRY: THE NEED FOR HIV TESTING*

HIV (Human Immunodeficiency Virus) can infect anyone, of any age, race, ethnicity, or sexual orientation. While people with the virus can look and feel healthy for years, they can still infect others, and HIV can damage their immune systems, even when they feel well. The only way to know if you have the virus is to take an HIV test. While the test will not protect you from HIV, the process of taking it can provide you with information to make safer choices.

WHY SHOULD I BE TESTED? I'M CAREFUL!

Have you . . .

... had unprotected anal or vaginal sex (no condom)?

... shared a needle, syringe, or other drug paraphernalia?

... had sex with more than one partner?

... had sex with a partner who has had sex with others or shared drug paraphernalia?

... had a sexually transmitted disease?

... had a blood transfusion before 1985.

... been raped or didn't know your partner?

... questioned your possible exposure?

Are you . . .

... a man or woman who has had unprotected anal sex with another man?

... a health care provider who may have been exposed to someone else's blood through a needlestick injury or other medical procedure.

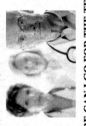

If you can answer yes to any of these questions, then it could be good to be tested to be sure that you haven't been exposed to HIV.

WHERE CAN I GO FOR THE TEST?

The tests are given at most doctors' offices, hospitals, family planning clinics, county health departments, drug treatment facilities, and even some university health care centers. Call your local health department for the testing center nearest you.

I HATE TESTS! WHAT DOES THIS ONE INVOLVE?

An HIV test looks for antibodies to the virus in your body. Your health care provider will help you determine which test suits your needs. Common ones include:

Blood test – You have these at the doctors during physicals. They will take a sample of your blood and run an antibody test on it.

Oral test – This one involves no needles. A cotton swab is wiped inside your cheek to collect cells for the test.

Rapid test – The test involves a needle prick or oral swab. Initial test results come back within 20 minutes.

Home based test – For anonymity, a home testing kit may be purchased. You prick your own finger and draw the blood. The test is sent to a lab and results come to you by calling a telephone number in about a week.

AND THE TEST RESULTS ARE . . .

POSITIVE!

Don't panic! The results do not mean you have AIDS. Your body has the virus that can lead to AIDS. There are treatment options available.

SO WHAT DO I DO NOW?

Figure 4.3—continued

Therefore, there is neither mandatory name reporting nor contact tracing at an anonymous test site. The HIV+ person receives his or her results with an explanation of what they mean and then leaves. Depending on the ATS, the person may receive additional literature about an HIV+ diagnosis and where to receive medical, legal, or sociopsychological care. There is no follow-up at an anonymous test site.

Confidential HIV test sites deliver HIV+ results differently than at an ATS. Mandatory name reporting is increasingly common in the United States (CDC 2003a; Body 2003b; Kaiser Family Foundation 2005). In these states, all the demographic data collected during the pretest counseling—name, address, age, gender, and mode of transmission—are reported to the state department of health (Body 2003b). A few states have mandatory non-name reporting. Mandatory non-name reporting includes the above demographic data without the person's name. Individuals are traced by a code number to avoid duplications of the same person (*Policy Watch* 2003a; Kaiser Family Foundation 2005).

In those states with mandatory contact tracing, the HIV+ person is required to give the names of his or her sexual and needle-sharing partners. Notification of these people can be done in several ways. The HIV+ person can tell his or her partners that they may be at risk for HIV. In New York state, the HIV+ person can bring sexual and needle-sharing partners individually to the HIV test site and discuss test results with the HIV test counselor.

Alternatively, the state department of health may notify the person's partners. The state of New York has a program known as **P-NAP**. P-NAP stands for **Partner Notification Assistance Program**. The New York State Department of Public Health runs this program. Someone from the program notifies the individual's sexual and needle-sharing partners that they may have been exposed to HIV. No identifying information about the original contact, the date of possible exposure, or the mode of transmission is given, to protect the contact. HIV testing is recommended for the sex- and needle-sharing partners.

New York State has a caveat for mandatory contact tracing. If the client who has received an HIV+ test result believes that there is a risk of danger to himself or herself or his or her children from contact tracing, contact tracing can be postponed. The risk of contact tracing is reviewed periodically, and contact tracing will be done only if the person and the person's children are believed to be safe. New York State also allows "good faith" reporting. People who test HIV+ are trusted to inform their sexual and needle-using partners if they choose (HIV Education and Training Programs 2000).

Mandatory name reporting for people who test positive for HIV and mandatory contact tracing are controversial aspects of HIV testing. Both the CDC and the states that require them believe that these practices will

allow for more-accurate accounting of incidence and prevalence rates;

allow for more-effective allocation of prevention, testing, and treatment resources with more-accurate demographic information;

allow for earlier intervention with HAART, since people who are HIV+ can receive information and medical help earlier in the course of infection; and

allow for more-accurate knowledge and ability to reduce **perinatal transmission** of the virus from mother to fetus during pregnancy and childbirth and after birth during breast-feeding (CDC 2003a, 2003b, 2005b; Kaiser Family Foundation 2005).

There are advantages and disadvantages to, as well as similarities and differences between, anonymous and confidential testing. Both forms of testing require pre- and posttest counseling. Both are voluntary. Both can provide prevention information and explain the benefits of HIV testing and what test results mean. Both involve informed consent. Informed consent means that the patient/client is aware of the risks and benefits of a given medical test or procedure before agreeing to it and has a right to refuse the test or procedure (Geller and Kass 1991; Blankenship 1997).

The major differences between anonymous and confidential testing involve who has access to the test results and what kind of follow-up is available if the person tests HIV+. There is no way to trace or identify the person who takes an anonymous test. The person's anonymity and confidentiality are protected. No one, other than the individual and the HIV test counselor, knows the person's test results. There is neither identifying information nor a way to trace the individual to the test results. This is important for people who fear negative economic, legal, or social consequences if their test result became known. It also reduces fear or suspicion that authorities, such as government agencies, would know the identities of people who test HIV+ (Powers 1991; see chapter 8).

People who support anonymous testing and oppose confidential testing with mandatory name reporting believe that accurate demographic data for intervention and resource allocation are important. They believe that information such as age, gender, ethnicity, general geographic location (as opposed to a specific address), and mode of transmission are valuable data. But they also believe that providing an individual's name violates the person's privacy and could deter people from having a confidential HIV test (HIV Education and Training Programs 2000). These privacy concerns can extend to mandatory contact tracing for people who test HIV+.

Anonymous testing cannot provide follow-up for people who test HIV+. They are given their test results and an explanation of them. After that, they are essentially on their own to find medical, psychological, or other types of care. Because mandatory name and contact tracing apply only to people receiving confidential testing, there is a lack of accurate demographic reporting about HIV incidence. This can impact resource allocation and help for people who test HIV+.

In contrast, a confidential test maintains a record of who was tested and their results. Because blood samples are sent with the demographic data included on the lab requisition slip, the people who draw the blood, run the analysis, and conduct the HIV test counseling know the person's HIV status. The results become part of the person's medical record as well as being reported to the state department of health and the CDC. There is a paper trail of the person's HIV status that can be accessed by insurance companies and by others with written consent from the individual.

Confidential testing, however, provides people with additional help upon hearing their test results. The person can be referred for additional tests and medical care, recommended for psychological counseling to deal with the news of an HIV+ status, and offered access to resources that can help with daily life. The HIV+ person can be contacted to see how she or he is coping with HIV and can be referred to support groups.

Confidential test result disclosure takes on different connotations in a hospital setting. HIV test results for inpatients may have broader dissemination than usual. To coordinate and administer care, the team of physicians, nurses, residents, and interns all may have access to the person's medical records and HIV information (CDC 2003a; Bader 2002; Powers 1991).

I have experience with confidential testing. I am a certified HIV test counselor in both New York and California. I have worked at both anonymous and confidential test sites prior to and after name-reporting policies went into effect.

Since 1995, I have conducted HIV test counseling at my campus's student health center. This student health center conducts confidential HIV testing, complying with New York State's name-reporting and mandatory contact-tracing regulations.

Most of the students with whom I conduct HIV test counseling request testing for one of three reasons. One, they want a baseline HIV status assessment. Two, they are involved in a relationship that they define as monogamous and want an HIV test to make decisions about practicing safer sex. Three, they have engaged in behaviors they define as risky and want to know their HIV status. Since this is a confidential test site, I provide students with pre- and posttest counseling, informational brochures about HIV testing and results, and information about name reporting and contact tracing before the students sign the consent form. These procedures help to ensure informed consent.

There are costs and benefits to both anonymous and confidential HIV testing. For people who are considering having an HIV test, it is important to weigh the pros and cons of each kind of testing, to find out what kinds of testing are available where they live, and to assess their own level of risk prior to signing an HIV test consent form.

Mandatory and Voluntary Testing

HIV testing involves issues of consent, volition, and coercion, as well as the circumstances under which testing occurs and who has access to the results. In general, HIV testing in the United States is voluntary. There are, however, situations of mandatory testing. The military requires HIV testing prior to acceptance, blood and organ donors are tested, and there can be **mandatory HIV testing** under court order for certain offenses (Bayer 2000; McGuire 2000; Kaiser Family Foundation 2005). Mandatory or voluntary prenatal testing and testing of newborns are two areas of controversy.

Pre- and postnatal HIV testing are attempts to reduce HIV transmission before and during birth. The controversies around who should receive prenatal HIV testing increased after 1994. Since 1994, AZT076, an antiretroviral drug, has been given to HIV+ pregnant women in the United States during pregnancy and birth. Administering AZT076 during this period dramatically reduces the incidence of babies born truly

HIV infected. The decrease has been from 16–25 percent of newborns who are HIV+ to 2–3 percent (Anderson 2001). Initially, only "high-risk" women were encouraged to have an HIV test during pregnancy. "High-risk" women include those who are IDUs, the sexual partners of IDUs, or those with "a number of sexual partners." This recommendation has changed since the 1990s to include all pregnant women (CDC 2003a).

Informed consent and volition are vital to the controversies surrounding prenatal HIV testing (Kendall 1996; Kass and Faden 1996a, 1996b; Geller and Kass 1991). By 2000, pregnant women who received prenatal care at a clinic, women's health center, or physician's office were encouraged but not required to have an HIV test. Those giving birth at birthing centers or hospitals were asked to have an HIV test during labor if they had not had one already, but they could not be forced to do so. Health-care facilities could not refuse to treat a pregnant or birthing woman if she refused an HIV test (Bayer 2000; Anderson 2001; Bennett 1999; Geller and Kass 1991). Women agreeing to have an HIV test were to receive appropriate pre- and posttest counseling and were to experience no discrimination in care based on their test results (Bayer 2000; Bennett 1999; Kendall 1996).

The CDC recommendations in 2003 changed some of these practices. The previous policies were "**opt-in**" practices, in which pregnant women elected to have an HIV test. The new recommendations are for an "**opt-out**" choice. Pregnant women will receive an HIV test as part of routine prenatal care. If they do not want to have the test, they must sign an opt-out waiver (CDC 2003a, 2005b; Bayer 2000; Chase 2006; Kaiser Daily AIDS Report 2006g). It is unclear what kinds of pre- and posttest counseling will accompany these new recommendations and what kinds of training are in place for health-care workers to provide HIV counseling and testing to pregnant women. Prenatal testing falls under the rubric of **pronatalism**. Pronatalism is a concern for procreation and fetuses as the center of interest, not the woman (Patton 1994; Faden et al. 1996).

Women do not want to contract HIV, regardless of whatever risks they take, nor do women want to transmit HIV to their fetuses or infants. If given the option, most women would agree to take a HIV test (Allen 1996; Auer 1996; J. Anderson 1996) (see also chapter 7).

Opt-out prenatal testing, does, however, raise several questions having to do with informed consent, volition, and quality of care. First, how is informed consent obtained? Do women know that they are specifically being tested for HIV in advance, or does it become part of "routine" blood work? At what point in the pregnancy does a woman receive an HIV test? Gestation is nine months; window periods for seroconversion are thirty days, three months, and six months. Does she receive multiple HIV tests during pregnancy, and if so, do these occur with multiple counseling sessions? What kinds of pre- and posttest counseling occur, and by whom? Is "opt out" truly voluntary and fully explained to women? Who has access to her test results if she tests positive, since prenatal testing would be confidential? If a woman opts out of testing, is the rest of her prenatal care guaranteed to be of the same quality as if she had the test? Does the question of testing come up again when she gives birth?

These questions are of particular concern in the United States. Since 83 percent of women with AIDS here are either Latina or African American, and most are poor, HIV testing cannot be used discriminatorily against low-income ethnic women (CDC 1999, 2001a, 2003a; Anderson 2001; Loue 1999; Hutton and Wissow 1991; LeVine 1996; Powers 1991).

4.3

The CDC's September 2006 decision about opt-out testing for pregnant women now states that "high-risk" women are to be tested at least twice during their pregnancies. If they have not been tested before they go into labor, they are to be tested then without informed consent and counseling. If women do not want to be tested, their health-care provider is to question them about that decision and is supposed to "try to convince them to get tested." This new policy seems to contradict a general medical policy of informed consent for tests and procedures and could potentially be sexist (the babies' fathers, who could have infected the mothers, are not tested) and racist, given that most pregnant women with HIV are from ethnic minority groups (Kaiser Daily HIV/AIDS Report 2006g; Kropp et al. 2006).

The state of New York has the highest incidence of AIDS in the United States. Given the incidence of AIDS, the state has mandated HIV testing of babies born in hospitals or birthing centers since 1987. This is a sero-status test of the mother because an infant is born with its mother's antibodies. Therefore, if the baby tests HIV+, the mother is likewise HIV+ (see chapter 7). For many years in New York, HIV testing of newborns was double-blinded. That means that the test results were known, but neither the mother nor her baby was identified. Mothers did not know that their babies were being tested, and the results were unidentifiable to them and the researchers. Neither the mothers nor the babies received medical follow-up, and the mothers did not receive care for their HIV infection (HIV Education and Training Programs 2000).

New York State decided to legalize unblinding these HIV tests after intense debate over the ethics of double-blind HIV testing of newborns. As of 2000, newborns in New York state still receive an HIV test. But their test results and identities and the identities of their mothers can now be known (HIV Education and Training Programs 2000). This change in policy means that women can now know their and their babies' initial HIV status. HIV health care for both the mother and infant, if truly HIV+, thus can begin early.

Providing newborns' HIV test results has other consequences. It means that those health-care facilities that see infants and children need trained staff to perform HIV tests and to provide HIV+ infants with follow-up care (Gerbert et al. 1999). That requires providing additional economic and possibly personnel resources to these offices.

4.4

Currently, this practice is not limited to New York State. Although New York was one of the first states to adopt mandatory testing of newborns, other states are now either considering this or requiring it as well (Kaiser Family Foundation 2005).

Ethics and Controversies of HIV Testing

Ethics and HIV Testing in the United States

What constitutes confidentiality and informed consent, who is tested, how often, where, and how test results are processed form ethical controversies in the United States. Before HAART became available in the United States in 1996, drugs to prevent and treat opportunistic infections (OIs) were prescribed. However, few drugs increased T-cells or reduced viral load for any length of time. People who developed AIDS lived on average about four years if they had access to medical insurance and health-care providers who were knowledgeable about HIV and AIDS. Without effective drugs to prolong life and with discriminatory insurance practices toward people who tested positive, many people refused to get tested. It was psychologically easier to practice safer sex and not know one's HIV status than to learn that one was HIV+ with limited help available (Odets 1995; Strauss and Falkin 2001; Anderson and Barrett 2001; Dean 1995; Doll et al. 1991).

With the development of HAART, the medical community began to recommend an expansion of HIV testing (CDC 2003a, 2005b; Bartlett 2002; Stryker and Coates 1997). The medical community views HIV testing and early intervention with HAART for those who test positive as life enhancing and extending (CDC 2003a; Bartlett 2002). However, these recommendations are not universally followed. The Department of Health and Human Services estimates that about 25 percent, or about 250,000 people who are HIV+, do not know their HIV status (CDC/HHS 1999; CDC 2005b).

The percentage of HIV+ people who do not know their status, the mutability and potential resistance of HIV, and the availability of HAART (which can dramatically improve people's health for at least several years) have led the CDC to recommend routine testing of everyone between the ages of thirteen and sixty-four (CDC 2005b; Kaiser Family Foundation 2005). The recommendation reflects data and assumptions that indicate that people who know they are HIV+ will modify their behavior to reduce transmitting the virus, to obtain treatment, and to take care of their health (Stryker and Coates 1997; CDC 2005b; Kaiser Family Foundation 2005). This recommendation includes the opt-out testing option, no written informed consent, and minimal pre- and posttest counseling (CDC 2005b). As such, this recommendation can pose several problems:

HIV/AIDS still carries stigma, and there are places in the United States where HAART is unavailable (see chapters 8 and 9).

HIV/AIDS is a serious medical condition. Being tested for it involves an awareness of this. Written informed consent helps to ensure this awareness.

Pre- and posttest counseling provide valuable opportunities to educate people about risk and prevention and to refer people for treatment if they test positive with confidential testing.

Generalized HIV testing at clinics and doctors' offices eliminates anonymous testing and raises issues about confidentiality of patients' records.

Medical and life insurance companies can ask whether a person has had an HIV test or has been diagnosed with an immunosuppressant disease. Legally, insurance companies can deny insurance, raise premium rates, and drop insurees who answer yes to either of these questions.

There is debate about whether universal, routine testing is a misuse of HIV resources, particularly in areas of low seroprevalence.

There are controversies involving having an HIV test and knowing one's HIV status. There is the fear of knowing that one has a fatal disease. HAART does not cure AIDS. It works to reduce viral load and increase T-cells for about 50 percent of the people who take it. HAART has serious side effects, and adhering to the rigidly scheduled regimen for taking the drugs can be difficult (*HIVPlus* 2002b). Consistently practicing safer sex and safer needle usage does reduce the risk of transmission. However, most people do not consistently practice either of these. Of the two behaviors, research indicates that it is easier to practice safer needle usage than it is to practice safer sex (see chapters 5 and 6).

While it is illegal to discriminate against someone who is HIV+ or has AIDS in employment, housing, or education, the fear or reality of subtle and overt discrimination exists. Ostracism, denial of raises or promotions, firings, and evictions have happened to people with HIV/AIDS (Powers 1991; Bray-Preston et al. 2007; Bucher et al. 2007).

Privacy is highly valued in U.S. culture. Dissemination of someone's HIV status or test results is a violation of privacy. Yet public health concerns enter into the discussion of privacy. At what point and under what circumstances does someone have the "right" to know another's HIV status (see Mayer and Pizer 2000; Powers 1991; Chase 2006)?

There have been lawsuits between health-care workers and clients over the "right to know" the patients' and providers' HIV status. The controversy centers on the "right" to individual privacy versus knowing a patient's or provider's HIV status to reduce the risk of infection from invasive medical procedures (Rom 1997; Rotheram-Borus et al. 2001; Gerbert et al. 1999; Gostlin and Lazzarini 1997; Shilts 1987). There have also been controversies and lawsuits about disclosure of one's HIV+ status to sexual and needle-using partners. These health-care and personal situations and controversies persist and generally seem to be decided legally on a case-by-case and state-by-state basis (Shernoff 1999; Reilly and Woo 2001; Bingman et al. 2001) (see chapter 6).

HIV Testing and Ethics Cross-Culturally

Cross-culturally and among nonassimilated ethnic groups in the United States, HIV testing and results occur in the context of specific cultural behaviors and beliefs. Our concepts of "rights," "privacy," "individuality," and "confidentiality" may not have the same meanings in other societies and subcultures. The ethical concerns about consent, confidentiality, HIV test counseling and results, and who is tested filter through each culture's structures and values (Faden et al. 1991; Loue 1999; UNFPA 2007a).

The ethics of HIV testing outside Euro-American societies have generated international controversy (Bennett 1999; Bennett and Erin 1999). Generally, concepts of family, confidentiality, privacy, and decision making include more people cross-culturally than in industrialized societies. Decisions are less individualistic. Members of extended kin groups or husbands often make the decisions about sexuality and reproduction in much of sub-Saharan Africa, for example. When women do not have control over their sexuality, their ability to practice safer sex diminishes, putting them at higher risk for HIV and other STIs (Machekano et al. 2000; Setel 1999; Orubuloye, Caldwell, and Caldwell 1994; McGrath et al. 1993; Varga 1999; UNFPA 2007a, 2007b).

HIV/AIDS is stigmatized in societies where it occurs. Obtaining an HIV test raises questions about possible infection, violation of the group's sexual norms, and fear of reprisal from the individual's kin group (Solomon et al. 2000; Pankhurst 2006). As in the United States, there is the question of why someone would have an HIV test unless the person either is infected already or is behaving in a risky manner (Solomon et al. 2000; Pankhurst 2006).

There is little that occurs in small communities that is private. Gossip is common and often serves as a primary means of social control. Daily life activities generally are known by neighbors and the family (Solomon et al. 2000; Coodvadia 2000). In Chennai, India, for example, the stigma of HIV puts people in precarious social situations. They may be ostracized and lose support from the community and family if HIV+. Going for an HIV test raises questions about one's morality and behavior (Solomon et al. 2000; UNFPA 2007a). Social ostracism in small, traditional communi-

---

4.5

Recommendations by the CDC have international implications, as they can be adopted as protocol by other countries. The CDC's recommendation for universal testing without informed consent and with a "streamlined" counseling process has raised concern among people who conduct HIV testing in nonindustrialized societies. The AIDS Asia Internet forum presented a variety of responses to the recommendations, ranging from acceptance to serious concerns about violations of human rights (AIDS Asia 2006).

---

ties may threaten people's survival. In this situation, the availability of the rapid HIV test, OraQuick®, would help to reduce suspicion because only one medical appointment is necessary.

Another variable is polygyny. Polygyny, having more than one wife, is common in parts of sub-Saharan Africa such as Tanzania, Kenya, and Zimbabwe. Men can have multiple sexual partners and make the sexual decisions for themselves and their partners, including whether or not to have an HIV test (Machekano et al. 2000; Marck 1999; Orubuloye et al. 1994; Varga 1999). While the men are polygynous, the women are expected to be monogamous; therefore, the women are at greater risk for infection than are the men. The levirate, a practice where women marry their deceased husband's brother, often occurs in situations of polygyny.

The levirate traditionally provided continuity in economic resource distribution and contributed to the social integrity of the extended family. It provided for the ongoing socialization of children within the kinship group and maintained the values of the social unit. Practicing the levirate currently also means that the woman may be simultaneously exposed to HIV from her new husband and subject to his decisions about sex (Malungo 1999).

Because of economic factors, many men who practice the levirate and polygyny travel far from home to work to support their families. As part of their economic geographic mobility, these men have sex with women along trade routes and in the cities where they work (Orubuloye et al. 1994). These women may be mistresses, girlfriends, or prostitutes.

Both men and women distinguish between sex with a casual partner, such as a prostitute or brief encounter, and sex with a primary partner such as a spouse or lover. Worldwide, men and women rarely practice safer sex with a primary partner and are more likely to do so with a casual partner (Cohen, Sande, and Volberding 1999; Balmer et al. 2000; Sanguiwa et al. 2000; Saul et al. 2000; Volk and Koopman 2001; Klein-Alonso 1996).

When men travel and have sex with prostitutes, safer sex is negotiable. Female prostitutes generally work in order to survive economically, particularly in nonindustrialized societies (Bond et al. 1996; Basu, Mate, and Farmer 2000; Anon. 2000a; Beyrer 1998; Kane 1998). As discussed in chapter 7, prostitutes' ability to use condoms consistently with clients is highly variable. Condom usage depends on their financial situation, whether they have support from their place of employment, and the availability of condoms. In much of sub-Saharan Africa, female prostitutes are geographically stable; it is the men who travel, resist condom use, and are the potential sources of infection (Balmer et al. 2000; Marck 1999; Malungo 1999). Given cultural sexual practices, social patterns of interaction in daily life and economic pressures, what is the context in which HIV testing occurs?

Cultural sexual practices and economic resources affect who is at risk for HIV, recommendations for testing, and how testing occurs. In general, couples are more willing to have an HIV test than are individuals. Couples are less willing than individuals to modify their behavior, but they may engage in less risky behavior than do individuals (Bakari et al. 2000; Sanguiwa et al. 2000; Machekano et al. 2000). With the availability of rapid HIV testing in Zambia, couples who are assured of confidentiality per their culture's definition of it are willing to be tested (Bakari et al. 2000). Rapid testing reduces kin and community suspicion, gives them immediate results, and saves travel time, time away from work, and money (Bakari et al. 2000; Coodvadia 2000).

When establishing voluntary HIV test sites outside the United States, organizations must consider indigenous beliefs about sexuality, gender relations, economics, and access to test sites (Vollmer 2000). Having to travel too far or too often to get tested and receive results can be an economic drain and also can raise suspicions within the community. For these reasons, rapid HIV testing (OraQuick®) may be a viable screening alternative to standard confidential and anonymous test sites. As stated earlier, rapid HIV testing is relatively inexpensive and easy to administer. Results are available quickly. The individual testing saves time and money and deflects suspicion from family and the community because only one visit to the health clinic is required. OraQuick® can also be helpful to women who are pregnant or breast-feeding. If they are HIV+, they may be able to reduce the risk of perinatal or postnatal transmission if they can receive either **Nevirapine** (an antiretroviral drug) or AZT076 prenatally and reduce the amount of time they breast-feed. However, if people test positive on OraQuick®, they do need a confirmatory Western Blot test.

As in industrialized societies (specifically, the United States), the availability of ARVs in nonindustrialized cultures has promoted HIV testing. Knowing one's test results when there are medicines to take if one is HIV+ provides hope and a sense of control over the situation. Increasingly, countries such as Botswana and Lesotho in sub-Saharan Africa, both with high HIV/AIDS incidence and prevalence rates, are considering more-widespread testing of their populations (Kaiser Daily HIV/AIDS Report 2005, 2006d).

Case Studies of HIV Testing Cross-Culturally

The complexities of HIV testing cross-culturally are illustrated from research by anthropologists and others conducted in Cuba, Brazil, and Mozambique. HIV testing in Cuba challenges concepts of ethnocentrism, cultural relativism, and the idea of "universal human rights." Cuba's HIV policies receive international attention (Scheper-Hughes 1994; Manlowe 1997). Because Cuba is a communist country, the government makes decisions for groups and individuals. Although economically poor, Cuba has one of the highest literacy rates in the world and universal health-care coverage. Voluntary HIV testing occurs in Cuba (Manlowe 1997; Parameswaran 2004). People who tested positive or who had AIDS were quarantined until 1993 (Parameswaran 2004). While quarantined, they received food, medical care, housing, and conjugal and family visits for the rest of their lives. People with HIV/AIDS in Cuba are cared for. They are not abandoned by their families (Manlowe 1997). The separation of people with HIV or AIDS from the rest of the community, even though they were cared for, raises questions about privacy, confidentiality, and human rights (Scheper-Hughes 1994; Manlowe 1997).

Under what circumstances are the needs and rights of the individual subsumed to the needs and welfare of the group (see Mayer and Pizer 2000)? Are there universal standards for human rights, and if so, who defines them? Whereas Cuba views the welfare of the whole and rights of the state to supersede those of the individual, others felt differently and challenged Cuba's HIV/AIDS policies. The United States and the World Health Organization were vociferous in their criticisms (Parameswaran 2004). HIV is infectious, but it is not contagious. It is not spread through casual contact; therefore, why would people need to be isolated?

While human rights activists criticize Cuba's AIDS policies, there are culture-specific factors to consider:

> Because Cuba is a communist country, the needs of the group take priority over the needs of the individual.
>
> Cuba has one of the lowest incidence rates of HIV in the world.
>
> Given that Cuba is a Latino culture with attitudes about privacy, confidentiality, and individualism that differ from those in the United States, criticism of Cuba's policies in those respects may be ethnocentric.
>
> People with HIV/AIDS receive medical care, housing, and have contact with their families. They are not homeless or ostracized, per se.

In the discussion of Cuba, comparison with other societies may be illuminating. The United States, for example, prides itself on its human rights record, as well as the value it places on individuality, self-determination, autonomy, and privacy. However, since the first wave of the epidemic in the United States, various members of Congress and some fundamentalist religious groups have suggested either mandatory HIV testing or quarantine for people with HIV/AIDS (Loue 1999; Bayer 2000; McGuire 2000). In addition, for much of the world that lacks access to socialized medicine or national health care, medical treatment of HIV/AIDS is highly variable. People with HIV/AIDS in Cuba receive medical care.

Cuba's positions on HIV testing and care for HIV-infected people became a lightning rod of controversy over the questions of cultural relativism, ethnocentrism, and universal human rights. Anthropologists became embroiled in a heated discussion over this issue (Scheper-Hughes 1994). How relativistic can individuals and societies be? Are there limits to cultural relativism, and if so, who decides what these limits are?

Brazil is a Latin American country that has managed its HIV/AIDS epidemic proactively and with recognized success (Okie 2006). However, some critics of Brazil's HIV testing policies say that it favors the middle class and the worried well over those who are more at risk for HIV and therefore in greater need of testing (Biehl et al. 2001). Critics believe that the biomedical approach and social groups created the need for HIV testing among those with resources, rather than directing those resources toward those who are more at risk and their communities (Biehl et al. 2001).

Mozambique, a country in sub-Saharan Africa with an adult HIV/AIDS prevalence rate of 13.6 percent as of 2002, is conducting research into the feasibility of generalized HIV testing. Anthropologist Esmeralda Mariano is working on this project and is particularly interested in the ethical considerations of HIV testing. Her goals are to train HIV test interviewers to be sensitive to the group's values, beliefs, and behaviors and to develop protocols that clearly protect the participants' confidentiality, privacy, and access to informed consent (Mariano 2005).

HIV testing can be a valuable screening device. When done correctly, it can provide essential epidemiological data about incidence and prevalence of infection. These data can then be used in developing preventive and treatment intervention programs. However, an HIV test is not benign; there are risks associated with testing and receiving results. HIV/AIDS is stigmatized wherever it occurs. There are social, political, and economic ramifications of conducting and having an HIV test.

HIV testing programs need to consider cultural variables and respect local norms. They need to incorporate group norms about privacy, confidentiality, and decision making. HIV testing is one aspect of intervention. Accompanied with ongoing, culturally sensitive HIV education, it has the potential to reduce infection and to provide information to determine allocation of resources.

SUMMARY

HIV antibody testing has been available since 1985.

An HIV test detects antibodies to the virus. It is *not* an AIDS test. There is no AIDS test.

HIV testing can be confidential or anonymous. There are benefits and drawbacks to both methods of testing.

Mandatory versus voluntary testing and the reporting of names of people who test HIV+ are controversial issues.

There are ethical issues associated with confidential and anonymous testing and with voluntary versus mandatory testing.

The CDC currently recommends HIV testing for the general population. There are advantages and disadvantages to this recommendation. HIV testing cross-culturally needs to consider and include the society's views about consent, confidentiality, and decision making. The advent of OraQuick® may increase the feasibility of HIV testing cross-culturally.

Thought Questions

What does a culturally sensitive and culture-specific approach to HIV testing entail? Why is this approach important?

How do the needs of the individual versus the needs of the group impact the decision to get an HIV test, the interpretation of confidentiality and informed consent, and the dissemination of the results?

Resources

Articles

Bray-Preston, Deborah, Anthony R. D'Augelli, Cathy D. Kassab, and Michael T. Starks. "The Relationship of Stigma to the Sexual Risk Behavior of Rural Men Who Have Sex with Men." *AIDS Education and Prevention* 19, no. 3 (June 2007): 218–30.

O'Leary, Ann, May Kennedy, Katina A. Pappas-DeLuca, Marlene Nkete, Vicki Beck, and Christine Galavotti. "Association between Exposure to an HIV Storyline in the 'Bold and the Beautiful' and HIV-Related Stigma in Botswana." *AIDS Education and Prevention* 19, no. 3 (June 2007): 209–17.

Yanushka-Bunn, Janice, Sondra E. Solomon, Carol Miller, and Rex Forehand. "Management of Stigma in People with HIV: Re-examination of the HIV-Stigma Scale." *AIDS Education and Prevention* 19, no. 3 (June 2007): 198–208.

Books

Treichler, Paula. *How to Have Theory in an Epidemic: Cultural Chronicles of AIDS.* Durham, N.C.: Duke University Press, 1999.

Suggested Hotlines

CDC Hotline Number for General Information about HIV and HIV Testing:
English: 1-800-342-2437
Spanish: 1-800-344-SIDA
Hearing Impaired: 1-800-243-7889

National AIDS Hotline Number:

English: 1-800-342-2437 (24 hr.)

Spanish: 1-800-344-7432 (5 a.m.–11 p.m.)

Hearing Impaired: 1-800-243-7889 (M–F 7 a.m.–7 p.m.)

New York State HIV Testing Guidelines Hotline: 1-800-962-5063. A Telecommunication Device for the Deaf (TDD) hotline is available at (585) 423-8120.

Web Sites

Bucher, J. B., K. M. Thoma, D. Guzman, E. Riley, N. DelaCruz, and D. R. Bangsberg. "Community-Based Rapid HIV Testing in Homeless and Marginally Housed Adults in San Francisco." Electronic document, http://www.medscape.com/viewarticle/554783_1, accessed April 24, 2007.

Chase, Marilyn. "Plans to Expand AIDS Testing Alarm Activists." Electronic document, http://www.ph.ucla.edu/epi/seaids/plansexpandtesting.html, accessed July 5, 2000.

General HIV Information, Including HIV Testing. Electronic document, http://www.HIVInSite.com, accessed June 26, 2004

HIV/AIDS Hotline Numbers Web Sites for the United States. Electronic document, http://www.mentalhealth.org/hotlines/hiv.asp and http://www.ashastd.org, accessed November 23, 2003.

Holtgrave, David R. "Costs and Consequences of the U.S. Centers for Disease Control and Prevention's Recommendations for Opt-Out HIV Testing." PLoS Med 4, no. 6: e194. (June 12, 2007) Electronic document, http://medicine.plosjournals.org/perlserv/?request=get-document&doi=10.1371/journal.pmed.0040194, accessed June 12, 2007.

New York State HIV Testing. Electronic document, http://www.health.state.ny.us/diseases/aids/index.htm, accessed February 15, 2005.

SUNY Potsdam AIDS Education Group (PAEG). Electronic document, http://www.potsdam.edu/content.php?contentID=E9CABAC13BFD227 A43FF1BE205B2B184, accessed April 28, 2005.

UNFPA. "Gender Responsive Budgeting and Women's Reproductive Rights: A Resource Pack." Electronic document, http://www.unfpa.org/upload/lib_pub_file/686_filename_gender_eng.pdf, accessed August 16, 2007.

———. "Culture in the Context of UNFPA Programming: ICPD+10 Survey Results on Culture and Religion." Electronic document, http://www.unfpa.org/upload/lib_pub_file/528_filename_culture_religion.pdf, accessed August 16, 2007.

5

Sex and AIDS

Definitions of sexuality, gender, and sexual orientation in the United States and cross-culturally

Discussions of the limitations of a Euro-American approach to sexuality, gender, and sexual orientation in relation to the risk for HIV

Explanations of the sexual risk continuum, including distinctions between safe and safer sex

Discussions of sociocultural factors that either support or impede safer sex practices in the United States and cross-culturally

Controversies regarding HIV and sex education programs in the United States and cross-culturally

> Understanding the AIDS epidemic as a medical phenomenon involves understanding it as cultural phenomenon.
>
> Treichler (1999)

Concepts of sex/**sexuality, gender**, and **sexual orientation** are central to discussions of HIV/AIDS. Sexuality is one of the most basic, personal, and intimate aspects of our humanity. As basic as sexuality is, the definition and expression of it are culturally defined. Sexual expression varies across cultures and through time.

As primarily a sexually transmitted disease worldwide, HIV/AIDS elicits deep cultural beliefs about sexuality. These beliefs involve not only the specific sexual behaviors that can transmit the virus but also values about the age, gender, and circumstances under which sexuality is expressed. The need for culture-specific knowledge and sensitivity to the definitions and expressions of sexuality across the life cycle is a focus of this chapter.

Sexual and ethnic groups in the United States and cross-culturally provide examples of the need for culturally sensitive approaches to HIV prevention.

Sexuality

Sexuality is part of our evolution and species. We evolved as sexual beings. A highly complex phenomenon, sexuality is defined, mediated, and expressed through culture. Sexuality is a broad term that includes specific behaviors, sexual attraction, concepts of maleness and femaleness (gender), and foci of desire (orientation). Sexuality exists across the life cycle from conception through old age and is biocultural. This means that sexuality is an interaction of biology (genes and chromosomes, hormones, anatomy and physiology) and learned behaviors. The boundary between what is biological and what is learned is fluid and not clearly defined (Rogers 2001). Sexuality can be reproductive or recreational, voluntary or coerced, and can be used for social, economic, political, and emotional purposes. Although the kinds of sexual behavior that are possible run the gamut of the human imagination, this chapter is concerned primarily with those behaviors that are most likely to transmit HIV. These include unprotected (that is, without latex barriers) penetrative penile-vaginal intercourse (**p-v**), penile-anal intercourse (**p-a**), and to a much lesser extent, oral sex, both fellatio (oral sex on a man) and cunnilingus (oral sex on a woman) (Bartlett 2006).

Cultures determine the age, numbers, and genders of one's sexual partners, the frequency and kinds of sex that occur, and the contexts in which it occurs. Although sexual behavior occurs among individuals, it is shaped by community and larger societal expectations and beliefs (Rhodes and Quirk 1998). People are members of families, ethnic groups, communities, and societies. These larger social entities transmit values, beliefs, and behaviors to individuals. Through both overt and covert mechanisms and through positive and negative support, these larger groups influence individual sexual behavior, including decisions about **safer sex** practices. The rules and values about sexuality can be highly visible in society (such as those about dress) or covert (such as norms and beliefs about nonmarital sex). Marriage and kinship systems are two ways in which cultures regulate sexuality.

Marriage and Kinship Systems

Marriage and kinship systems serve a number of functions. These include the continuation of the group through reproductive practices; formal socialization of new members into the group through either birth or adoption; and access to and distribution of resources within and between groups. Marriage practices imply and allow for sexual behavior between spouses.

Structurally, marriages can be either **monogamous**, defined as having one partner for life, or **polygamous**, having several partners at a time. Behaviorally, most people worldwide have more than one sexual partner, a practice that is often referred to as **serial monogamy** when one relationship follows another. The fact that most people have more than one sexual partner during their lifetime indicates a potential risk for HIV infection (Bolin and Whelehan 1999; Whelehan 2001b; Green 2003; Hughes 2004; Morof et al. 2004).

The preferred form of marriage worldwide is polygamy, specifically polygyny. (Polygamy is distinct from the popular term *polyamory*, which means an individual's ability to love and be sexually involved with more than one person at a time.) Polygyny formally allows males more sexual freedom and expression than it does females, who are expected to be monogamous (Orubuloye et al., eds. 1994; Feldman 2003b; Hogle et al. 2002; Schoepf 2003b, 2004). Since polygyny can be expensive, men may not have multiple wives, but they may have mistresses and girlfriends and have internalized the belief in having multiple sex partners (Orubuloye et al. 1994; Setel 1999).

Kinship systems complement preferred forms of marriage. Most kinship systems around the world require known paternity for children to have a recognized place in the society (see chapter 1). As with polygyny, **patrilineal descent** (through the father's side of the family) and **bilateral descent** (through both the father's and the mother's side of the family) systems grant men more sexual expression and a greater number of partners than they do females. Granting females the same sexual freedom would threaten known paternity and thus the lineage. Usually, bilateral and patrilineal descent societies repress female sexuality and maintain double standards of sexual behavior.

In contrast, **matrilineal decent** societies can allow females a greater range of sexual behavior. In these societies, kinship is traced through the mother's side of the family, and children belong to their mother's kin group. Double standards of sexual behavior are either less salient or their effects are reduced compared to those in bilateral/patrilineal descent societies (Whelehan 2001a; Bolin and Whelehan 1999).

Kin groups (that is, families) provide the basis of social, psychological, and economic support in most cultures. They are an individual's survival mechanism in many societies. In a number of societies, it is the kin group, not the individual, that makes major life decisions, such as whom to marry, use of birth control, where the person lives, what kind of work the person does, and where and how an individual's resources are distributed.

Marriage and kinship systems generally complement each other. The predominant marriage, kinship, and family forms worldwide support polygyny, multiple sexual partners for men, descent through males, and extended kin group decision making. These systems all impact safer sex practices and the sexual risks of HIV transmission (McGrath et al. 1993).

Culture change has affected indigenous kinship, marriage, and sexual practices. Precontact patterns of patrilineal and bilateral descent that favored males as well as initiation practices that elucidated accepted male and female sexual behaviors and gender roles were impacted by colonialism. Colonialism tended to reinforce the patricentricity or male-centeredness of these societies. In places such as Tanzania (see Setel 1999; Dilger 2007), European influence ended or changed initiation practices that had previously given women some control over their sexuality (Svensson 2007; Pfeiffer 2004: 88; Rasing 2003). In addition, changing world markets, war, and globalization have all contributed to changing gender roles, sexual behaviors, and women's sexual decision-making ability (Mufune 2003).

Gender

Our sense of who we are as male, female, or another gender (such as *mahu* among Hawaiians or *hijras* in India) is a deep part of our identity as individuals. Gender is yet another biocultural phenomenon. Gender refers to the designation and sense of being male, female, or categorically **third and fourth genders**. Among the Zuni in the southwestern United States, people identifying as something other than male or female are referred to as "**Two Spirits**" (Roscoe 1998). Gender includes biological characteristics such as chromosomes, hormones, and primary and secondary sex characteristics. These involve sexual and reproductive anatomy such as penises and clitorises, scrotums and labia majora, as well as breasts in women and muscle development in men.

Gender is also cultural. Cultures decide what constitutes gender and assign gender(s) to its members. One's sense of gender develops within a community that defines and influences its expression. The United States officially recognizes only two genders, male and female, based on sexual and reproductive anatomy. People in the United States are expected to accept and conform to one of these two gender identities and the corresponding masculine or feminine gender role. **Gender role** is the expression of culturally defined male and female behaviors and norms in relation to activities such as emotional displays, speech, dress, work, and body language. Anthropologists generally adopt a social constructionist approach to gender issues, believing that gender role in particular is largely learned. In contrast, essentialists believe that gender, gender identity, and gender role are largely determined by biology: chromosomes and hormones (Dowsett et al. 2006; Rubin 1997).

A **gender identity** other than male or female is pathologized and stigmatized in the United States (Bockting and Kirk 2001; Herek and Greene 1995). People in the United States who are etically classified as **transvestites (TVs)** (the emic term is *cross-dressers*) and/or **transsexuals/transgenders (TSs/TGs)** are medically defined as having a "disorder" and often are ostracized socioculturally (Bockting and Kirk 2001). Etically, transvestites generally are men who dress in women's clothes. From an etic perspective, transgenders/transsexuals are people who believe that they are the other gender, either **MTF/M2F**, male to female, or **FTM/F2M**, female to male. Emically, many TSs/TGs may either identify as the other gender or adopt a gender identity that is outside the larger societal binary male-female dichotomy. For reasons discussed later in this chapter, transgendered people have multiple risks for HIV infection.

In contrast to the United States, many other cultures traditionally recognized more than two genders prior to European contact (Robertson 2005; Blackwood and Wieringa 1999). More than five hundred Native American groups, including Hawaiians, as well as groups in Brazil, India, and Thailand and other parts of South and Southeast Asia accepted more than two genders (Roscoe 1998; Nanda 2000; Vernon 2001; Inciardi et al. 2001; Cáceres et al. 2006; Dowsett et al. 2006). These "third and fourth" genders (or "Two Spirits" among southwestern U.S. Indian cultures) generally were well-integrated members of society. Biological males and females, these individuals often adopted the roles of the other gender, were sometimes seen to possess spiritual powers, and embraced a fluid sexuality. As a result of European contact and colonization, many of these roles and the people who filled them lost status, became stigmatized, and were banned or persecuted (Nanda 2000; Roscoe 1998; Vernon 2001; Dowsett et al. 2006; Cáceres et al. 2006). In the age of AIDS, people who identify as third or fourth gender in these societies negotiate mixed cultural norms and messages about who they are, their sexuality, and safer sex (Vernon 2001; Dowsett et al. 2006; Cáceres et al. 2006).

Safer sex HIV education programs in these cultures need to develop programs that respect the history of multiple gender roles as well as the current situation. Intervention programs need to include specific sexual messages that address the needs of people with alternative genders in these societies (Sittitrai et al. 1991; Oetomo 1991; Cáceres et al. 2006; Dowsett et al. 2006).

5.1

The open resurgence of Two Spirits in Native communities has received a mixed reaction there and in the non-Native world. These individuals may experience acceptance or rejection by their own communities, emulation by lesbian-gay-bisexual-transgendered (LGBT) groups, or dismissal by the larger society (Canadian Aboriginal AIDS Network 2000; Jacobs et al. 1997; Roscoe 1988). Where structural factors such as discrimination, poverty, or **syncretic** beliefs interact to reject Two Spirit Native peoples, the stigma and rejection can increase risky sex and needle usage, as it has for other transgendered and gay populations (Walters and Simoni 2004, 2005).

Sexual Orientation

As with gender, what constitutes sexual orientation is culturally defined and expressed. The causes and expressions of sexual orientation are complex. Generally, sexual orientation refers to the sex of one's sexual and romantic love partners. While cultures have long recognized that their members could be sexual with a variety of people, the idea of having an identity based on the sex of one's sexual partners is relatively recent and Euro-American (Aries 1989; Whelehan 2001b; Bolin and Whelehan 1999; Rubin 1997). Sexual orientation is not the same as sexual behavior. Sexual orientation refers to the sex of the person one is attracted to; sexual behavior refers to with whom a person has sex (Tielman 1991; Dowsett et al. 2006; Cáceres et al. 2006).

Culture contact and change over several hundred years between industrialized, Euro-American societies and nonindustrialized groups has had an effect on the conceptualizations and expression of sexual orientation cross-culturally. In some ways, this effect is similar to the effect of culture contact on the expression of third and fourth genders. Understanding the vagaries of sexual orientation will help to explain the sexual risk for and stigma accompanying HIV in the United States and cross-culturally.

Three major categories of sexual orientation have been recognized in Euro-American societies since the late nineteenth century. Etically, these are **heterosexual** (or "**straight**"), sexual attraction to the other sex; **bisexual** (or "**bi**"), sexual attraction to both one's own and the other sex; and **homosexual**, attraction to one's own sex (designated as "**gay**" if male and open about it and "**lesbian**" if female and open about it) (Bolin and Whelehan 1999).

Heterosexuality is the only orientation in the United States that is culturally, legally, and socially recognized and protected on a federal/national level. This position reinforces a value on reproductive success and penile-vaginal intercourse. The federal position, however, does not speak to the statutes and laws within given states, within communities, or among some employers. In some major cities such as San Francisco and New York, people whose sexual orientation is other than heterosexual can receive domestic partner benefits at work and are protected from discrimination based on their sexual orientation. As of 2006, five states (California, Hawaii, New Jersey, Maine, and Massachusetts) have domestic partner laws. Vermont recognizes civil unions for people of the same sex, and Massachusetts began to recognize marriage between same-sex couples in May 2004. This decision has sparked a great deal of controversy. In 2004, President George W. Bush called for a constitutional amendment to ban same-sex marriages. This amendment was not supported by Congress in 2006.

The United States is dualistic about gender and sexual orientation. One is either male or female, heterosexual or not. The subtleties and nuances of what constitute gender and orientation, including psycho-emotional or ethnic factors, do not fit well with the approach to gender and orientation in the United States. As part of stigmatized groups, TVs, TSs, gays, lesbians, and bisexuals may engage in a variety of behaviors that can put them at risk for HIV. They may be in denial about who they are, conform to larger societal expectations overtly and engage in risky behaviors covertly, or inconsistently behave according to gender and sexual norms. Their own identities may not neatly fit researcher-based etic categorization and labels. This can be particularly true for women who identify as lesbians, as will be discussed later.

Sexual Orientation outside of the United States

Cross-culturally, concepts of orientation are as different as are concepts of gender (Tielman et al. 1991; Orubuloye et al. 1994; Whelehan 2001b; Levine et al. 1997; Dowsett et al. 2006; Cáceres et al. 2006). As with gender, culture contact with Euro-American cultures has altered indigenous beliefs about orientation. China is a good example of this. The earliest Taoist beliefs in China accepted same-sex sexual behavior and relationships (Ruan 1991). Contact with Europeans over several hundred years and the communist Cultural Revolution of the twentieth century changed China's relatively sex-positive views and acceptance of same-sex sexuality.

The Cultural Revolution in China imposed a rigid birth control policy and a sex-negative policy that reinforced the primacy of sex for reproduction. Same-sex sexual relations became illegal, could be punished if discovered, and were stigmatized (Ruan 1991). These policies and views increased the risk for HIV infection by driving sexual behaviors underground and impacted China's response to AIDS in its culture. Only recently have some of China's policies toward same-sex relationships, sex, and HIV changed to be more open and accepting (Wang and Ross 2002; Becker 2003; Stanmeyer 2003).

Same-sex relationships traditionally were accepted in other parts of the world, including Africa, Japan, Thailand, Bangladesh, Indonesia, and India (Whelehan 2001b; Aing 1991; Oetomo 1991; Tielman et al. 1991; Dowsett et al. 2006; Robertson 2005; Blackwood and Wieringa 1999). Currently, however, most areas of the world stigmatize open expressions of same-sex sexuality, particularly male-male sex. Same-sex sexuality tends to be marginalized, which increases the risk of HIV infection (Aing 1991; Bailey 1995; Byrnes 1996; Chng et al. 2003).

Same-sex sexuality also takes on symbolic meanings that can affect HIV risk and prevention (Carrier 2001; Carrier and Bolton 1991). Mexico and Brazil present two examples of this. In both Mexico and Brazil, men who are the inserter in male-male sex maintain their sense of maleness, masculinity, and heterosexuality (Doll et al. 1991). They are not considered to be homosexual.

Sexual behavior, gender identity, and sexual orientation are not synonymous. A woman who identifies as a lesbian may have sex with a man for economic reasons, to become pregnant, for fun, or to "pass" as straight to her family. An unassimilated Latino or Asian/Pacific Island male immigrant to the United States may have sex with men but not identify as gay, to preserve family harmony or save face (Carballo-Dieguez 1995; Chng et al. 2003; Blackwood and Wieringa 1999; Robertson 2005). An urban African American man who has sex with both men and women (known as "down low" behavior) may not let his female partners know this, to avoid rejection by his church and community (Clay 2002; Peterson 1995). It is important to know and understand these distinctions and how they are manifested in each targeted group when developing safer sex intervention programs (Bolton 1994).

The Sexual Risk Continuum

The previous overviews of sexuality, gender, and orientation provide a background for examining the sexual risks for contracting HIV. Not all sexual behaviors are equally risky for contracting HIV. HIV can only be transmitted sexually through infected blood, semen, or vaginal fluids. Any sexual behavior that does *not* put someone in contact with these infected body fluids will *not* transmit HIV. In addition, if sexual partners test negative for HIV and agree to a monogamous relationship, they can engage in any sexual behavior with each other and neither transmit nor contract HIV (see chapter 4).

The sexual risk for HIV exists along a **sexual risk continuum** (Bolin and Whelehan 1999; http://www.gmhc.org). This risk continuum is based on Euro-American Anglo concepts of sexuality. It indicates risk from the riskiest sexual behavior to the least risky (CDC 2003b; PAEG 2002).

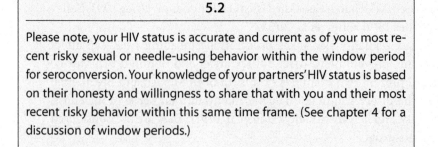

5.2

Please note, your HIV status is accurate and current as of your most recent risky sexual or needle-using behavior within the window period for seroconversion. Your knowledge of your partners' HIV status is based on their honesty and willingness to share that with you and their most recent risky behavior within this same time frame. (See chapter 4 for a discussion of window periods.)

Risky Sex

In general, the sexual partners whose mucous membranes—anal, vaginal, or oral—are being touched are at higher risk for infection than is the person who is touching them. Semen contains higher concentrations of HIV than do vaginal fluids (Tortu et al. 2000; Bartlett 2006). Therefore, men are more infectious with HIV than are women. Receiving penises into anuses, vaginas, and mouths is riskier than inserting them. Men are more likely to transmit HIV to their partners in penetrative sex than women are to men or to other women (Padian et al. 1991; Padian 1998; Cohen 1999; DeGraaf et al. 1997; Bartlett 2006).

The riskiest sexual behavior is unprotected receptive anal intercourse; the next is unprotected receptive vaginal intercourse. On the sexual risk continuum, these behaviors are considered unsafe or risky. The chance of contracting or spreading HIV with unprotected anal or vaginal sex depends on a number of factors that will be discussed later in the chapter. Oral sex can transmit HIV, but it is much less risky than anal and vaginal intercourse (McIlvenna and Taylor 1999; Bartlett 2006). The risk from oral sex is not from saliva; saliva does *not* transmit HIV. The risk from oral sex is from having cuts or sores inside your mouth or on your lips and gums and having those exposed areas come in contact with infected blood, semen, vaginal fluids, or breast milk.

5.3

People are curious about the mathematical odds for contracting HIV through protected and unprotected sex with people whose HIV status is unknown. According to John Bartlett, an HIV/AIDS specialist and physician at Johns Hopkins Medical Center, the risk of contracting HIV from unprotected sex is twenty times higher than that of any particular protected sexual behavior, regardless of whether it is anal, vaginal, or oral sex on a man. He does not give information for oral sex on a woman. For specific sexual behaviors, here is a list of the risk of contracting HIV in one act of unprotected sex per 10,000 exposures (Bartlett 2006: 11; Farook 2007: 1–2).

Insertive fellatio	0.5
Receptive fellatio	1
Insertive vaginal sex	3
Receptive vaginal sex	5–9
Insertive anal sex	9
Receptive anal sex	27

The odds of contracting HIV are based on mathematical models calculated in reference to populations whose serostatus is unknown, not individuals. Other factors such as genital sores, STIs, or other health situations that might compromise the immune system are not considered. In addition, these models do not consider the loading dose, that is, how many exposures a given individual requires before she or he is infected or how much virus may be present in infected semen, blood, or vaginal fluids. They also do not consider the prevalence of HIV in the geographic area where the sex occurs. Higher prevalence rates in an area increase the risk of contracting HIV from people in that area. Rather than playing safer sex roulette based on the "odds" of getting infected, another strategy may be to decide for yourself what your acceptable level of risk is, what sexual behaviors you are comfortable with and want to use protection for when engaging in them, and then following through on that.

Safer Sex

The term *safer sex* denotes using some form of latex barrier when engaging in penetrative anal, vaginal, or oral sex. These barriers include various forms of latex: male and female condoms for vaginal and anal intercourse; unlubricated male condoms for oral sex on a man; dams (latex squares) for oral sex on a woman and for rimming (analingus or oral-anal sex); and finger cots or gloves for any contact with infected semen, blood, or vaginal fluids, including anal or vaginal fisting (inserting fingers or hands into the rectum or vagina).

It is important to use latex condoms rather than skin condoms such as Naturalamb®, as HIV can pass through the pores of skin condoms. The CDC recommends the use of water-based lubricated condoms for vaginal and anal intercourse; oil-based lubricants such as those found in lotions, creams, massage oils, and vegetable and mineral oils break down the latex in the condoms. The CDC recommends against using spermicidal condoms, as they may irritate vaginal and anal mucosa, providing a portal of entry for HIV or other pathogens (CDC 2003b).

To be effective in preventing HIV, using these latex barriers as consistently as possible during penetrative sex reduces one's risk for contracting HIV and other STIs (Bartlett 2006; UNAIDS 2006; Institute of Medicine 2001). Some activists and safer sex educators refer to using "layers of protection" to reduce the risk of transmitting or contracting HIV. This means, for example, to use latex gloves or finger cots for vaginal and anal fist-ing and fingering in addition to using latex male and/or female condoms for anal and vaginal intercourse. It refers to using nonlubricated, flavored condoms for oral sex on a man and dams for oral sex on a woman or for rimming (oral-anal stimulation) (McIlvenna and Taylor 1999; Taylor and Lourea 1992).

The more layers of protection that are used with penetrative sexual en-counters, the safer that sexual behavior is. The fewer layers used (or if they are used inconsistently, incorrectly, or not at all), the riskier the specific sexual behavior is. The only exception to this is not using both the male and female condom together. Use one or the other; using both simulta-neously increases the chance of tearing the condoms. If a sexual partner is allergic to latex, polyurethane condoms can be used. The female con-dom, for example, is made of polyurethane, as are several brands of male condoms. Since most people worldwide and in the United States do not know their HIV status, the recommendation is to practice safer sex with anyone whose HIV status is unknown or with whom monogamy cannot be guaranteed. The pamphlets shown in figures 5.1 and 5.2 describe the sexual risk continuum and illustrate how to correctly use a male condom and dam.

Safer sex practices extend to the use and sharing of sex toys. Preferably, sex toys such as dildos (rubber phallic-shaped devices) are not shared. Sex toys should be cleaned after each use. If dildos are used for both anal and vaginal penetration, safer usage includes washing them and covering them with a new, lubricated condom between anal and vaginal stimulation.

5.4

Sex toys are easy to care for and maintain. If you have battery-oper-ated sex toys, remove the battery before cleaning them with soap and warm water and dry them away from heat and light. Do not use abrasive cleansers on sex toys. Use water-based lubricants with sex toys (Sex Toys 2006).

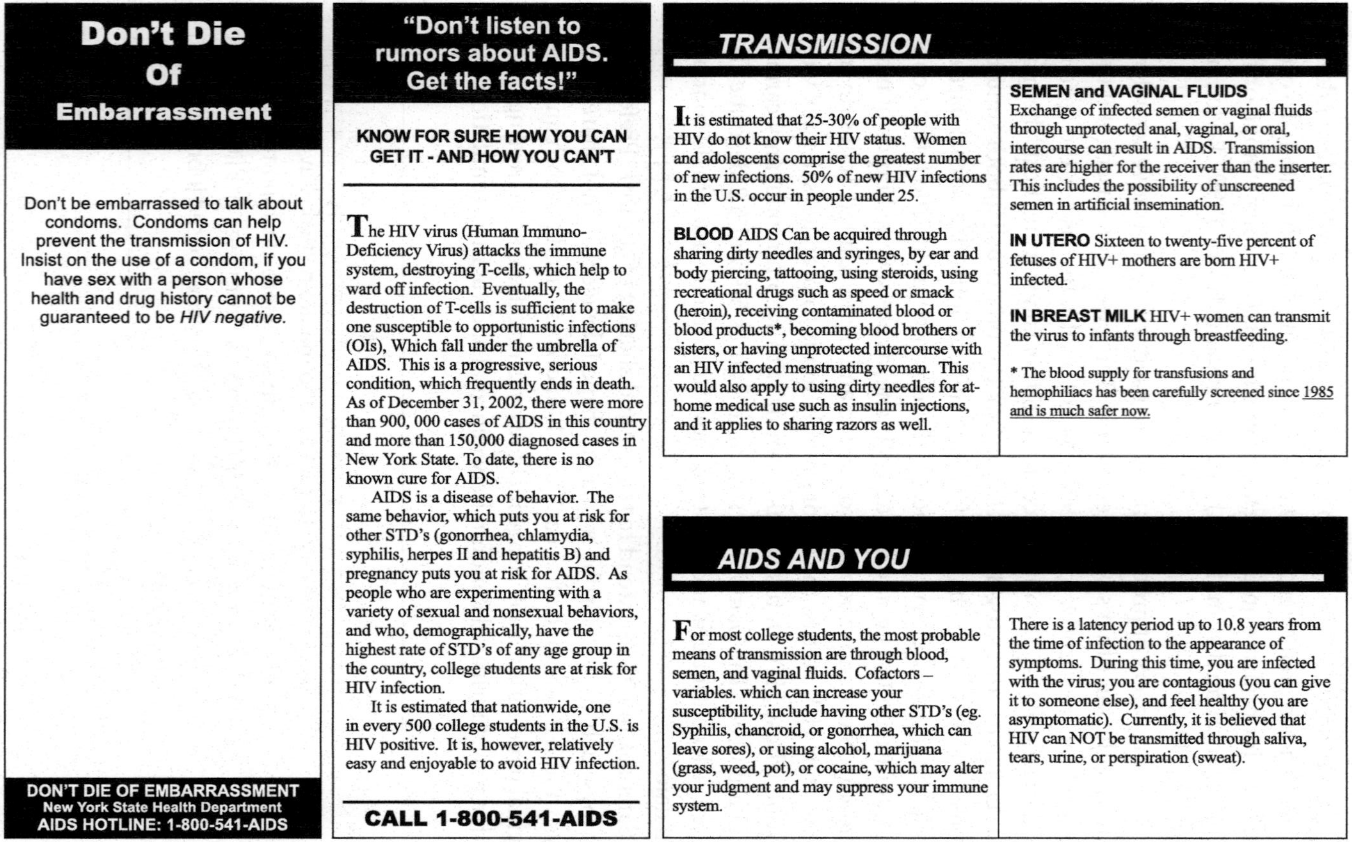

Don't Die Of Embarrassment

Don't be embarrassed to talk about condoms. Condoms can help prevent the transmission of HIV. Insist on the use of a condom, if you have sex with a person whose health and drug history cannot be guaranteed to be *HIV negative*.

DON'T DIE OF EMBARRASSMENT
New York State Health Department
AIDS HOTLINE: 1-800-541-AIDS

"Don't listen to rumors about AIDS. Get the facts!"

KNOW FOR SURE HOW YOU CAN GET IT - AND HOW YOU CAN'T

The HIV virus (Human Immuno-Deficiency Virus) attacks the immune system, destroying T-cells, which help to ward off infection. Eventually, the destruction of T-cells is sufficient to make one susceptible to opportunistic infections (OIs), Which fall under the umbrella of AIDS. This is a progressive, serious condition, which frequently ends in death. As of December 31, 2002, there were more than 900, 000 cases of AIDS in this country and more than 150,000 diagnosed cases in New York State. To date, there is no known cure for AIDS.

AIDS is a disease of behavior. The same behavior, which puts you at risk for other STD's (gonorrhea, chlamydia, syphilis, herpes II and hepatitis B) and pregnancy puts you at risk for AIDS. As people who are experimenting with a variety of sexual and nonsexual behaviors, and who, demographically, have the highest rate of STD's of any age group in the country, college students are at risk for HIV infection.

It is estimated that nationwide, one in every 500 college students in the U.S. is HIV positive. It is, however, relatively easy and enjoyable to avoid HIV infection.

CALL 1-800-541-AIDS

TRANSMISSION

It is estimated that 25-30% of people with HIV do not know their HIV status. Women and adolescents comprise the greatest number of new infections. 50% of new HIV infections in the U.S. occur in people under 25.

BLOOD AIDS Can be acquired through sharing dirty needles and syringes, by ear and body piercing, tattooing, using steroids, using recreational drugs such as speed or smack (heroin), receiving contaminated blood or blood products*, becoming blood brothers or sisters, or having unprotected intercourse with an HIV infected menstruating woman. This would also apply to using dirty needles for at-home medical use such as insulin injections, and it applies to sharing razors as well.

SEMEN and VAGINAL FLUIDS
Exchange of infected semen or vaginal fluids through unprotected anal, vaginal, or oral, intercourse can result in AIDS. Transmission rates are higher for the receiver than the inserter. This includes the possibility of unscreened semen in artificial insemination.

IN UTERO Sixteen to twenty-five percent of fetuses of HIV+ mothers are born HIV+ infected.

IN BREAST MILK HIV+ women can transmit the virus to infants through breastfeeding.

* The blood supply for transfusions and hemophiliacs has been carefully screened since <u>1985</u> and is much safer now.

AIDS AND YOU

For most college students, the most probable means of transmission are through blood, semen, and vaginal fluids. Cofactors – variables. which can increase your susceptibility, include having other STD's (eg. Syphilis, chancroid, or gonorrhea, which can leave sores), or using alcohol, marijuana (grass, weed, pot), or cocaine, which may alter your judgment and may suppress your immune system.

There is a latency period up to 10.8 years from the time of infection to the appearance of symptoms. During this time, you are infected with the virus; you are contagious (you can give it to someone else), and feel healthy (you are asymptomatic). Currently, it is believed that HIV can NOT be transmitted through saliva, tears, urine, or perspiration (sweat).

Figure 5.1. "Don't Die of Embarrassment" pamphlet (SUNY-Potsdam AIDS Education Group/SUNY-PAEG).

SAFER SEX...

**It's fun,
It's easy,
and
it may save
your life.**

Don't Die of Embarrassment

Don't be too embarrassed to talk about condoms. Condoms can help prevent AIDS. Insist on the use of a condom if you have sex with a person whose health and drug history cannot be guaranteed to be HIV negative.

The materials in this kit are provided to help you maintain your health. The pamphlet is graphic and explicit in explaining ways of reducing your risk of contracting or transmitting HIV. These materials are not meant to shock anyone. The goal is to encourage responsible behavior and decision-making relative to your sexuality and to keep you and your partner(s) safe and infection free.

AIDS HOTLINE
1-800-541-AIDS
Toll-free and confidential

For information, referral and support call your regional hotline and ask for the HIV counselor. This is a confidential service.

REGIONAL AIDS HOTLINES

Rochester area	585-423-8081
Syracuse area	315-475-2437
Buffalo area	716-847-4520
Suffolk County	800-462-6786
Northeastern NY	800-962-5065
Bronx	212-447-8200
Harlem	212-369-8378

Condoms, water-based lubricants, latex gloves, vaginal dams and fingercots are in this kit and can be purchased in drug stores and some grocery stores.

Condoms and safer sex kits can be obtained free from Student Health Services on campuses.

— SAFER SEX

Safer sex involves reducing your risk of contracting the HIV virus as well as enhancing your sexuality. Once one decides to have genital sexual contact with a partner, one moves from safe sex to the safer-to-risky continuum. Only you can decide what level of risk and trust are acceptable to your health. If a person lies to you about their HIV status, your life is at risk. Remember, PEOPLE LIE TO GET LAID, unfortunately. You are solely responsible for your decisions.

If you decide to become sexually active with a partner in which semen, blood or vaginal fluids could be exchanged, your behavior enters the realm of risk-taking. Safer sex is for anyone-male or female- who is sexually active with males and/or females. Safer sex practices that reduce the risk of infection are encouraged. It is recommended to use as many different forms of protection as possible: lubricated condoms for penetrative anal and vaginal intercourse; unlubricated, nonspermicidal condoms for fellatio (oral sex on a male) and vaginal dams for cumilingus (oral sex on a female) or any oral-perineal or perianal activity.

Cuts, scratches, scrapes on fingers, hands, lips, any broken skin surface may be a potential entry for infection. Therefore, finger cots and gloves are recommended in this situation. A glove can be turned into a vaginal/perineal dam by leaving the thumb intact for a finger cot and cutting open the rest of the glove. An unused unlubricated condom can also be used as a similar barrier by cutting it lengthwise.

In this pamphlet is a list of behaviors that are considered high-risk and absolutely unsafe. Most of the behaviors on the list you will probably recognize, but there are some that may be unfamiliar to you. By listing these, the editors of this pamphlet are neither condoning nor condemning them. But to be safe, you must have as much information as possible. It is important to remember that you must choose behaviors that are right for you, and you need not participate in any activity that you are uncomfortable with. Consider your own values carefully so you know how you feel before you find yourself in a situation that requires a decision about sex.

ABSTINENCE IS A PERFECTLY ACCEPTABLE, HEALTHY CHOICE TO MAKE

Figure 5.2. "Safer Sex" pamphlet (SUNY-Potsdam AIDS Education Group/SUNY-PAEG).

continued

The following information from:
1989 San Francisco AIDS Foundation, San Francisco
Our Bodies, Ourselves, Boston Women's Health Collective

CONDOM USAGE

Befriend your condom. You might want to buy some cheap ones and play with them. Get used to how they look, feel, smell and taste and how to open the package before you want to use them. They are awkward at first, so is riding a bike, learning how to use tampons, shaving, anything that is new and different.

How to put the condom on

Do retract (pull back) the foreskin if you are uncircumcised (uncut) before putting on the condom.

Do remove rolled condom from package.

Do roll condom down penis as soon as it is hard, before you start to make love (foreplay).

Do leave ¼ - ½ inch extra space at the tip of the condom to catch the ejaculate if the condom has no nipple.

Don't unroll the condom before using it. Instead carefully roll the condom down the erect penis toward the base.

Don't wait to put the condom on until you are ready to enter your partner- it may be too late. Drops of semen- precum- may drip from the uncovered penis before ejaculation, and may infect or impregnate your partner.

Don't twist or bite or prick the condom with a pin- this will damage it and allow fluid to leak out, possibly infecting your partner.

Don't use two condoms at once or the male and female condom at the same time. Double bagging can create friction that can cause tears in the condoms.

After ejaculating, hold the condom at the base of the penis and withdraw immediately. Unroll the condom from the penis and discard it.

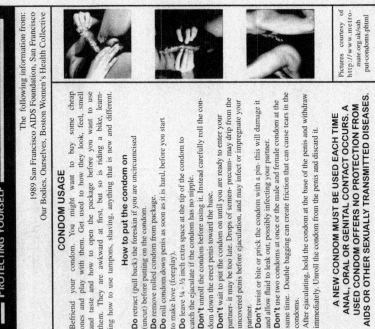

A NEW CONDOM MUST BE USED EACH TIME ANAL, ORAL OR GENITAL CONTACT OCCURS. A USED CONDOM OFFERS NO PROTECTION FROM AIDS OR OTHER SEXUALLY TRANSMITTED DISEASES.

Pictures courtesy of http://www.metro-mate.org.uk/sah put-condoms.phtml

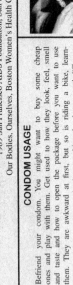

veneris mons
clitoral hood
clitoris
labia majora
labia minora
perineum

VAGINAL DAM USE

Vaginal dams are difficult to find here. They come in a variety of sizes, thickness, colors, tastes, and smells. Generally, they take more accommodation than do condoms. Vaginal dams are needed when performing oral sex on a woman, oral-perineal stimulation, and any kind of oral-anal contact.

Vaginal dams are placed over the genitals, perineum, or anal area before and during any oral contact. Stimulation is through the vaginal dam. Because vaginal dams are difficult to obtain, we are including a vaginal dam in the Safer Sex Kit.

A NEW VAGINAL DAM MUST BE USED EACH TIME ANAL OR GENITAL CONTACT OCCURS.

Picture courtesy of http://www.luckymojo.com/faqs/ altsex/vulva.html

■ HIGH RISK, UNSAFE SEX PRACTICES ■

• Multiple genital partners without using condoms or vaginal dams
• A single genital sex partner without using condoms or vaginal dams unless monogamy and HIV-status can be guaranteed now and in the future
• Oral genital (male or female) contact, anal penetration, vaginal penetration, without condoms and vaginal dams; or sharing sex toys
• Rimming (oral-anal contact) without a vaginal dam
• Fisting (finger-hand vaginal-anal penetration)
• Oral-perineal contact without a vaginal dam

(the perineum is the soft skin between the genitals and the anus)
• S/M (sado-masochism), B/D (bondage-discipline), tying up, spanking, M/S (master-slave) behavior that breaks the skin or deeply bruises it
• Sharing sex toys such as vibrators or dildoes with a partner
• Water sports (playing with urine) on broken skin and, possibly, internal water sports

Engaging in any or all of the behaviors in this group even once jeopardizes your own and your partner's health.

CO-FACTORS: NON-SEXUAL BEHAVIORS WHICH MAY INCREASE YOUR RISK

Using alcohol and other drugs may impair your judgment or lower your inhibitions and may cause you to behave unsafely

SAFER SEX GUIDELINES

Always use lubricated condoms for anal and vaginal sex

Don't get semen or vaginal fluids in your mouth.
Use a condom or vaginal dam for any oral sex. Unlubricated condoms may be used, if preferred, for oral sex.

Don't have mouth to rectum contact without using a latex barrier.

Figure 5.2. —continued

Safe Sex

The term *safe sex* entails a wide range of sexual behaviors. **Safe sex** includes people in monogamous relationships who know that their HIV status is negative. Monogamy denotes one partner for life. One definition of monogamy is as follows: you have had no partners other than your partner, neither before nor after, and your partner has had no other partners other than you, neither before nor after. The challenges of being truly monogamous in the United States and cross-culturally have been alluded to earlier in the chapter and will be discussed more fully later. Safe sex encompasses all those behaviors that do not exchange potentially infected blood, semen, or vaginal fluids. The range of these behaviors is vast. They can include, but are not limited to, fantasy, phone sex, masturbation and mutual masturbation with a partner, and erotica. To understand why people engage in risky sex or practice safer sex worldwide, one must look at those sociocultural values and behaviors that impact safer sex.

Safe sex and safer sex effectively reduce HIV transmission when practiced consistently and correctly. Abstinence from penetrative sex and guaranteed lifelong monogamy will reduce the sexual transmission of HIV. However, most people worldwide do not practice either abstinence or lifelong monogamy.

Consistent use of latex barriers for penetrative anal, vaginal, and oral sex is highly effective in preventing HIV transmission if used correctly with every sexual encounter (CDC 2003a, 2003b). The difficulties in consistently and correctly practicing safer sex will be discussed later in this chapter.

Sex and HIV in the United States

People in the United States receive very mixed messages about sexuality. Despite the degree of sexual explicitness that is available in the media and over the Internet or is visible in our daily dress or between people in public, this culture has highly conflicting views about sexuality, sex, and orientation. There are several reasons for this. First, we are a highly heterogeneous society in terms of socioeconomics, ethnicity, and religion. There are competing values about sexuality within and between ethnic and socioeconomic groups and differing religious views. Second, mainstream views about sexuality and gender carried over from our Puritan ancestors persist. These views, while embracing heterosexuality in the context of monogamous marriage, were largely sex negative (Bolin and Whelehan 1999; SIECUS 2001, 2003; *HIVPlus* 2002b; Aries 1989).

The sociologist Lilian Rubin describes our conflicting stands on sexuality as "public noise" and "private silence" (Rubin 1983). Public noise refers to the media portrayal of sex and the open displays of sexuality in public. Public noise presents the façade that people in the United States are comfortable with sexuality, are able to communicate with each other and their children about sexuality, and support comprehensive sex and HIV education in schools and communities.

Private silence, in contrast, is the difficulty people have in communicating about sexuality (Rubin 1983). This includes communicating one's sexual needs with partners, discussing and providing sex education for one's children, and supporting comprehensive sex and HIV education in schools and communities. Private silence carries over legislatively to the local, state, and national levels. Despite a recommendation from the surgeon general of the United States in 2001, it remains a challenge to provide sex and HIV education in public schools that includes information other than abstinence (Office of the Surgeon General 2001; SIECUS 2001, 2003, 2006; Waxman 2006).

Federal funding for public and private schools in the United States either mandates or strongly encourages abstinence-only sex education programs (SIECUS 2001, 2003, 2006; Waxman 2006; Mayer and Pizer 2000: section 3). Schools may jeopardize their funding if they offer comprehensive sex and HIV education. Despite U.S. federal endorsement of abstinence-only sex education programs, the efficacy of such programs is unproven; indeed, some research indicates that lack of knowledge about contraception and safer sex can increase people's, especially teens', risk for unplanned pregnancy and STIs, including HIV (Waxman 2006; SIECUS 2006; Kaiser Daily Women's Health Policy 2007; Underhill et al. 2007). Most researchers (including anthropologists) and agencies involved in preventing unwanted pregnancies and HIV endorse comprehensive sex education and comprehensive HIV prevention efforts (Feldman 2003b; Bolton 1992; McGrath et al. 1993; Schoepf 2003b, 2004; SIECUS 2006; Waxman 2006; www.agi-usa.org, UNAIDS 2004, 2006; UNAIDS/UN-FPA/UNIFEM 2004).

The firing of Dr. Joycelyn Elders is perhaps one of the more dramatic examples of our sex-negative views and governmental discomfort with comprehensive sex and HIV education in schools. Dr. Elders, a physician, was surgeon general of the United States under President Bill Clinton. Clinton and his Democratic administration were allegedly politically liberal. However, in 1994, President Clinton fired Dr. Elders for her recommendations about sex and HIV education for children. In a speech about HIV/AIDS for the United Nations, she recommended that children be informed that masturbation was the safest sexual behavior possible and that it was a "normal" activity. She did not say that teachers and parents should show their students and children how to masturbate, a statement she was accused of making. The controversy generated by her remarks resulted in her being fired (Elders 1994).

In contrast to abstinence-only sex and HIV education for children and adolescents, comprehensive programs include discussions of abstinence and monogamy in addition to information about contraception and safer sex in an age- and developmentally appropriate manner (SIECUS 2001, 2003, 2006; Waxman 2006). Comprehensive sex and HIV education programs more realistically reflect the sexual behavior of the people in the United States.

Regardless of people's actual sexual behavior, gender, and orientation in the United States, the government and mainstream Anglo culture uphold several sexual norms. These include the primacy of heterosexuality, penile-vaginal intercourse as the definition of sex, heterosexual marriage, and a value on monogamy. The farther away an individual's or group's behavior is from these norms, the less tolerance for and acceptance of it there is. The lack of tolerance is expressed in sodomy laws and nonfederal government protection in employment and housing. In a 2003 landmark decision, the Supreme Court overturned a Texas sodomy law that made it illegal for two "homosexual men" to have sexual relations (ironically, the Texas law had no restrictions on female-female sex and allowed oral and anal sex and bestiality among heterosexuals) (Lochhead 2003).

Despite restrictive legal statutes and political regulations about sexuality in the United States, people's behavior indicates a range of nonmarital and nonmonogamous sexual activity. The United States has the highest rates of unplanned and teenaged pregnancy, particularly for females under the age of fifteen, in the industrialized world. We have the highest rates of STIs and one of the highest rates of HIV/AIDS in the industrialized world (Planned Parenthood 2004; www.agi-usa.org; SIECUS 2001, 2006). As of 2002–2003, 50 percent of HIV infections in the United States occur in people under twenty-five (CDC/HHS 2003; UNAIDS 2006). According to the National Campaign to Prevent Teen Pregnancy, 20 percent of children between the ages of twelve and fifteen engage in intercourse, oral sex, or other sexual activities (Anon. 2003d).

Drug usage can also affect safer sex practices. Drug usage can be a co-factor in the sexual transmission of HIV. (The topic is introduced here; it is discussed in depth in chapter 6.) Generally, the use of legal and illegal recreational drugs such as alcohol may impact people's decision-making ability and may suppress their immune system, depending on the type and use of the drug. Variables such as age, gender, relationship status, and cultural acceptance of the gender of one's sex partners also influence safer sex practices.

In contrast, the use of injection drugs—particularly the use of illegal injection drugs such as heroin, cocaine, and speed—increases the risk of infection by transmitting the virus directly and by affecting the immune system (see chapter 6). Interestingly, as discussed in the next chapter, injection drug users (IDUs) will more readily change their needle-using behavior than their sexual behavior. This phenomenon reflects the depth, intimacy, and personal nature of our sexuality.

Sexual Communities in the United States

Despite lack of larger cultural support, various sexual communities exist in the United States. They include the gay, lesbian, and bisexual communities, transsexuals/transgendereds, and sex workers. These groups occupy marginalized and stigmatized, yet significant, places in U.S. society. In addition, ethnic groups such as Latinos, African Americans, Native Americans, and Asian/Pacific Islanders have their own interpretations about sex.

Gays

Gay communities, largely found in the epicenters of the epidemic in the United States, were on the forefront of developing safer sex materials and strategies. These included culturally sensitive and appropriate forums and meetings, campaigns, posters, and brochures with prevention and risk-reduction information. Initially, the gay community borrowed some ideas, such as using latex gloves for fisting, from the sadomasochism (SM) and bondage and discipline (B/D) communities, as well as those communities' openness in discussing sexual behaviors and flexibility in what they did sexually. Gay communities took a lead in the safer sex campaigns with the idea of using latex condoms, finger cots, and vaginal dams in their sexual activities (McIlvenna and Taylor 1999; Rubin 1997; Taylor and Lourea 1992). The gay community, through its social, political, and economic activism, was instrumental in encouraging research, prevention, and treatment efforts for HIV.

Lesbians

The cultural discomfort with open discussions of sexuality and the single-minded recognition of heterosexuality as the only "legitimate" sexual orientation extends to the CDC. The CDC establishes risk exposure categories for HIV/AIDS. Risk exposure categories refer to groups that reflect high incidence of HIV/AIDS. The CDC defines risk, the modes of transmission, and the category. According to the CDC, if a woman who identifies as a lesbian has had sex with a man even once since 1978, she is not a lesbian (Goldstein 1997; Campbell 1999; Aggleton 1994). In the United States, women who identify as lesbians are more likely to have sex with men than men who identify as gay are to have sex with women (Gomez 1995). As of 2003, the CDC still does not have an HIV risk exposure category for lesbians and **Women Who Have Sex With Women (WSW)**.

The CDC's position reinforces larger cultural values of what constitutes sex: p-v sex is the norm (Schneider and Stoller 1995; Gomez 1995; Stoller 1998). The CDC's position ignores what it means to be a lesbian in the United States. It reinforces the invisibility of women who identify as lesbians, and by doing so, it increases their risk for infection. Identifying as a lesbian is an interaction of sexual, sociopsychological, emotional, and political feelings and beliefs (Parker and Ehrhardt 2001; Parker, Barbosa, and Aggleton 2000; Hunter and Alexander 1996; Parker and Aggleton 1999; Rotheram-Borus et al. 1995). Lesbians may and do incorporate any or all of these beliefs as part of their identity; it is not just sexual (Gomez 1995; Roth et al. 1998; Bailey 1995; Goldstein 1997; O'Sullivan and Parmer 1992; Ramos 1997; Robertson 2005).

Ignoring the emic conceptualization of what it means to be a lesbian has consequences. First, there is inaccurate epidemiological data for WSW/ lesbians (Padian et al. 1991; Fethers et al. 2000; Kwakwa and Ghobrial 2003). Second, within the lesbian community, there is a sense of invulnerability to HIV infection (Roth and Fuller 1998; Chapkis 1997). Third, there is a lack of and sometimes misdirected HIV prevention efforts toward women who identify as lesbians (Gomez 1995; Parker and Aggleton 1999; Parker, Barbosa, and Aggleton 2000). To reduce the risk of sexual transmission of HIV to women who identify as lesbians, outreach efforts need to consider all of these components of a lesbian identity (Fethers et al. 2000; Kwakwa and Ghobrial 2003).

Bisexuals (Bis)

Bisexuals, those people sexually attracted to their own and the other sex, receive little support from the straight, lesbian, and gay communities in the United States (Rust 2000). Because Bis can behave both heterosexually and homosexually, they are accused of being fence sitters, passing (pretending in public to be straight to gain societal approval), immature, or indecisive (Bolin and Whelehan 1999). Bisexuals have been blamed for bringing HIV/AIDS to the heterosexual community (Doll et al. 1991). They have been among the scapegoats for HIV in the United States. Sexphobia, homophobia, and the belief that HIV is a "gay" disease persist in these views.

Unless sexual behavior is coerced (as in rape or other sexual assault), our culture perceives adult sexual behavior as consensual. People involved in consensual sex have responsibility for their behavior—the kinds of sex they are willing to engage in and whether or not to practice safer sex. Blaming bisexuals for "crossing over" and introducing HIV into the heterosexual community victimizes their partners rather than holding their partners responsible for the sexual decisions those partners made. In addition, blaming reinforces HIV as a "gay" disease and increases shame, guilt, and nondisclosure about one's sexual behavior. Blaming bisexuals also ignores the number of women, IDUs, children, and heterosexual couples infected with HIV since the beginning of the epidemic (Anderson 2001; Roth and Fuller 1998). Homophobia reinforces the tendency to deny one's sexual behavior and sexual orientation: "If I have sex with someone of the other sex, then I'm not gay, lesbian, or bisexual" (Clay 2002). Deceit, dishonesty, and lack of responsibility for one's sexual behavior are not the domain of one gender or orientation.

Transsexual/Transgendered People

Transsexual/transgendered people in the United States are a small subculture at risk for HIV infection (Bockting and Kirk 2001). The social ostracism from family and communities contributes to denial, a sense of isolation, feelings of low self-esteem, and risky sexual and needle-using behaviors (Bockting and Kirk 2001). Those who inject hormones may share needles. As a stigmatized population, TSs/TGs may engage in risky sexual behavior to gain acceptance for who they are. A recent report indicates that if they are HIV+, TGs/TSs are less likely to take HAART than are others with HIV (Melendez et al. 2006).

To pay for the hormones and sex reassignment surgery, TSs may engage in prostitution (Kammerer et al. 2001; Clements-Noelle et al. 2001). In general, clients of prostitutes pay more not to use condoms (Beyrer 1998; Thuy et al. 2000; Grandi et al. 2000; Basuki et al. 2002). Many clients of TSs are self-identified heterosexual men (Grandi et al. 2000; Kammerer et al. 2001; Reback and Lombardi 2001). Community responses to reduce risk for TSs include support for safer sex practices, petition for legal protection for their status, and acceptance from the medical community (see Bockting and Kirk 2001).

Sex Workers

Sex workers—a broad group that includes female, male, and transgendered prostitutes, strippers, dominatrices, pornography actors, and phone sex operators—constitute another category of scapegoats in the United States blamed for spreading HIV (Cohen 1999; Padian 1998; Padian et al. 1991). Of these sex workers, female prostitutes receive most of the blame (Whelehan 2001a; Alexander 1996; Cohen 1999). Women who identify as prostitutes and those who exchange sex for drugs or drug money are two distinct groups (Kwiatkowski and Booth 2000; Whelehan 2001a). Many prostitutes do not identify as drug users, and some women who exchange sex for drugs or drug money do not identify as prostitutes. Equating the two emic identities can negatively impact intervention efforts and the ability to obtain accurate epidemiological data (Whelehan 2001a; Waterston 1997). According to the CDC, about .04 percent of HIV transmission in the United States is attributable to men who contract it from female prostitutes (Cohen 1999; Whelehan 2001a). Four one-hundredths of one percent (4 per 10,000) is considered statistically insignificant in statistical analysis and quantitative research. Women's risk for contracting HIV and most other STIs from a man in unprotected p-v intercourse is much more significant.

In comparison to men, women are seven to nine times more likely to contract an STI other than nongonococcal urethritis (NGU) from a man in any given act of p-v intercourse (Tortu et al. 2000; Cohen 1999). They are three to eight times as likely to contract HIV from a man in any given act of p-v intercourse (Tortu et al. 2000; UNAIDS 2006). Biologically, women's increased vulnerability to STIs in general and HIV in particular is due to several factors. The woman's vaginal mucous membranes, rather than the man's surface penile skin, are abraded in p-v intercourse. The vagina has a much larger surface exposed to infection than do the urethra and the penis. There is a higher concentration of HIV in pre-ejaculatory fluid ("pre-cum") and ejaculate ("cum") than there is in vaginal fluids (Tortu et al. 2000; Osmond and Padian 1999).

Despite data that indicate that women, not men, are more at risk for HIV in p-v intercourse, the myth persists that women are the **vectors of transmission** (Stine 1997; Patton 1994; Orubuloye et al. 1994; Hunter and Alexander 1996; Treichler 1999). Prostitute women are particularly blamed for HIV transmission to men. The reasons for these views reflect deep cultural convictions about sexuality and women (Treichler 1999; see also chapter 7).

HIV, Sex, and Ethnicity in the United States

The categories of gender and orientation are largely based on middle-class Anglo norms and values. As such, they can be ethnocentric even within the culture. We are a highly ethnically diverse society. Latinos, African Americans, Native Americans, and Asian/Pacific Islanders who engage in same-sex sexual behavior or identify as other than male or female may not see themselves in Anglo terms (Vernon 2001; Diaz 1998; Clay 2002; O'Donnell et al. 2002; Choi et al. 2002; Peterson 1995; Carballo-Dieguez 1995, Choi et al. 1995).

Ethnic diversity is a major factor in the AIDS epidemic in the United States (see chapter 2). Proportionately, African Americans and Latinos have higher rates of HIV/AIDS than do Anglos and some other ethnic groups such as Native Americans. There are multiple reasons for the ethnic distribution of AIDS in the United States. These include cultural differences about sexuality, cofactors for infection related to STIs and overall states of health, poverty, drug usage, and differential access to health care. African Americans and Latinos comprise 15 and 12 percent of the U.S. population respectively but comprise about 57 percent of the people with AIDS (CDC 2003a). Of the women with AIDS in the United States, 83 percent are either African American or Latina (Robinson et al. 2002; Global Health Council 2005). Most of them are poor (Loue 1999).

People who are members of different ethnic groups in the United States

---

5.5

The actual prevalence of "down-low" behavior in the African American community is unknown. However, the lack of acceptance for same-sex behavior within the community in general can increase the "chances of being on the down low" (Howell 2007; Whitehead 1997: abstract; Peterson et al. 1996). Researchers believe that the reasons behind homophobia in the African American community are primarily a result of slavery, ongoing discrimination, and economic factors contributing to poverty, drug usage, and high rates of incarceration for young adult black males (Whitehead 1997). African American males internalize their own and the larger culture's values about maleness, masculinity, and the importance of heterosexuality. Intervention efforts need to be multidimensional and work with the community at the local level, including church leaders, while continuing to address issues of racism, discrimination, and employment. Responding to these issues can lead to reductions in incarceration and alter gender relationships (Howell 2007; Adimora and Schoenbach 2005; Barker et al. 1998; Torres et al. 1999).

---

may push gender boundaries and engage in same-sex sexual behavior for a variety of reasons. They may conform to larger Anglo societal labels and have an orientation as gay, bi, or lesbian. Or, following their own subculture's sexual beliefs, they may behave "bisexually" to avoid cultural rejection for having sex with members of their own sex.

In general, the African American community does not accept same-sex sex and sexual orientation. To avoid community censure, some African American men who have sex with men may keep this behavior hidden from their female partners to appear heterosexual (Clay 2002; Peterson 1995).

Sexual behaviors vary among African Americans. In African American religious communities, there are strong values on heterosexuality, monogamy, and sex within marriage (Clay 2002). Although African Americans begin having sexual intercourse earlier than Latinos and Anglos, their overall number of lifetime sexual partners is about the same as for Anglos.

The values on heterosexuality preclude community acceptance for people who identify as gay, bi, or lesbian (Peterson 1995; Clay 2002). The primary value on heterosexuality encourages African American men who have sex with men (MSM) to deny this sexual behavior and behave bisexually (Clay 2002). Therefore, it is not unusual for African American MSM to not inform their female partners about their male-male sexual behavior. Condom use with female partners can be inconsistent (Clay 2002).

Passing as heterosexual can result in an increase in HIV infection and AIDS in some parts of the African American community. It is estimated that 25–30 percent of urban African American MSM between the ages of eighteen and thirty-four are HIV+ or have AIDS (CDC 2001a; Clay 2002; Global Health Council 2005). Because same-sex sexual behaviors are stigmatized, men are reluctant to come out to their families, wives, and girlfriends.

Behaving heterosexually in the African American community involves a positive value on sexuality itself for both men and women. Women are recognized as sexual beings and are permitted and encouraged to express and enjoy their sexuality, particularly in the context of a relationship. African American women embrace the concepts of family, community, and sociopsychological support of their male partners (Robinson et al. 2002; Roth and Fuller 1998). They may engage in risky sexual behaviors to maintain these cultural values (Robinson et al. 2002).

Cultural and economic factors also influence the sexual risk for HIV/ AIDS for Latinos in the United States. Although generally regarded as one subculture in the United States, Latino populations come from diverse cultures in the Caribbean and in Central and South America. Common characteristics include values on *la familia* (family), *respeto* (respect), and *machismo*. Machismo values emphasize male sexual virility, risk taking, and honoring and protecting the family (Diaz 1998; O'Donnell et al. 2002). Machismo, racism, poverty, and a large number of high school female dropouts interact to contribute to the sexual risk for HIV infection.

Men from Latino subcultures may engage in same-sex sexual relations because of lack of female sexual partners owing to premarital sexual taboos. They may do this covertly to maintain the concept of respect for the family. Latino men in the United States may have sex with men as an initiation ceremony or rite of passage, to avoid having sex with a virgin female before marriage, or as a display of machismo if they are the inserter in sex. They will be discreet about this to protect the family's honor (Diaz 1998; Doll et al. 1991; Garcia et al. 1991; Carballo- Dieguez 1995). Depending on their age and degree of assimilation into mainstream U.S. society, these men may or may not identify as "gay" and may use Anglo terms to describe their behavior. Most identify themselves as straight men. HIV safer sex intervention methods need to recognize these variables.

La familia, the family, is the core value and social structure in Latino culture. Individual family members and their resources contribute to the maintenance of large, extended, multigeneration kin groups. Females, particularly the mothers, are the center of the family. Girls are socialized to believe that family responsibilities come first and that being good wives and mothers will earn them respect and status. Females depend on each other socially and psychologically to fulfill family obligations (Dugan 1988). Within the family, gender roles are well defined, even if the woman works outside the home. The home is female territory, and she is responsible for its functioning. Within the family and marriage, females are expected to be *marianismo*: chaste, deferential to males, and sexually passive (Saul et al. 2000; Campbell 1999).

While men and women discuss sexuality with members of their own sex, discussions of sexuality with spouses and children are rarer (O'Donnell et al. 2002). As in African American communities, same-sex sexual behavior is stigmatized (Ramos 1997). However, in Latino communities, if same-sex relationships and sexual behavior are discreet both in the community and at home, the person will receive acceptance within the kin group (Diaz 1998). Discretion is part of *respeto* (respect). The family is sacred and inviolate. Individuals maintain family respect by not openly expressing their sexual behavior (Diaz 1998).

Gender roles are clearly defined in Latino culture (Klein-Alonso 1996). The deferential female is balanced by the sexually open and initiating male. As long as the male is the initiator and inserter in penetrative sex, he retains his masculinity, maleness, and heterosexuality, regardless of the sex of his sex partner. If he is the receiver in penetrative sex, he jeopardizes his position as a male in society if his behavior becomes known. These values about maleness can lead to denial and risky behavior and can contribute to a man's being a "vector of transmission" to his wife and female lovers. Females, in contrast, put the male's needs above their own if they are "good women" (Klein-Alonso 1996).

Female same-sex and bisexual sexual behavior in Latino cultures tends to be diminished, denied, and stigmatized (Ramos 1997; Roth and Fuller 1998; Kaschak and Tiefer 2002). In general, Latinos' risk for HIV in the United States is related to their degree of assimilation. The less assimilated they are (that is, the more they uphold Latino norms and values), the higher the risk for infection (Diaz 1998; Tross 2001); the more assimilated into mainstream U.S. culture they are (particularly in relation to gender roles, sexual values, and behaviors), the lower the risk (Tross 2001; Ramos 1997).

Condoms have symbolic and preventive value in Latino cultures. Condoms are acceptable for men to wear with casual sex partners or with prostitutes. They are not acceptable to wear with one's wife, the mother of one's children (Diaz 1998; Ulin et al. 1996). Therefore, for a female to insist on a condom with her husband or lover implies distrust, that her sexual behavior is suspect, or that he will jeopardize his family's health by engaging in risky sexual behaviors. If she is economically dependent on him, she is also less likely to suggest using a condom or to challenge his sexual decisions (Ulin et al. 1996; Raffaelli and Suarez-Al-Adam 1998; Saul et al. 2000; Tross 2001). The interaction of these complex values, behaviors, varying degrees of assimilation, and economics are cofactors for HIV infection among Latinos in the United States.

A third ethnically diverse group affected by HIV is the Asian American/ Pacific Island (A/PI) community. Asian/Pacific Islander men who have internalized homophobia from the larger society and conform to their subculture's value of "face," that is, maintaining public decorum, may have sex with men discreetly. Discretion avoids bringing shame onto their families (Choi et al. 1995). As with Latino men, whether or not they identify themselves as gay depends on their degree of assimilation and support from their community.

Cultural values about sexuality, women, and men within these three groups influence risk for infection. Double standards of sexual behavior, sexism, disparate economic conditions, and greater biological susceptibility to the virus in penetrative sex increase the risk for women within these groups (Halperin 1999).

A group's rules and values are filtered through adaptation to the larger U.S. culture. They need to be considered when determining risk for HIV infection and developing intervention programs. The cultural components of language, behavior, identity, and orientation are all components of prevention efforts. Using Anglo models of sexuality, gender, and orientation can be problematic when developing HIV education and prevention programs among the ethnic and sexual subcultures in the United States. Safer sex programs need to incorporate the community's values and beliefs of the target population during the development of HIV prevention strategies for individuals. HIV prevention efforts are most effective when they are community-based and use peer educators (LeVine 2000; Wilson and Miller 2003; Amirkanian et al. 2003; Waterston 1997; Varga 1999).

The constructions of sexuality in the United States (and our deeply based discomfort with sex as expressed through homophobia and double standards of sexual behavior) affect safer sex practices. The CDC estimates that about 25 percent of the people who are HIV+ do not know their HIV status. There is an upsurge in syphilis rates and HIV for young, eighteen- to-twenty-four-year-old MSM and much higher incidences for African American MSM within the United States (CDC 2003a, 2001a, 2005b; Clay 2002). Fifty percent of new HIV infections in the United States occur in people under twenty-five years old (CDC 1999, 2003a; Kaiser Family Foundation 2005). The safer sex practices that worked in the 1980s among communities of MSM to reduce the incidence of HIV are no longer being practiced as they were (Parker and Ehrhardt 2001; Mc-Farland et al. 2004; Low-Beer and Stoneburner 2003). There are reasons that safer sex messages that promoted behavior change in the 1980s are less effective now.

First, HAART was unavailable in the 1980s. The death rate from AIDS was high, and people with AIDS visibly appeared to be very ill. Kaposi's sarcoma, an OI, caused purplish lesions and blotches on people's skin. Several bouts of **Pneumocystis carinii pneumonia** (another OI) and gastrointestinal problems left people wasted and skeletal looking. There were very clear signs that AIDS was fatal and took a toll on the body. Additionally, with so many Anglo MSM infected in the 1980s, there was a strong sense of community and purpose among them to control the epidemic and reduce infections. There were clear incentives to remain HIV negative if one was so and not to transmit the virus if one was HIV positive. Safer sex practices were developed within affected communities, and they worked. New and creative ways of using condoms and other latex barriers prevented infection and allowed people to be sexually active (Taylor and Lourea 1992; Rubin 1997). HIV incidence rates declined among MSM in the late 1980s and early 1990s. During this time, **survivor guilt** among HIV- MSM did not appear to negatively affect safer sex practices. Those who were HIV- remained so, and those who were HIV+ did not pass on the virus (Johnston 1995; Odets 1995).

HAART became available in the United States in 1996. Until 2003, taking HAART resulted in both fewer cases of full-blown AIDS and fewer deaths (Anon. 2003a). Taking HAART correlates with a decrease in safer sex practices (Parsons et al. 2003). Safer sex is difficult to maintain consistently, particularly with steady partners (Furlonge et al. 2000; Pilkington et al. 1994). With fewer cases of AIDS and fewer deaths from it, the need to consistently use condoms becomes less apparent. Pharmaceutical companies advertise the dramatic effectiveness that HAART can have for people who can afford the drug: take it regularly, and live with the side effects of the regimen. Overall, the risk from HIV/AIDS therefore does not seem as serious as it once was. There is a generation of people coming of sexual age in the era of HAART. They did not experience the devastation of the first wave of the epidemic. They are also in our culturally defined period of rebellion, risk taking, and figuring out who they are as individuals and sexual beings. If an eighteen- to twenty-four-year-old does become HIV infected, there are drugs to help.

5.6

People engage in a wide range of sexual behaviors for a variety of reasons: it feels good, it's forbidden, it's an expression of caring for someone, it's coerced, there's peer pressure, or to make babies. Under circumstances of consensual sex, the correct and consistent use of condoms can reduce the risk of pregnancy to 3 percent and the risk of HIV to less than 1 percent (WHO 2004a).

If HIV/AIDS can become a "chronic but manageable" disease that can be controlled by taking HAART, how risky is it not to practice safer sex and possibly become infected? We are a society of drug users. We regularly ingest over-the-counter, herbal, prescription, recreational, legal, and illegal drugs. Think of the aspirin, coffee, vitamins, alcohol, or other drugs or drug-containing products you take daily. In addition, many chronic and incurable diseases are treated by drugs: diabetes, arthritis, and high blood pressure, for example. When HAART works, it reduces viral loads and increases T-cells, improving immune function and making the person less infectious (see chapter 3). The availability of HAART in industrialized and some nonindustrialized societies combined with its efficacy and the difficulty in consistently maintaining safer sex practices over a long period of time contribute to decisions to engage in riskier sexual behaviors.

Long-term survivors or nonprogressors (that is, people who have been HIV+ for more than fifteen years without developing AIDS) have their own safer sex issues to address. Practicing safer sex reduces the chances that they will infect anyone else or be reinfected with another strain of the virus. However, consistently practicing safer sex is difficult, regardless of whether a person is HIV+ (Meyer-Bahlberg et al. 1991; Reilly and Woo 2001), largely because there are emotional factors involved in sexual decision making that enter into noncasual sexual relationships (Pilkington et al. 1994). For example, HIV+ women or women with HIV+ male partners must practice unprotected sex to get pregnant. There are also ethical dilemmas involved in the decision to practice safer sex. These include disclosure of HIV status and decisions about when to initiate and modify safer sexual behavior in relationships.

In the United States, safer sex messages need to change to accommodate changes in the "face of AIDS." During the first wave of the epidemic, the insistence on using condoms for every penetrative sexual act was relatively authoritarian in approach. For some, mandates about practicing safer sex and views that "no one is monogamous" and "you are sleeping with everyone your partner has slept with" evoked rebellion, denial, and shame in the targeted groups. This dogmatic approach resulted in imperfect and inconsistent safer sex practices for some people (Johnston 1995; Dowsett 1999).

Safer sex messages since the mid-1990s are changing. The importance of practicing safer sex and engaging in less-risky behaviors remain. However, there is a shift away from an authoritarian approach toward a **harm-reduction model**, adapted from safer needle usage and drug rehabilitation programs. This new model of safer sex emphasizes awareness, conscious decision making, and acceptance of responsibility for sexual risks and whatever safer sex practices are used (McIlvenna and Taylor 1999).

5.7

Barebacking is a sexual practice engaged in by some MSM where a conscious decision is made not to use condoms, generally during anal sex. Barebacking involves negotiated risk, responsibility for the behavior, and a heightened awareness of what the sexual partners are doing and of the increased eroticism (Bolton 2000; Halkitis 2003; Dawson et al. 2005).

Abstinence-only messages persist, however. Abstinence is a guaranteed method of not contracting or transmitting an STD or HIV and is very effective. For those couples who want to be abstinent before having an HIV test or who believe in being sexually active only after marriage, it is also effective in preventing HIV and other STDs. Abstinence is a reasonable, safe, healthy choice for some individuals and couples.

It is a personal decision and sexual choice, heavily influenced by one's cultural and religious background. However, research indicates that it is not the most effective applied behavioral intervention to prevent HIV transmission or unplanned pregnancies. Many anthropologists, medical groups, and other organizations have criticized federal support of abstinence-only programs, particularly those that use scare tactics or provide inaccurate and misleading information about the efficacy of condoms to prevent HIV (Pastore et al. 2001; Waxman 2006; Bolton 1992; Feldman 2003a, 2003b; Hammar 2004; Hogle et al. 2002; McGrath et al. 1993; SIECUS 2005; www.agi-usa.org; Underhill et al. 2007).

Sex and HIV/AIDS outside the United States

Sub-Saharan Africa

Outside the United States, HIV/AIDS poses serious threats to the continuation of some groups (UNAIDS 2002a; Barnett and Whiteside 2002). With 70–80 percent of the world's AIDS cases in sub-Saharan Africa and a male to female ratio there of 1:1.5–2.1, the impact of this disease is different in this area than in industrialized societies (Barnett and Whiteside 2002; Stine 1997; UNAIDS 2006). Although HIV is primarily a sexually transmitted infection, the culture-specific behaviors and values defining sexuality vary widely. In sub-Saharan Africa, as with ethnic groups in the United States, poverty is a cofactor in the risk of infection and the course of the disease (Basu, Mate, and Farmer 2000; Stine 1997; Schneider and Stoller 1995).

Poverty influences safer sex practices and access to prevention, testing, and treatment. Poverty creates a thriving subculture of female prostitution along trade routes and in cities in Africa (Marck 1999; Outwater 1996; Orubuloye et al. 1994; White 1990; Schoepf 2003b). As discussed previously, traditional sexual behaviors are varied and extend over the life cycle. They can include male and female circumcision; dry sex, in which women use vaginal astringents to dry the vagina to make intercourse tighter; polygyny; **sexual cleansings of widows**, whereby widows have ritual symbolic or real intercourse with their dead husband's male relatives; the levirate; and various premarital behaviors that have been influenced by Christianity, including the placing of value on abstinence and monogamy (Orubuloye et al. 1994; www.aarg.org 2003; Obermeyer 2003; Malungo 1999; Dilger 2007; Mufune 2003). Christianity encourages female chastity and monogamy. Double standards of sexual behavior between men and women exist, because men are culturally allowed to have multiple sexual partners whereas women are encouraged to be monogamous (LeClerc-Madlala 2001; Varga 1999). Traditionally in the levirate, women brought their wealth to the new marriage and controlled the distribution of it. With culture change, women have lost control of the decision making and their wealth in some situations, putting them at further sexual and financial risk for HIV (Orubuloye et al. 1994; Gender-AIDSeForum 2003; McGrath et al. 1993; Schoepf 2003b, 2004).

The culture changes that have occurred in sub-Saharan Africa present structural cofactors for HIV infection. Men continue to have multiple sexual partners, and the responsibility for practicing safer sex is largely made the women's, as it is in industrialized societies. Women have lost much of their economic base and, with that, decision-making power. In much of sub-Saharan Africa, men make the sexual and economic decisions for the kin group (Outwater 1996; Varga 1999; McGrath et al. 1993; Malungo 1999; UNAIDS 2006). With the loss of economic autonomy and increasing poverty, many women engage in prostitution and survival sex. Women's abilities to negotiate safer sex are limited (Machekano et al. 2000; Varga 1999).

In addition, traditional prostitution practices changed in some parts of Africa, such as Nairobi, Kenya, with European contact (White 1990). Prior to colonization, prostitutes in Nairobi operated and controlled the assets of comfort houses to men traveling on the trade routes. Women kept the money they earned, often using it to support the kin group in rural areas. Comfort houses provided men with food, shelter, companionship, and negotiated sex (White 1990). After colonization and the impact of World War II, women lost control of the comfort houses, violence against them increased, and street prostitution began to flourish with the adoption of Euro-American views of sexuality (White 1990). European concepts of women, sexuality, and prostitution became more firmly established. Loss of economic and political power increased women's susceptibility to sexual exploitation and sexually transmitted infections, including HIV.

Overall states of health—including other sexually transmitted infections (STIs), nutrition, and genital sores—are cofactors in HIV infection and impair the immune system. Other STIs and genital sores are pathways for HIV. These health problems are common in sub-Saharan Africa (Barnett and Whiteside 2002; UNAIDS 2002a). The use of spermicidal condoms, once recommended as part of safer sex and for prostitutes in Africa, is no longer recommended. The nonoxynol-9 used in the spermicide can irritate vaginal mucosa, increasing the risk for HIV. As of 2003, the CDC no longer recommends the use of spermicidal condoms to prevent HIV (CDC 2003b).

Male and female circumcision are controversial variables in HIV infection. **Male circumcision (MC)** is common in West Africa and less common in East Africa. HIV infection is less common among circumcised males and their partners in West Africa. This leads many researchers to believe that circumcising males in Africa could be one way to reduce female-to-male HIV transmission (and ultimately male-to-female transmission). The CDC, WHO, and UNAIDS have all endorsed MC as *one* preventive strategy in reducing HIV transmission (Orubuloye et al. 1994; Halperin and Bailey 1999; Halperin and Williams 2001; USAID/AIDS-Mark 2003; Bailey, Neema, and Othieno 1999, 2001; Halperin, Steiner et al. 2004; WHO 2007).

However, while many researchers support male circumcision to reduce female-to-male transmission of HIV, others point to the problems involved in changing this practice; the erroneous belief that male circumcision alone without also practicing safer sex would prevent HIV transmission; and that MSM in the United States, most of whom were circumcised, constituted the greatest number of people with HIV/AIDS in the first two waves of the epidemic (www.aarg.org; Bailey, Neema, and Othieno 1999; Weiss et al. 2000; Cold and Taylor 1999; de Vincenzi and Mertens 1994; Inungu et al. 2005; Gray 2003). Nor does MC appear to protect women from STIs, a cofactor for the sexual transmission of the virus (Holmes and Miller 2007: abstract). In addition, anthropologist Peter Aggleton discusses how MC has been used for several thousand years to differentiate and distinguish groups from each other politically, socioeconomically, and religiously. He believes that any decision to implement wide-scale male circumcision to prevent female-to-male transmission of HIV in sub-Saharan Africa needs to examine and incorporate these aspects of circumcision as part of the process (Aggleton 2007: 18, 20).

5.8

While current research indicates a 70 percent reduction of female-to-male transmission of HIV among circumcised males in East and South Africa over a short period of time, there are concerns about the long-term efficacy and wisdom of this approach to reducing HIV incidence (Inungu et al. 2005; Williams et al. 2006). One of the primary concerns is that circumcised men will either stop using condoms or refuse to use condoms. Condoms are 80 to 90 percent effective in preventing HIV transmission in real usage terms, as opposed to theoretical or perfect usage terms (UNAIDS 2006; Feldman 2003a). Promoting condom usage remains a noninvasive primary prevention tool.

The AIDS and Anthropology Research Group (AARG) has been conducting a spirited debate about the role of male circumcision in reducing HIV transmission since early 2003. That debate can be found on their Web site: www.aarg.org.

The role of female circumcision in HIV infection is unclear. Female circumcision of varying degrees of severity—from removal of the prepuce, or clitoral hood, to infibulation (removal of the clitoris and labia minora, scraping, and then closing the labia majora)—is common among a number of Islamic groups in Africa (Lightfoot-Klein 1989; Obermeyer 2003). This practice occurs for a number of reasons, including marriage eligibility (since only circumcised women can be married), preservation of chastity, cultural perceptions of beauty and hygiene, and as a source of status and economics for the women who perform the circumcisions (Lightfoot-Klein 1989). Controversial and banned by the World Health Organization (WHO) in the 1980s, the practice continues and is made more dangerous by the circumcisions being performed "underground" with dirty equipment and lack of recourse if infections, trauma, or other complications develop (Lightfoot-Klein 1989). The concerns regarding HIV transmission include transmitting the virus during the procedures as well as women becoming infected from the procedure and transmitting HIV to their sexual partners. The latter is probably less of a risk than the former, given that female-to-male transmission in p-v intercourse is less efficient (Padian et al. 1991).

5.9

Virginity testing has been initiated among the KwaZulu-Natal in South Africa as a way to prevent HIV. Virginity testing of girls from six years old to marriageable age is supported by mothers and grandmothers to prevent and curb "sexual licentiousness." External genital exams and inspections are publicly performed by village women, who use the same latex glove for each exam and grade the girls on their degree of virginity. Girls who "pass" are cheered and given a certificate; girls who "fail" are publicly shamed. Anthropologist Suzanne LeClerc-Madlala notes that this practice, while not traditional to the group in its present form, upholds deeply held patriarchal views about women's worth and sexuality among the Zulu. LeClerc-Madlala discusses the potential health risks, the false sense of security that derives from passing the exam, the double standards about sex, and the culturally structured beliefs about female sexuality that exist among this group. Boys are not tested since "they wouldn't come anyway" and "are like animals; they can't control themselves" (LeClerc-Madlala 2001: 547). These practices can foster the spread of HIV because they reinforce larger views about disease, blame, and women as vectors of transmission.

In proposing international and indigenous responses to HIV intervention, local customs, behaviors, and beliefs need to be known and programs developed that work within these beliefs. Uganda is an example of how holistic indigenous programs can help to reduce HIV infection. Uganda's response to its epidemic includes

Early recognition and acknowledgment in the 1980s of the presence of the virus in Uganda's population.

A president, Yoweri Kaguta Museveni, who openly addressed the problem.

The establishment of **The AIDS Support Organization (TASO)**. TASO is an HIV/AIDS organization that provides treatment and services to those infected and their families. It works with local groups to educate and to support safer sex practices that include condom usage, reduction of the number of sexual partners, encouragement of monogamy, and provision of HIV testing. TASO addresses both the disease and illness aspects of HIV/AIDS (www.tasouganda.org).

An ABC model of safer sex. Abstinence (A) is encouraged for pre- and early adolescents. It entails delayed onset of penetrative sex. Be faithful (B) is encouraged for married couples. Condoms (C) are available for those who have multiple sex partners, concurrently or serially. It is not an abstinence-only approach, although recently A has been emphasized, with resulting criticism of this move (see chapter 8).

Improved education for girls and economic opportunities for women that contribute to their independence and economic security.

Development of social networks to spread information and encourage safer sex practices.

A die-off rate from AIDS that decreases the prevalence rate.

These efforts drastically reduced the prevalence of AIDS in Uganda from about 25 percent to 6–8 percent (UNAIDS 2002a, 2006). Controversy exists over which of these strategies had the most impact on reducing Uganda's AIDS prevalence (Feldman 2003a; Schoepf 2003b, 2004; Green 2003; Hogle et al. 2002; Low-Beer and Stoneburner 2002). Because there is some evidence that Uganda's AIDS cases are increasing and that abstinence-only policies are being promoted by the government to achieve funding from the United States, there is debate concerning whether reduced numbers of partners, an early die-off rate, or increased use of condoms had significant relevance to preventing an upsurge in the country's epidemic (Kaiser Daily HIV/AIDS Report 2006e, 2006f; see chapter 8).

Iran, Zambia, Sierra Leone, and Senegal have either shown decreases in the incidence and prevalence of HIV/AIDS or have kept their rates of HIV/AIDS relatively low (UNAIDS 2006; Low-Beer and Stoneburner 2003; Allam 2006; Larsen 2003). Although these societies are very different from each other, there are some common factors that contribute to their successes. In addition to strategies similar to those that contributed to Uganda's reduced prevalence rate, these countries' efforts stemmed initially, at least, from grassroots organizations. In Senegal, for example, sex workers formed support groups that encouraged condom use with clients (Low-Beer and Stoneburner 2003; Renaud 1997). Iran provides clean needles for its prison population and encourages safer sex as part of its contraceptive planning services (Allam 2006; Larsen 2003). A comprehensive, culturally sensitive, and multifaceted approach can reduce the impact of HIV/AIDS in communities.

Brazil, India, and Thailand

Brazil, India, and Thailand have long histories of culturally recognized multiple genders and broader definitions of gender than exist in the United States (Inciardi et al. 2001; Parker and Aggleton 1999; Nanda 2000). With culture contact and change, people in these roles have also lost status and a recognized place in society.

BRAZIL

Until recently, Brazil had one of the highest rates of HIV/AIDS in Latin America. Prevention and treatment efforts over the past few years are helping to slow the incidence of HIV/AIDS in Brazil (UNAIDS 2002a; Okie 2006). For example, more than 80 percent of Brazil's HIV+ population has access to ARVs (Okie 2006). Brazil also refused to accede to pressure from the United States to stigmatize organizations that provided services to sex workers (Ditmore 2005). In Brazil, HIV is largely attributable to unprotected sex both between men and between men and women.

Brazilian culture is a mix of Portuguese, African, and indigenous populations. Officially a Catholic, Latino society, Brazil incorporates Catholic values about women's sexuality and machismo values about men, gender, orientation, and sexual practices (Parker and Aggleton 1999; Parker, Barbosa, and Aggleton 2000). Heterosexuality is the norm and expected, with gender-appropriate roles and sexual behavior valued. Nevertheless, Brazil also openly recognizes transvestite and transgendered communities (Aggleton 1994; Parker and Aggleton 1999; Inciardi et al. 2001).

Female virginity is valued, and overt female sexuality is discouraged in Latino Brazil. Abstinence is the only form of birth control sanctioned by the Catholic Church. For heterosexual Brazilians who engage in premarital sex as well as for married couples in Brazil, anal sex is an acceptable sexual behavior (Halperin 1998, 1999). Unprotected anal sex preserves virginity and chastity, reinforces gender roles, and prevents pregnancy. Condoms, used with prostitutes, do not need to be used with penile anal sex to prevent pregnancies in one's girlfriend or wife. This behavior and value system increases the risk for HIV infection and other sexually transmitted diseases, particularly if males engage in anal sex with other males (Klein-Alonso 1996).

Brazilian culture also permits socially defined alternative gender roles. This is particularly evident during *Carnaval*, the festival immediately preceding Lent. *Carnaval* is a time of revelry and the inversion of traditional gender roles. Flouting norms about sexuality and modesty occurs during this time. Brazil also has a large transvestite (*transvesti*) population, men who dress in women's clothes and may engage in prostitution. A part of the culture, they can also be stigmatized, and as a stigmatized group, they engage in risky sexual behavior.

Brazilian men are encouraged to have many sexual partners. As discussed previously, as long as they are the inserter in sex regardless of the gender of their sexual partners, they retain their male status, masculinity, and heterosexuality. They are *hombre hombre*—a "man's man." Men who engage in oral, anal, and vaginal sex also achieve high sexual status as having "done it all" (Halperin 1998, 1999).

As it did in Africa, the Catholic Church influenced Latin American sexuality. The church's influence on proscribing birth control other than abstinence and on prohibiting nonmarital penile-vaginal intercourse and its symbolic portrayals of women as either virtuous, nurturing mothers or tempting, sexual wives are considerable (Parker, Barbosa, and Aggleton 2000; Miguez-Burbano et al. 2002). Violating church doctrine constitutes sin, possible condemnation to hell for unconfessed and unrepented sins, and shame on one's kin group if transgressions become known. This belief system may lead to riskier sexual behavior to maintain beliefs and norms that penile-anal sex between men and women prevents pregnancy or preserves chastity. Men who have sex with men in both Mexico and Brazil retain their masculinity, maleness, and heterosexuality as long as they are the inserters. There is thus no perceived need to use condoms for penetrative sex with either a man or a woman.

Over the past several years, Brazil, aware of its increasing HIV/AIDS incidence rate, began educational and treatment programs for its Portuguese population (Andrade et al. 2001; d'Adesky 2002b). These programs use a variety of venues such as the media, clubs, and small groups to educate and reinforce the value of safer sex within established cultural norms. Their generic antiretroviral drug treatment program is able to provide HIV-infected people with drugs and slow down the progression of AIDS. It is considered by some to be a model of such efforts for nonindustrialized societies (d'Adesky 2002b; Okie 2006). Knowing, respecting, and incorporating cultural definitions of gender and orientation are crucial in developing safer sex programs (Reilly and Woo 2001; Carrier 2001; Dowsett 1999; Bolton 1994).

INDIA

India traditionally recognized the existence of multiple genders. Three of the most common are male, female, and *hijras*. *Hijras* are biological males who are castrated and adopt a cultural gender identity that is neither male nor female (Nanda 2000). This identity took on spiritual connotations in Hindu India prior to colonization. *Hijras* held sacred places in indigenous Indian culture. Often they were seers and prophets, called upon during propitious events such as births and weddings to make prophecies about the lives of the newborn or newly married couples. With culture change and Westernization, *hijras* still exist. But their status has fallen, and currently they often survive as street prostitutes (Nanda 2000).

THAILAND

Indigenously, Thailand has a rich and varied sexual culture. Multiple gender roles exist in Thailand, and female prostitution is a cultural norm as a rite of passage for Thai men (Seabrook 2001; Sittitrai et al. 1991; Phanuphak and Serwadda 1998; Nanda 2000). Prostitution was a part of Thailand's economic structure. In traditional Thai culture, prostitution provided peasant women with a source of income and was an introduction into manhood for village men. As a traditional practice, it differs from much of the urban prostitution in Thailand that developed in the 1980s as part of the sex tourism trade (Beyrer 1998; Seabrook 2001; Bond et al. 1996; Lyttleton 2000).

With the impact of Euro-American contact and globalization, Thai sex practices and gender role interpretations changed. Traditional roles and practices, particularly those involved in sex tourism, have become part of economic survival and in some cases are stigmatized (Seabrook 2001; Nanda 2000). Moving prostitution to urban areas meant not only that women left their villages but also that the sexual behaviors expected of these women could differ from traditional practices, because the clients are primarily non-Thai. It also meant that women who moved to the cities worked primarily in brothels, where brothel owners made decisions about sex practices, the number of clients, and who was seen.

Sex tourism generally involves middle- and upper-middle-class businessmen from Europe, North America, and Japan who book sex tours to Thailand. These trips are expensive, averaging US$10,000–15,000 (Seabrook 2001). The men arrange to have sex with male and female prostitutes, who usually work in brothels. The brothel owners can arrange ahead of time the terms for the sexual behavior of the prostitutes, including whether or not condoms are used. Although there is an active sex workers' rights organization in Thailand, many women working in the brothels have little role in decision making about their hours, working conditions, the number of clients they see, or safer sex practices. Often, clients will pay more not to use a condom or to have sex with a virgin, believing that that will protect them from HIV and other STDs. This can lead to the sexual exploitation of children (Beyrer 1998; Bond et al. 1996).

Rural, impoverished families in Thailand will accept payment for their children to be sent to the cities to work. Families believe that their children will receive an education and employment and will be able to help support the extended kin group in the countryside. These payments may mean the difference between survival and starvation (Beyrer 1998; Bond et al. 1996). Frequently, the children do not return to their villages, do not have contact with their families, and end up working in sex-tourism brothels in the cities (Beyrer 1998; Seabrook 2001).

From the late 1980s to the mid-1990s, activist groups in Thailand, including sex workers' rights groups, organized to protest the working conditions in these brothels. Protests addressed the lack of safer sex practices and the use of child prostitutes to avoid practicing safer sex. Widespread educational and reform efforts in Thailand reduced the incidence of HIV/AIDS (Seabrook 2001; Ninth International Conference on AIDS 1993; Bhutani and Khanna 2001; Bond et al. 1996; Low-Beer and Stoneburner 2003).

What are the larger sociocultural factors that influence sex tourism in Thailand? The tourists have economic resources to spend, and they perceive Asian women to be passive, nurturing, and willing to please and dote on a man. Some of these tourists expect emotional attachment and involvement from the women. They believe Thai and other Asian women to be able to take care of men's sexual and daily needs (Seabrook 2001; Whelehan 2001a). The sex tourists do not perceive that this is work for the women they hire. Sex tourists' use of brothels that do not require safer sex and that support sexual behavior outside of missionary-style, man-on-top, penile-vaginal intercourse allows men to fulfill their fantasies, reinforces their views of Asian women, and absolves them of responsibility for their behavior (Seabrook 2001). Sex tourism also allows these men to engage in behavior that is probably illegal or stigmatized in their home countries:

sex with minors, sex with male or female prostitutes, and same-sex sex (Seabrook 2001).

For Thai culture, sex tourism generates much-needed income (Beyrer 1998). Thai definitions of what constitutes childhood are not necessarily the same as Euro-American concepts. Families who sell their daughters do this out of economic need and survival. With relatively little political authority locally, nationally, and internationally, Thai villagers have little recourse in this situation. Their choices are practical: to starve and possibly break up the kin group, or to send their children to the city for a "better life." As an activist Thai prostitute who emigrated to the United States told me, "Until you have seen family members thrown to sharks off lifeboats [to prevent the overcrowded lifeboat from capsizing] trying to escape political regimes, you have no right to judge us" (Whelehan 2001a: 84).

The general ethnocentric misperception of Thai and Asian women as passive and docile also exists. As the same Thai activist said, "Nice is not passive. Passive is not submissive" (Whelehan 2001a: 87). Thai women working in brothels or other venues serving sex tourists interpret their behavior differently than do the tourists. For them, this is work, and work that pays more with overall better working conditions than other forms of employment given their education and skills (Seabrook 2001). These women are playing out a role. Most of them are neither emotionally attached to nor interested in tourists as either partners or protectors. Most of their income is spent on supporting their own nuclear and extended families. They have few illusions about their work or their clients (Seabrook 2001; Whelehan 2001a).

The ethnocentrism, sexism, and racism underlying the sex tourists' beliefs and expectations are rampant. Perceptions of Asian women as passive and submissive to men reinforce fantasies and Euro-American concepts of gender, men, women, and sex. It provides a contrast to the sex tourists' perceptions of Euro-American women as more independent, more assertive, and less nurturing. Sex tourists can attribute their behavior to cultural differences and promotion of the Thai economy and thereby rationalize their behavior (Seabrook 2001). They can deny that their behavior contributes to the risk of contracting HIV infection from prostitutes or infecting their partners at home by the fees paid to have sex with virgins or "clean" prostitutes (Ninth International Conference on AIDS 1993). Both international sex workers' rights organizations (International Committee for Prostitutes' Rights 1987) and human rights groups such as Amnesty International and Gender AIDS speak out against exploitation and coercion, and for the support of consensual, adult sex that protects against HIV/STI transmission and unwanted pregnancy (Bond et al. 1996). Activist work includes advocating for safer working conditions, providing educational and economic opportunities for women, and developing safer sex programs to encourage men to use condoms.

Sexual behavior and beliefs constitute some of the most deeply structured views about gender, sexuality, men, and women that exist in a society. Cultural assumptions about these topics need to be known, examined, and understood before HIV intervention programs are implemented. Program acceptance and implementation increase with an awareness and avoidance of ethnocentrism and bias, and with sensitivity to the cofactors involved in the sexual transmission of HIV. Societies are not static; they exist in a state of flux. In both the United States and elsewhere, there are behaviors and beliefs that both impede and support safer sex. The impact of culture change, heterogeneity within groups, and the influence of religious, political, and economic factors in sexual behavior are important in preventing the sexual transmission of HIV.

Focusing on individual sexual behavior change, particularly from an authoritarian and judgmental perspective without attending to community and larger societal political, economic, and cultural factors, will have limited long-term effect in reducing risk and changing behavior. Those groups and societies that have reduced the incidence and prevalence of HIV/AIDS in their communities have done so largely from an emic, relativistic, and interdisciplinary approach to sexuality.

SUMMARY

Worldwide, 80 percent of HIV is transmitted sexually.

Factors that promote safer sex practices include awareness of a culture's beliefs and behaviors, avoidance of ethnocentrism, and use of a group's symbolic system and indigenous beliefs to encourage safer sex.

Economic, social, and political structures affect the ability to practice safer sex.

Gender inequality affects the ability to practice safer sex.

Factors that impede safer sex practices include a one-standard-fits-all approach, programs that do not incorporate a culture's beliefs and values, judgmental attitudes, and biases that program implementers bring with them.

Thought Questions

What variables are involved in providing sex and HIV education? How do they affect decisions to practice safer sex in the United States and cross-culturally?

What approaches increase the chances that safer sex will be adopted and practiced within a group and among individuals?

What are the ethical problems with not providing comprehensive sex education to people?

Resources

Articles

Adimora, Adaora A., and Victor J. Schoenbach. "Social Context, Sexual Networks, and Racial Disparities in Rates of Sexually Transmitted Infections." *Journal of Infectious Diseases* 191 (2005): S115–S122.

Barker, Judith C., Robynn S. Battle, Gayle L. Cummings, and Katherine N. Bancroft. "Condoms and Consequences: HIV/AIDS Education and African-American Women." *Human Organization* 57, no. 3 (1998): 273–83.

Dilger, Hanjorg. "Healing the Wound of Modernity: Salvations, Community and Care in a Neo-Pentecostal Church in Dar Es Salaam, Tanzania." *Journal of Religion in Africa* 37, no. 1 (February 2007): 59–83.

Holmes, King, and William C. Miller. "Circumcision Status Does Not Affect Women's STI Risk." Paper presented at the 17th Meeting of the International Society for Sexually Transmitted Diseases Research, July 30, 2007. Abstract 449.

Howell, Amy. "UC Studies HIV Patients: Religious Support, Alienation Scrutinized." *Enquirer,* Friday, August 10, 2007.

Mufune, Pemplani. "Changing Patterns of Sexuality in Northern Namibia: Implications for the Transmission of HIV/AIDS." *Culture, Health, and Sexuality* 5, no. 5 (September 2003): 425–38.

Peterson, John L., Susan Folkman, and Roger Bakeman. "Stress, Coping, HIV Status, Psycho-social Resources, and Depressive Mood in African-American Gay, Bisexual, and Heterosexual Men." *American Journal of Community Psychology* 24, no. 4 (1996): 461–87.

Pfeiffer, James. "Condom Social Marketing, Pentecostalism, and Structural Adjustment in Mozambique: A Clash of AIDS Prevention Messages." *Medical Anthropology Quarterly* 18, no. 1 (2004): 77–103.

Svensson, Jonas. "HIV/AIDS and Islamic Religious Education in Kisumu, Kenya." *International Journal of Qualitative Studies on Health and Well Being* 2, no. 3 (2007): 179–92.

Torres, M. I., S. Tuthill, S. Lyon-Callo, C. M. Hernandez, and P. Epkind. "Focused Female Condom Education and Trial: Comparison of Young African-American and

Puerto Rican Women's Assessments." *International Quarterly of Community Health Education* 18, no. 1 (1999): 49–68.

Walters, Karina L., and Jane M. Simoni. "Trauma and HIV Risk among Urban Gay/Bisexual/Two Spirit American Indian Men: Research Findings and Decolonizing Practice Strategies." National HIV Prevention Conference, June 12–15, 2005. Abstract #M2–D 1402, pp. 1–2.

———. "HIV Prevention Issues among American Indian and Alaska Native 'Two Spirits': The Linkage." *Newsletter of the Behavioral and Social Science Volunteer Program* (Summer 2004): 1, 3.

Whitehead, Tony. "Urban Low-Income African-American Men, HIV/AIDS, and Gender Identity." *Medical Anthropology Quarterly*, n.s., 11, no. 4 (December 1997): 411–47.

Books

Adams, Vincanne, and Stacy Pigg, eds. *Sex in Development: Science, Sexuality, and Morality in Global Perspective.* Durham, N.C.: Duke University Press, 2005.

Jacobs, Sue-Ellen, Sabine Lang, and Wesley Thomas, eds. *Two Spirit People: Native American Gender Identity, Sexuality, and Spirituality.* Urbana: University of Illinois Press.

Parker, Robert, and Peter Aggleton, eds. *Culture, Society and Sexuality: A Reader.* London: UCL Press, 1997.

Renaud, Michelle Lewis. *Women at the Crossroads: A Prostitute Community's Response to AIDS in Urban Senegal.* Amsterdam: Gordon and Breach Publishers, 1997.

Roscoe, Will, ed. *Living the Spirit—Gay Indians Tell Their Own Stories: A Gay American Indian Anthology.* New York: St. Martin's Press, 1988.

Seabrook, J. *Travels in the Skin Trade: Tourism and the Sex Industry.* 2nd ed. Sterling, Va.: Pluto Press, 2001.

Videos

Kleiman, V. 1992. *My Body's My Business.* Berkeley, Calif.: Cultural Resource and Communication.

Web Sites

AIDS and Anthropology Research Group: "AIDS/Side Effects." http://www.puffin.creighton.edu/aarg.

BAYSWAN (a sex workers' rights group in the United States): http://www.bayswan.org.

Body, The: http://www.thebody.com.

Canadian Aboriginal AIDS Network. http://www.caan.ca, accessed August 2, 2007.

Eve's Garden: http://www.evesgarden.com.

Gay Men's Health Crisis: http://www.gmhc.com.

GaySex.com: http://www.gaysex.com.

Good Vibrations: http://www.goodvibrations.com.

Guttmacher Institute: http://www.guttmacherinstitute.com.

Kaiser Daily HIV/AIDS Report. "Lack of Sex Education in U.S. Increases Vulnerability to Sexual Assault, STIs, Former Surgeon General Elders Says." http://www.kaisernetwork.org/daily_reports/rep_index.cfm?DR_ID=46943, accessed August 17, 2007.

Planned Parenthood Federation of America: http://www.plannedparenthood.org.

Rasing, Thera. 2003. "HIV/AIDS and Sex Education among the Youth in Zambia: Towards Behavioural Change." http://www.ascleiden.n4pdf/paper09102003.pdf, accessed July 31, 2007.

SIECUS (Sex Information and Education Council of the United States): http://www.siecus.com.

SUNY-PAEG (Potsdam AIDS Education Group): http://www.potsdam.edu/content.php?contentID=E9CABAC13BFD227A43FF1BE205B2B184.

SWOP (Sex Workers Outreach Project—Australia): http://www.swop.org.au/.

Underhill, Kristen, Paul Montgomery, and Don Operario. "Sexual Abstinence-Only Programmes in High Income Countries: A Systematic Review." *British Medical Journal* (July 26, 2007). http://www.bmj.com/cgi/content/full/bmj39245.446586.BEv1, accessed August 14, 2007.

World Health Organization. "WHO and UNAIDS Announce Recommendations from Expert Consultations on Male Circumcision for HIV Prevention." http://www.who.int/hiv/mediacentre/news68/en/index.htm, accessed April 12, 2007.

6

Drugs and AIDS

CHAPTER HIGHLIGHTS INCLUDE

Definitions and categories of drugs

Discussions of drug usage as either a cofactor or a direct cause of HIV infection

Discussions of needle usage related to HIV infection in both medical and nonmedical settings

Discussions of blood-supply safety

Explorations of drug usage cross-culturally as a risk for HIV infection

---

Social justice means, above all, unflagging concern for those who have gained least from modern prosperity, education and democracy. Social justice takes seriously the rightful claims of all persons to life, health, dignity, and hope.

Philip Selznick (Buchanan et al. 2004)

The staggering inequities of the intertwined epidemics of AIDS and substance abuse borne by poor people and people of color are the moral wrongs we seek to address.

Buchanan, Shaw, Ford, and Singer (2004)

While HIV/AIDS is primarily a sexually transmitted disease globally, infection from drug/needle usage can be either a cofactor in or the primary means of contracting the virus (Beyrer 1998; Andrade et al. 2001; Marins et al. 2000). Drug/needle usage was the second major source of HIV infection in the United States, India, parts of Southeast Asia, and Brazil during the early days of the HIV epidemics in those regions (Marins et al. 2000; Brimlow and Ross 1998; Francis and Cargill 2001; CDC 2001b). At the beginning of the twenty-first century, it is the primary cause of infection in China, Russia, Vietnam, Puerto Rico, and Spain (Thuy et al. 2000; Choi et al. 2000; Somlai et al. 2002; Stimson et al. 1998; Stimson and Choopanya 1998; Colón et al. 2005; Gamella 1994; Roberts and Cohen 2006). As with sexuality, the conceptionalization and use of drugs are culturally contexted, being politically, economically, and symbolically structured and encompasses ethnicity and gender.

Generically, drugs are substances that alter body chemistry and physiology when taken into the body (Weil 1998). Altering body chemistry through either drugs or mental states is an ancient and culturally widespread practice (Weil 1998, 2004). Cultures determine and define what constitutes a drug, acceptable and unacceptable usage of drugs, the circumstances under which drugs are used, and the role of needles in drug use.

Drugs and the United States

Drug usage is common in the United States. Most people in the United States use a variety of drugs daily (Francis and Cargill 2001). There are several subjective, value-laden categories of drugs and drug usage in the United States, including prescription, over-the-counter (OTC), herbal, recreational, legal, and illegal drugs. Many of these categories overlap. For example, alcohol is legal and recreational; speed is illegal and recreational. We further categorize drugs as either "good" (as in prescription drugs) or "bad" (as in illegal recreational drugs). We may also categorize drugs as not drugs: caffeine, vitamin pills, and nicotine are drugs but generally are not perceived as such. "Drug and alcohol usage" is a common phrase in United States, obscuring the drug aspect of alcohol. "Good drugs" can include OTC drugs when used medicinally, and "bad drugs" can include legally purchased herbal drugs used medicinally but without a physician's supervision or FDA approval. This chapter explores the different contexts of drug and needle usage as they affect the risk of HIV transmission.

The debate over illegal recreational drug usage can be more emotional than scientific, as exemplified by the use of medical marijuana to ease pain, control nausea and vomiting, and stimulate the appetite for people with HIV/AIDS, cancer, or glaucoma. Despite endorsement of its value in treating some medical conditions by such groups as the Institute of Medicine and the American Medical Association, the politics surrounding medical marijuana keep it illegal (Institute of Medicine 2001; DesJarlais et al. 1998; Kane and Mason 2001; Buchanan et al. 2004).

Alternative and Complementary Drugs and Therapies

Alternative/complementary forms of health care, including the use of herbal drugs, are popular in the United States. Many of these alternative/complementary forms of healing, such as acupuncture and meditation, derive from ancient Chinese and Indian medical and drug philosophies, and their efficacy is currently under study by the National Institutes of Health (Weil 1998, 2004; Singer 2005; http://www.vitaminshoppe.com). Relative to HIV, they are primarily used to treat symptoms of HIV infection and side effects of HAART such as depression, nausea, and vomiting, or to stimulate the appetite.

Pharmaceutical companies fear loss of income if people use alternative/complementary therapies, and medical doctors can be ethnocentric toward health care other than biomedicine. However, there are legitimate concerns about the use of alternative therapies and drugs relative to HIV disease. The primary concern is the overall lack of regulation and standardization for herbal drugs, as well as the unknown effects they may have on HIV and the potential for deleterious drug interactions with HAART. Herbal drugs in particular receive a mixed reaction from the biomedical community, since some herbal drugs, such as St. John's wort, used to treat mild to moderate depression, can negatively impact the efficacy of HAART.

Recreational Drug Use and HIV

Recreational drug use and the availability of certain drugs generate a great deal of controversy in the United States. These drugs can either be legal, such as alcohol, or illegal, such as marijuana, cocaine, heroin, and illegal designer drugs such as methamphetamines (various forms of speed), Ecstasy, and crystal meth. Legal recreational drugs such as alcohol and nicotine are culturally accepted in many industrialized and nonindustrialized societies. Their manufacture, sale, and distribution may be governmentally regulated and may generate considerable income for governments, producers, and distributors (Francis and Cargill 2001; Singer 2005; Kane and Mason 2001; Waterston 1997).

In general, recreational drug usage can be a cofactor in HIV infection for several reasons. First, these drugs may impair the immune system if they are abused. Second, drugs such as alcohol and Ecstasy may affect decision making. The combination of drugs used also affects the risk for HIV infection. For example, using alcohol with other drugs such as heroin can have synergistic effects and increase the physiological effects of each drug's individual properties.

Alcohol is one of the most popular and widely used recreational drugs. The role of alcohol as a risk factor for HIV infection is controversial, and the evidence is contradictory (Bolton et al. 1992). Alcohol use may be a cofactor in HIV since it can impair the immune system and affect decision making. However, alcohol's specific role as a cofactor in HIV infection depends on the population studied. The strongest support for alcohol as impacting decision making about safer sex exists for late-adolescent heterosexuals and college students; it is less consistent for other groups (Hingson et al. 1990; Francis and Cargill 2001; Stall and Purcell 2000; Ross et al. 2001).

Injection Drug Use (IDU) and Needles

Much of the recreational illegal drug usage associated with HIV infection involves needles (see figure 6.1). This includes heroin, injectable cocaine, and some methamphetamines. Needle usage involves blood contact and exchange, making it a direct mode of transmission for HIV and a focal point of prevention efforts. Not only do these drugs share risks such as impairing the immune system and decision making, as discussed above, but their illegality and expense and the difficulty that users have in obtaining and maintaining a steady supply of them increase the risk of contracting HIV. These additional risk factors include the use of dirty needles, exchanging unprotected sex for drugs or drug money, and not knowing the purity of the drugs used.

Much of the research about HIV and drug usage involves needle-based drugs (Kwiatkowski and Booth 2000; Williams et al. 2001; Andrade et al. 2001; Anon. 2000b; Singer 2003a; Stimson et al. 1998; Stimson and Choopanya 1998). In the United States, about 25 percent of HIV/AIDS transmission is attributable to injection drug use (IDU) (CDC 2001b; UN-AIDS 2006; Clatts 1999). Since most injection drug usage in the United States is illegal (outside of that used in medical situations), stigma, violence, crime, and ostracism of injection drug users (IDUs) accompany this behavior (Francis and Cargill 2001; Brimlow and Ross 1998; Stimson, DesJarlais, and Ball 1998; Anon. 2000b; Goden et al. 2001). As an illustration of the cultural stigma surrounding IDU in the United States, about 80 percent of incarcerations are drug related, with many of these cases

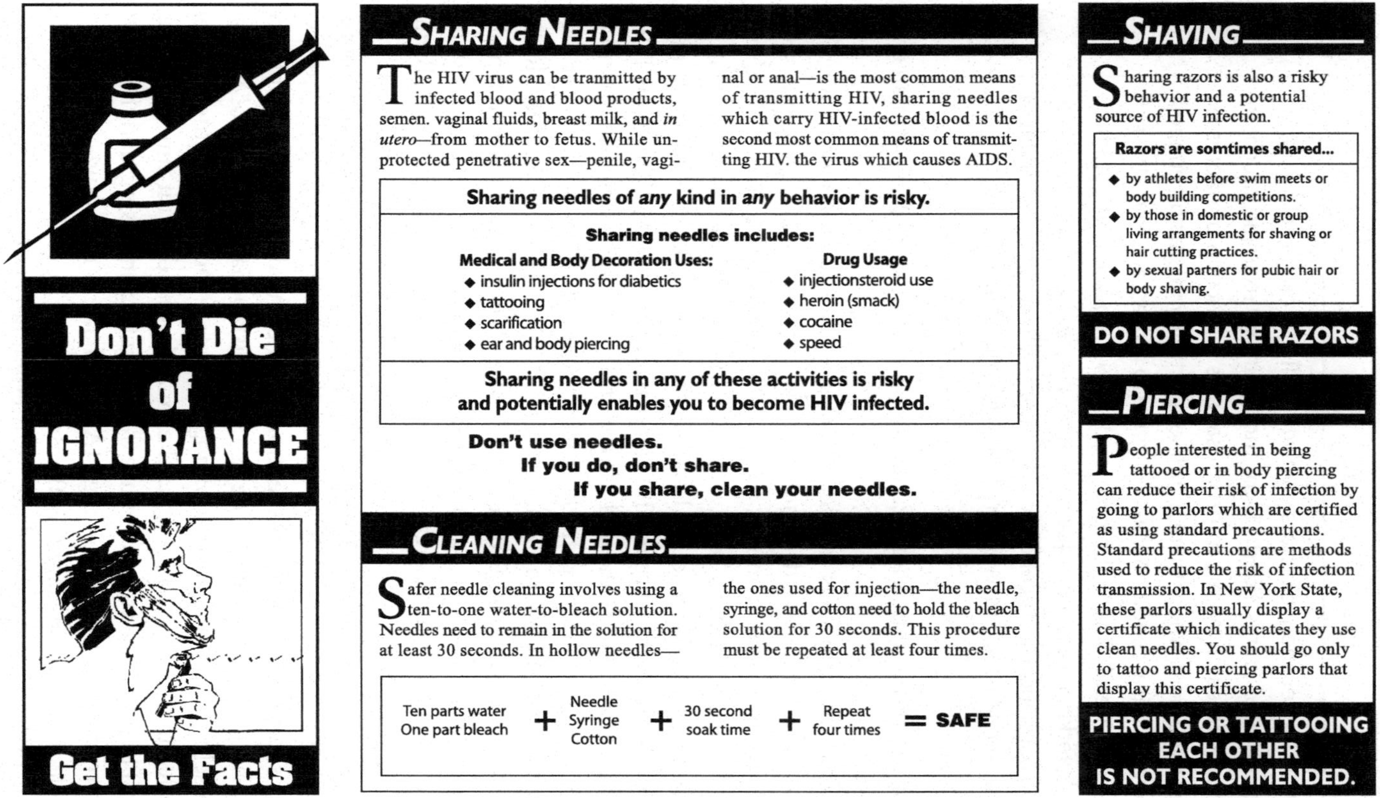

SHARING NEEDLES

The HIV virus can be transmitted by infected blood and blood products, semen, vaginal fluids, breast milk, and *in utero*—from mother to fetus. While unprotected penetrative sex—penile, vaginal or anal—is the most common means of transmitting HIV, sharing needles which carry HIV-infected blood is the second most common means of transmitting HIV: the virus which causes AIDS.

Sharing needles of *any* kind in *any* behavior is risky.

Sharing needles includes:

Medical and Body Decoration Uses:
- insulin injections for diabetics
- tattooing
- scarification
- ear and body piercing

Drug Usage
- injection-steroid use
- heroin (smack)
- cocaine
- speed

Sharing needles in any of these activities is risky and potentially enables you to become HIV infected.

Don't use needles.
If you do, don't share.
If you share, clean your needles.

CLEANING NEEDLES

Safer needle cleaning involves using a ten-to-one water-to-bleach solution. Needles need to remain in the solution for at least 30 seconds. In hollow needles— the ones used for injection—the needle, syringe, and cotton need to hold the bleach solution for 30 seconds. This procedure must be repeated at least four times.

| Ten parts water
One part bleach | + | Needle
Syringe
Cotton | + | 30 second
soak time | + | Repeat
four times | = | **SAFE** |

SHAVING

Sharing razors is also a risky behavior and a potential source of HIV infection.

Razors are somtimes shared...
- by athletes before swim meets or body building competitions.
- by those in domestic or group living arrangements for shaving or hair cutting practices.
- by sexual partners for pubic hair or body shaving.

DO NOT SHARE RAZORS

PIERCING

People interested in being tattooed or in body piercing can reduce their risk of infection by going to parlors which are certified as using standard precautions. Standard precautions are methods used to reduce the risk of infection transmission. In New York State, these parlors usually display a certificate which indicates they use clean needles. You should go only to tattoo and piercing parlors that display this certificate.

PIERCING OR TATTOOING EACH OTHER IS NOT RECOMMENDED.

Don't Die
of
IGNORANCE

Get the Facts

Figure 6.1. "Don't Die of Ignorance" pamphlet (SUNY-Potsdam AIDS Education Group/SUNY-PAEG).

6.1

The political and economic factors involved in illegal drug use are important. In the United States, Puerto Rico, and Spain, for example, much anthropological research points to drug usage as a function of depressed
economic conditions where there is little opportunity for gainful employment and of political conditions that continue to protect and favor the rich
over the poor. Merrill Singer also points out how drug scares about immigrant and working-class individuals and groups are used to maintain the
status quo of political and economic structures in the larger society (Singer
2005; Kane and Mason 2001; Waterston 1997; Needle et al. 1998).

---

involving IDU (Francis and Cargill 2001; Ross et al. 2001; Friedman et al.
1999).

Although numerous medical groups, such as the American Medical
Association, state that drug addiction is a disease and not a crime, most
IDUs are treated as criminals rather than people with a disease. IDUs are
one-third less likely to receive medical intervention and treatment for
their drug addiction and are less likely to receive HAART than are non-
IDUs (Francis and Cargill 2001; Friedman et al. 1999; Waterston 1997;
Carlson et al. 1996; Kane and Mason 2001). Health-care workers tend to
perceive IDUs more negatively and judgmentally than other people they
treat (Francis and Cargill 2001; Anon. 2000b; McCaul et al. 1996; Rothenberg 1996; Kass and Faden 1996b). Most IDUs—particularly if female,
poor, African American or Latino—do not receive drug treatment and rehabilitation but instead are incarcerated (Francis and Cargill 2001; Brimlow and Ross 1998; Anon. 2000b; Acuff 1996; Waterston 1997).

The stigma, illegality, censure, and lack of adequate treatment and rehabilitation services for IDUs increase the risk of contracting HIV by creating shame, secrecy, and deception around the drug usage. People are
less willing to get tested, since assessing risk behavior is part of pretest
counseling. They may be less willing to disclose their HIV status to other
needle-sharing or sex partners. They may have a difficult time accessing
help if they want to stop or reduce their injecting and using; and they have
a more difficult time obtaining HAART than do non-drug-using HIV+
people (Francis and Cargill 2001; Brimlow and Ross 1998; Anon. 2000b;
Acuff 1996; Strauss and Falkin 2001; Friedman et al. 1999; Singer 2005;
Needle et al. 1998; Rhodes and Quirk 1998).

HIV infection from IDU occurs within a sociopolitical and economic setting in the United States. A double standard exists toward drug users here, even within the subcategory of IDUs. Those IDUs who are poor, female, and from ethnic minorities receive a different cultural response to their drug usage than do those who are middle class and Anglo, regardless of sex. Middle-class drug users are more likely to find drug treatment and rehabilitation programs, rarely have their children taken from them, and seldom lose their employment and economic base. They are more likely to be accepted back into their peer group upon completion of a drug treatment program as well (Schneider and Stoller 1995; Brimlow and Ross 1998; Kane and Mason 2001; Waterston 1997).

6.2

An ongoing conflation exists between women IDUs and prostitutes in many models of female drug usage. This etic perspective tends to be punitive, inaccurate from an emic perspective, and counterproductive to changing behavior (Waterston 1997; Kane and Mason 2001; Parker, Barbosa, and Aggleton, 2000).

Needle/syringe exchange programs (N/SEPs) and prevention and intervention efforts for IDUs in the United States are controversial. This includes programs for female IDUs as well as for incarcerated and non-incarcerated populations (Institute of Medicine 2001; Anon. 2000b; McCaul et al. 1996; Goden et al. 2001; Buchanan et al. 2004). IDU intervention efforts can share characteristics of other programs but also have distinct differences because IDU is illegal. Both kinds of programs require peer-based, nonjudgmental, grassroots efforts to increase the chances of success (DesJarlais et al. 1998; Clatts and Sotheran 2000; Andrade et al. 2001). Bringing intervention efforts to the neighborhoods, shooting galleries, and hangouts where IDUs live and meet works much better than expecting IDUs to come to an outside locale (Clatts and Sotheran 2000; Carlson et al. 1996; Trotter et al. 1995). Consistent, patient, reliable efforts by the intervention community staffed with recovering IDUs increase the chances of success (Abeni et al. 1998; Ball 1998; Bastos et al. 1998; Cash 1996; Jenkins et al. 2002; Khoshnood and Stephens 1997).

Harm reduction models, initiated within the IDU community and adopted into safer sex messages, are more effective than all-or-nothing authoritative approaches for IDUs (DesJarlais 1998; Rhodes and Quirk 1998; Needle et al. 1998). Harm reduction involves reducing risks for HIV infection. For IDUs, this includes cleaning needles and syringes, reducing needle sharing, and N/SEPs (DesJarlais et al. 1998; Anon. 2000b). An example of harm reduction from a 1988 "Harm Reduction Card" produced by the San Francisco AIDS Foundation follows:

> If you use, don't share
> If you share, clean your needles

Harm reduction models recognize and accept the behavior, believe that behavior change can and will occur, and place responsibility on the user to modify his or her behavior. In general, harm-reduction programs tend to be well accepted in communities where they exist (Stoller 1998; Roberts and Cohen 2006).

N/SEPs tend to be among the most controversial forms of harm reduction models in the United States (Institute of Medicine 2001; Buchanan et al. 2004). They may operate in a legal limbo. Cities such as San Francisco, New York, and Miami have N/SEPs that are well established and operate without legal interference within fairly rigid boundaries of time and place. N/SEPs exchange used needles for clean needles. Needles are counted and recorded; it is a 1:1 exchange.

I worked at an established N/SEP in San Francisco in 1988 with my husband, a Peruvian outreach worker for Latino AIDS and the Mission Neighborhood Health Clinic. Needle exchanges occurred between 8 and 10 p.m. twice a week, on the same blocks in two different neighborhoods where there was a lot of injection drug use. Records were kept of the number of needles exchanged. Demographic information for age, gender (only in San Francisco is there a third category for "other"), and ethnicity was collected. During these two-hour exchanges, a human cross section of the city appeared. Homeless people, men, mink-wrapped women arriving in limousines, teenagers, TGs/TSs, and African Americans came to this particular neighborhood to exchange needles.

N/SEPs serve to reduce HIV transmission and encourage clean needle usage (Guydish et al. 2000; Friedman et al. 1999; Francis and Cargill 2001; Khoshnood and Stevens 1997). Then what is the controversy around these programs? National and local conservative political groups strongly oppose legal needle exchange programs. They believe that N/SEPs promote and accept IDU (Ostrow 2000; McGuire 2000; Buchanan et al. 2004).

> ## 6.3
>
> Despite empirical evidence that shows the efficacy of needle/syringe exchange programs, President George W. Bush does not support them nationally or as part of his international efforts to reduce HIV infection (Singer 2005; Parker, Easton, and Klein, 2000). Some conservative groups phrase needle/syringe exchange programs and harm-reduction models in moralistic terms. Buchanan and colleagues (2004) have offered suggestions about ways to counter these objections with moral arguments about compassion and the benefits to the individual and society that can derive from these intervention programs.

Although those programs in the epicenters of the epidemic operate with little legal interference, there are risks of arrest and being shut down. The Institute of Medicine and the American Medical Association support N/SEPS and harm-reduction programs (Institute of Medicine 2001).

Intervention programs with IDUs in the United States indicate greater success in harm reduction with cleaning and not sharing needles than with changing sexual behavior (Metsch et al. 2001; Williams et al. 2001; Anon. 2000b; Brimlow and Ross 1998; Friedman et al. 1999; Francis and Cargill 2001; Rhodes and Quirk 1998). Drug users have more difficulty in modifying their sexual behavior and practicing safer sex than in modifying their drug/needle-using behavior. Among IDUs in the United States, 87 percent of HIV infection occurs from unsafe sex rather than from sharing dirty needles or syringes (Friedman et al. 1999: 157).

There are several possible explanations for why harm-reduction programs work better to change drug and needle usage than to modify sexual behavior. First, people learn their values, attitudes, and behaviors about sexuality from birth. These are very deeply held and personal views that are overtly and covertly reinforced by family, peers, the community, and larger society (see chapter 5). The sense of one's self as a sexual being is holistic. It incorporates biological, cognitive, rational, emotional, and psychological dimensions. Drug-using behavior appears later in a person's life, after one's sexual identity is established. Drug-using behavior and the values supporting it are probably not as deep a part of someone's identity as is one's sense of who the person is sexually. One can modify drug-using behavior without questioning one's sense of gender, orientation, or what constitutes being sexual.

Second, needle-sharing relationships tend to be more goal-directed (with the goal being to obtain drugs) than are sexual relationships, which tend to be more comprehensive in the person's life. Studies involving the social networks of IDUs indicate a variety of interactions and relationships—or lack of them—among these groups of people (Trotter et al. 1995; Gamella 1994; Needle et al. 1998; Carlson et al. 1996).

Third, drug/needle-using intervention programs aim at harm reduction, a graduated model of reducing risk. Until very recently, safer sex messages tended to be absolutist and authoritarian: always use a condom; always practice safer sex. It may be easier to adhere to messages that support gradual changes in behavior than those that are more authoritarian and emphasize 100 percent adherence.

Fourth, culturally the United States accepts former drug users back into society at work and in the community more readily than it accepts people who behave sexually outside the norm. Former drug users can work in drug rehabilitation centers or engage in street outreach with society's blessings. One's sexual behavior is more private, more secret, and elicits different societal responses. As discussed in chapter 5, Lillian Rubin's research indicates that the private silence around sexuality makes it difficult for people to discuss their sexual needs and wants and to practice safer sex (1983).

Fifth, as a society, we are more willing to openly educate people about drug use than about sexuality. There is more societal acceptance for discussing drugs in public forums, in educational systems, and with government support than there is for the same kind and quality of sex education (Friedman et al. 1999; Anon. 2000b; SIECUS 2003).

Needles and Health-Care Settings

Injection drug use is merely one of several contexts in which needle usage occurs. People use needles for medical and legal recreational activities: for example, insulin-dependent diabetics inject insulin, and some HIV therapies require injections. Tattooing and piercing, popular forms of body adornment, involve needles or other piercing implements. In the United States, it is common for tattoo and piercing parlors to follow **universal precautions or standards**. These are practices adapted from medical environments that involve using gloves and new equipment as well as careful disposal of used needles to reduce the risk of HIV transmission through needles. Following these procedures entails minimal risk of contracting HIV or hepatitis when getting a tattoo or piercing. In both New York and California, for example, tattooers and piercers may prominently display cards that state that universal precautions are followed. It is medically sound to check out a tattoo or piercing parlor regarding their practices before getting a tattoo or piercing. Things to look for include cleanliness, waiting areas that are separate from where tattooing and piercing occur, and no rugs or carpets on the floor that may trap bacteria.

Given that HIV is blood-borne, the sharing of toothbrushes or razors is inadvisable. Although toothbrush and razor sharing may seem unlikely to many people in the United States, it can occur in residential living situations, on swim teams, or on camping trips. There has been one documented case of HIV transmission between brothers who shared a razor (Body 2003a). While there are no documented cases of HIV transmission through shared toothbrushes, the general recommendation is to only use your own toothbrush and razor (Body 2003a).

6.4

Malawi is a sub-Saharan African country beset with poverty and a relatively high prevalence of HIV. Dental hygiene is largely unavailable and dental health is poor, with many people having mouth and dental sores and infections. The director of the school of dentistry at the University of North Carolina at Chapel Hill has organized sending both dental students and toothbrushes to Malawi to help alleviate the situation. The peer educators in my Campus AIDS Education Group organized "Toothbrushes for Malawi" drives during the fall of 2005, and these efforts are ongoing. If you are interested in learning more about this project, please contact me at whelehpe@potsdam.edu.

A divisive and debated area of needle and blood transmission of HIV occurs in health-care settings. In the first wave of the epidemic, there were concerns about the safety of the blood supply, as hemophiliacs who needed Factor VIII, a blood product, to help clot their blood became infected (Shilts 1987; Leveton et al. 1995). There is also concern about HIV transmission during medical and dental procedures, either from an infected health-care worker to a patient or from an infected patient to a health-care worker. These concerns continue to the present, generate a lot of anxiety, and have resulted in at least one dramatic lawsuit and congressional action.

HIV infected blood contains high concentrations of the virus. Before an HIV antibody test became available in 1985, hemophiliacs and people receiving transfusions or organ transplants during surgery were at particular risk of infection. Transfusions and use of Factor VIII are efficient means of transmitting the virus. People infected with HIV in these ways quickly developed AIDS, and many of them died (Shilts 1987; CDC 2001b; Leveton et al. 1995). There were intense debates among health-care professionals, patients and their families, activists, and the Red Cross about the safety of the blood supply and the cost of testing blood for contamination (Shilts 1987; Leveton et al. 1995). The use of HIV infected blood in Paris in the 1980s brought the safety of the blood supply into an international context (Thomas 2001).

With the development of the HIV antibody test in 1985 and its widespread use since then, instances of HIV infected blood from transfusions, transplants, and use of Factor VIII are rare. Currently in the United States, the blood supply is considered statistically safe. This means that while it is possible to receive HIV infected blood through a blood transfusion, the probability of doing so is very low. Estimates range from 1/85,000 to 1/250,000 units of blood that are HIV infected (CDC 2001b). Ways to decrease the chances of receiving HIV infected blood from a transfusion include donating your own blood for scheduled surgery and having a family member who has compatible blood and an HIV negative blood test donate blood.

The American Red Cross imposes several restrictions and measures to increase the chances of receiving HIV negative blood. First, donating blood is guaranteed to be safe. Following universal precautions, a clean blood collection kit is used with each donation. There is *no* chance of infection to the person who is donating blood. People who draw blood (phlebotomists) wear gloves. Second, each unit of donated blood undergoes an ELISA HIV test (see chapter 4). All units of blood testing positive on the ELISA are thrown out. Please note, the Red Cross will only notify you if your blood tests positive on the ELISA; it will not contact you if your blood tests negative. This is not an alternative to HIV testing and counseling.

Third, the Red Cross engages in highly discriminating screening of potential donors. Entire groups may not donate blood. This includes Haitians, men who have sex with men (MSM), needle users, and people from Great Britain or people who have visited there or several countries in sub-Saharan Africa (see the Web site, http://www.redcross.org).

The ethics of these screening policies raise questions. The American Red Cross bases policies on membership in a risk group, not risky behavior per se. That position can contradict safer sex and needle usage messages that focus on behavior, not group identity or membership. There is

---

6.5

Gay and student groups around the country have protested the position taken by the Red Cross about refusing blood donations from MSM. In response, the Red Cross shifts the blame for the decision to the FDA, which decides blood donation policy (Bodzin 2005).

---

no litigation against the Red Cross's policies, however, because the organization maintains them to help protect the blood supply.

Donating blood to the Red Cross requires several steps. There are pages of excluding questions to answer about your risk behaviors and identities. Most of the questions refer to the donor's current and recent health history; sexual behavior regarding the number, gender, and sexual/drug/needle-using behavior of one's sex partners; and the donor's use of a variety of drugs and needles. Answers to these questions can exclude potential donors. If the donor passes the questionnaire, a finger prick of blood is taken to determine the presence of anemia, or lack of iron in the blood. These screening procedures exist to assess the health of the donor and reduce the risk of HIV or other diseases such as hepatitis from entering the blood supply.

Can HIV infected blood slip through these screening processes? Yes, *rarely,* but it can happen. An HIV infected donor unaware of his or her status could be in the window period before antibodies appear. This scenario explains why the blood supply is statistically but *not* absolutely safe and explains the statistic given above about the incidence of infected blood. The range of infected blood varies based on whether or not the blood collection is located in an epicenter, since epicenters have a higher prevalence of HIV/AIDS than do other areas of the country (see chapter 2).

The risks for HIV transmission during health-care procedures engender much debate. The risks apply to both the patient and the health-care provider. Perhaps the most well known case of health-care provider—to-patient transmission of HIV involved Dr. Acer, a dentist, and Kimberly Bergalis, one of his patients. Both of these individuals have died of AIDS. Kimberly Bergalis's situation attracted Congress's attention, resulting in federal recommendations about reducing HIV transmission in health-care settings through following universal precautions, including safe disposal of needles and other "hazardous wastes" (Rom 1997; Bartlett 2006).

Kimberly Bergalis accused her dentist of infecting her through dental procedures. Five other patients of Dr. Acer's also became HIV infected. Dr. Acer stated that he followed universal precautions/standards. He maintained that his dental procedures were not the source of his patients' HIV infections. Although the CDC decided that these individuals became infected as a result of Dr. Acer's practices, no one knows how this occurred (Rom 1997). After the controversy surrounding this case, congressional hearings, and Ms. Bergalis's death, new information appeared. Ms. Bergalis presented herself as sexually abstinent and a nondrug user. However, her sexual behavior became known after her death. No one knows for sure whether her sexual behavior or the dental procedures were the source of her infection. The results of this well-known case included stricter adherence to medical and dental protocols and tremendous legal, ethical, and social debate over disclosure of HIV status in health-care situations. These debates centered on privacy and confidentiality issues, what constitutes "acceptable risk," informed consent for medical procedures, and adequate sterilization procedures (Rom 1997).

These concerns extend to the risk posed to both the patient and the health-care provider in medical and surgical situations. Do health-care workers who perform invasive procedures that range from drawing blood and inserting IV lines to performing bloody orthopedic surgeries have the right to know their patient's HIV status? Do they have the right to refuse care to these patients out of fear of infection? Under what circumstances may they do so? In the 1990s, the AMA issued a statement that said that physicians could *not* refuse to provide care to an HIV+ patient when the medical condition was within their realm of competence (Feldman 1995; Bayer and Oppenheimer 2000).

Conversely, do patients have the right to know the HIV status of their health-care workers to avoid possible transmission during invasive medical procedures? There was a dramatic case addressing this issue as well.

Patients generally do not know the health status of their physicians. If HIV+ physicians and other health-care providers practice universal precautions during invasive procedures or are not in fields of medicine where they perform invasive procedures (these noninvasive fields of medicine include radiology, psychiatry, and pathology), there is not a risk to the patient. Does the patient, therefore, have the right or need to know the physician's HIV status and refuse to accept care from that person?

This situation occurred near Buffalo, New York. The HIV+ physician did not perform invasive procedures, followed universal precautions, and notified his patients of his status. He was fired by the hospital where he worked (Kirkland 1998). None of the patients he treated became HIV infected as a result of seeing him.

Between 1981 and 2002, 111 health-care workers whose only risk for exposure was work-related have been infected with HIV (CDC 2002; Bartlett 2006: 78, 79). Since 1987, with the wide availability of the HIV antibody test, very few patients have become infected by their health-care providers (Shernoff 1999). Yet the fear of possible transmission is very real from both sides, and the controversies continue. There are social, legal, ethical, and emotional issues involved regarding liability, intent, informed consent, and treatment.

If patients and health-care workers are HIV+, under what circumstances do they disclose their status? Is disclosure mandatory or voluntary, without coercion, threat of litigation, or denial of care? These questions take on particular salience in the United States. We value privacy and the integrity of medical confidentiality, and we are litigious. Many medical procedures incur some risk to the patient. That is why there are consent forms and informed consent for a number of medical tests and surgeries.

Invasive medical and surgical procedures may also involve some risk to the health-care provider, particularly if universal precautions are not followed. If health-care workers do not practice universal precaution, who is responsible if they become HIV infected? Who decides what an acceptable risk is?

I am my campus's HIV/AIDS education coordinator. As part of my responsibilities in this role, I have brought HIV+ speakers to campus. One such speaker refused to have a blood test at an area hospital because the phlebotomist would not wear gloves. The patient's HIV status was known to the phlebotomist. The HIV+ person asked me to check on the hospital's policy regarding wearing gloves during blood draws. When I checked with the hospital about this practice, I was told that gloves were recommended but not required to draw blood. However, if the phlebotomist did not wear gloves, the hospital was not liable for any infection the phlebotomist might incur in that situation.

Since the Middle Ages and the Black Death, doctors have faced the risks of infection from various pathogens. Under what circumstances are the risks too great? Attempts to legislate or regulate these fears beyond the use of universal precautions remain controversial (Shernoff 1999; Feldman 1995).

Statistics are based on populations and probabilities, not individual behavior. Culture defines what a risk is and influences an individual's decisions. Statistics may mean very little in the daily lives of individuals, their fears, and their concerns. Addressing people's fears about the risk for HIV infection in medical settings is one way of resolving them.

One way of addressing the concerns of health-care workers is through having PEP available. PEP is recent. It is available to health-care workers who experience needle-stick injuries or other exposure to body fluids during blood draws and surgical procedures. The person first takes a rapid ELISA HIV antibody test (see chapter 4) to establish a baseline HIV status at the time of exposure. The person can then begin a thirty-day course of HAART to prevent possible infection if she or he tests HIV negative. As of 2006, only six people who were put on a course of PEP have become HIV+ (Bartlett 2006: 79). Whether this low rate of seroconversion is due to insufficient exposure to the virus or because PEP worked remains unknown (Bartlett 2002, 2006).

As part of STI/HIV prevention, PEP is also offered in some health-care settings to people who have been raped. There is debate over whether PEP should be made available to people who forget to practice safer sex; this is similar to having emergency contraception (EC) available to women who fear pregnancy after intercourse without using contraception (Bartlett 2002, 2006). PEP, however, is a potent drug combination and has potentially serious side effects such as liver or kidney damage, and it can cause anemia, nausea, and vomiting (Bartlett 2002, 2006). The benefits of taking PEP to avoid possible HIV infection need to be weighed against the risks of the drugs and their potential side effects. For both providers and patients who are HIV negative, the concern is to remain negative. Given the real but statistically rare occurrence of health-care transmission of HIV to either patient or provider, the need-to-know arguments are laden with emotion. Physicians no longer are required to take the Hippocratic

---

6.6

Studies on the use of ARVs preventively to reduce the sexual transmission of HIV in nonindustrialized societies have come under intense controversy. One drug trial in Southeast Asia where Tenofovir, an ARV, was to be given to sex workers has been halted over issues regarding informed consent and provision of care if participants become infected while in the study. People in industrialized societies have different access to resources, better overall health, and generally more recourse when their rights are violated than do people in many nonindustrialized societies. At issue is the extent to which drug companies are responsible for their research subjects, particularly when those subjects are disenfranchised (De la Gorgendière 2005; Parker, Easton, and Klein 2000; Forbes 2006).

Oath upon graduation from medical school. Most physicians, however, honor and take the injunction to "do no harm" seriously (Feldman 1995).

During the first decade of the epidemic, many physicians refused to see people with HIV, for fear of becoming infected. Although this behavior was legal, it has since been found to be unethical by the AMA and many physicians (Shernoff 1999; Feldman 1995). As more information about the virus and the modes of transmission became available and adherence to universal precautions became stricter and more consistent, refusal to see HIV+ patients decreased. Increasingly, there are physicians in various medical disciplines who specialize in HIV (Feldman 1995; Shernoff 1999).

The blood supply in the United States became statistically safe because of activists during the 1980s who petitioned for HIV antibody testing of the supply. Most industrialized societies have the resources and capabilities for screening their blood supplies for HIV. Outside of industrialized societies, screening is variable, largely dependent on both the perception of risk and the resources available to screen the blood.

HIV, Blood, Drugs, and Needles Cross-Culturally

The role of drugs, needles, and HIV infected blood in the transmission of HIV varies cross-culturally. As in the United States, norms, behaviors, and beliefs about drugs and the use of needles influence the risk of infection, modes of transmission, and the safety of the blood supply.

The safety of the blood supply in nonindustrialized societies is difficult to determine accurately. Overall, between 5 and 10 percent of HIV transmission is estimated to occur through contaminated blood supplies (UNAIDS 2006). As of 2003, about 5 percent of the HIV infections in sub-Saharan Africa are estimated to be due to contaminated blood (http://www.scidev.net/). One of the concerns about circumcising adolescent and adult males in East Africa to reduce HIV transmission involves the risk of transmitting HIV during the surgery. Will clean needles be used to administer local anesthetics? How will the cleanliness of scalpels and other surgical instruments be ensured? What will be the additional expense entailed in ensuring clean equipment and operating conditions, as well as the implementation of universal precautions when performing circumcisions (Inungu et al. 2005)?

The security of the blood supply outside the United States depends on several factors. One is the prevalence of HIV/AIDS in the population. The higher the prevalence of HIV, the more difficult obtaining a safe blood supply in that group becomes (Bartlett 2002; CHIRON 2003. According to Chiron, a company that screens blood for HIV internationally, it is very difficult to test all of the world's blood supply and to enforce universal standards for donating, testing, and transfusing blood (CHIRON 2003).

A second factor in the safety of the blood supply is the availability of sterile needles both to draw blood and to transfuse blood and blood products. I am a member of an extended Peruvian kin group that spans from Lima, Peru, to the Dominican Republic to Miami, Florida. I conducted fieldwork regarding HIV education and prevention efforts with my husband in Lima and Santo Domingo (in the Dominican Republic) in the late 1980s. Part of this fieldwork entailed obtaining information about the availability of needles in health-care situations. At that time, Lima and Santo Domingo had insufficient needles and inadequate sterilization facilities to guarantee a readily available supply of clean needles. Middle-class families bought needles at pharmacies. Needles inserted as part of IVs remained unchanged during the course of therapy. This practice minimized the number of needles used and reduced the risk of HIV transmission and the need for either trying to clean the needles or reuse them. The use of clean needles outside of industrialized countries involves several factors. The per capita health-care costs, the availability of clean needles, and the urgency of other health crises such as malaria or tuberculosis impact the ability to realistically use clean needles.

Asia and India

Currently, the primary means of HIV transmission in China and Vietnam is through IDU. As discussed in chapters 4 and 5, until recently China's policies toward AIDS were repressive and based in denial. China has a historical foundation for drug usage through opium. Therefore, IDU in China occurs within an established drug subculture. IDU stands in contrast to the more widely known rich medical tradition based on beliefs in Chi (Qi), or vital energy, the use of various herbal and meditative practices to maintain health and treat illness, and the use of acupuncture. Chinese medicine also incorporates biomedicine into its health-care beliefs and practices. In China, condom usage is primarily for contraception, rather than HIV/STI prevention (Choi et al. 2000). Condom usage supports the one child per family policy established during Mao Zedong's rule.

China also has a double standard of sexual behavior. Men can have more sexual partners than women. Female sex partners of male IDUs in China are at greater risk of HIV than are the men, because of needle usage and multiple sex partners (Choi et al. 2000). In general, women IDUs whose male sex partners also inject drugs face a greater risk of contracting HIV from unprotected sex than from their own needle-using behavior (Francis and Cargill 2001). The official denial of AIDS in China until recently inhibited education and treatment programs for IDUs (Stanmeyer 2003).

Southeast Asia

In Bangladesh and Laos, **nongovernmental organizations (NGOs)** established N/SEPs (Beyrer 1998; Jenkins et al. 2001). N/SEPs in two cities in Bangladesh reduced needle sharing (Jenkins et al. 2002). Laos is officially an Islamic country. Current interpretations of Islam prohibit the government from establishing educational safer sex and needle/syringe exchange programs. However, **community-based organizations (CBOs)** can and do offer these programs, with sexual and needle-using risk reduction reported (Beyrer 1998).

In other parts of Southeast Asia, including Thailand, Vietnam, Myanmar, and other Indonesian cultures, the linkages between drugs and needles and risk for HIV are complex. Medical and injection drug usage for a variety of drugs is traditional in many Southeast Asian cultures (Stimson and Choopanya 1998). In Vietnam in particular, IDU is the major mode of transmission for HIV. The use of injection drugs increased after the Vietnam War, owing to the easy availability of heroin from Myanmar and the burgeoning tourist industry (Thuy et al. 2000). Injuries incurred during the Vietnam War increased drug usage as a treatment for pain and disability (Stimson and Choopanya 1998).

Vietnam is also undergoing rapid economic, political, and social change. The tourist industry provides significant economic resources. Tourists bring in their ideas about sex and drugs and know that drugs are relatively easy to obtain in Vietnam. Drug usage becomes part of social networks, garnering individual economic gain and facilitating personal relationships (McKeganey et al. 1998; Stimson and Choopanya 1998).

In other parts of Southeast Asia, such as Thailand and Myanmar, HIV infection attributable to IDU is rising (Stimson and Choopanya 1998). These areas are major tourist attractions. As discussed in chapter 5, Thailand has a thriving sex tourism industry. The relative availability of sex and drugs, low prices for drugs, social networks that foster drug usage, and the tourists' interest in the exotic encourage the desire and acceptability of drug usage in these areas (Stimson and Choopanya 1998; DesJarlais et al. 1998). In the earlier stages of the epidemic, drug and needle sharing occurred. Needle sharing fostered rapid transmission of HIV within these drug-using social networks (DesJarlais et al. 1998).

While 74 percent of HIV is sexually transmitted in India, the second major source of transmission is through IDU (Solomon et al. 2000). Most IDU occurs in northeastern and southern India (Solomon et al. 2000). The stigma attached to HIV discourages people in India from seeking help. Although men are the primary IDUs in India, their female sexual partners are at greater risk of infection from unprotected sex (Solomon et al. 2000; Francis and Cargill 2001). British colonization of India drastically changed India's social and economic patterns, relationships between men and women, and the status of women. Overall, women's status and power fell, and they lost economic control of households as a result of colonization. Freedom from British rule in 1947 did not significantly improve the status of women, nor did it grant them autonomy. Women have little overt say in sexual decisions and practices. HIV is stigmatized, and gossip is a major source of social control (Solomon et al. 2000). Therefore, women's risk of contracting HIV through sex is greater than that of their male partners, particularly if he injects drugs (DesJarlais et al. 1998, GenderAIDSeForum 2003).

Brazil

In Latin America, Brazil is one country where IDU is the second major means of contracting HIV (Andrade et al. 2001; Marins et al. 2000). Twenty-one percent of Brazil's AIDS cases are attributable to IDU (Andrade et al. 2001). As in the United States and parts of sub-Saharan Africa, Brazil's HIV epidemic began within the middle and upper-middle classes, eventually moving downward to include the poor and disenfranchised (Andrade et al. 2001). IDU and unprotected sex with multiple partners were the initial modes of HIV transmission (Andrade et al. 2001; Marins et al. 2000).

As discussed in chapter 5, Brazil is a highly complex society, with numerous sexual, gender, and several orientation subcultures and interactions. Drug-using and sexual behaviors combined to make Brazil the society with the highest HIV/AIDS rates in Latin America (UNAIDS 2002a).

Encouragingly, nongovernmental organizations (NGOs) and community-based organizations (CBOs) in Brazil, India, and parts of Southeast Asia, including Thailand, developed prevention and intervention programs in the 1980s that continue to the present to address the epidemic in their cultures. They are proving to be effective in reducing incidence rates. Although needle exchange programs (N/SEPs) are illegal in Brazil, CBOs established grassroots organizations to deliver clean needles to drug users. CBOs work with local police to prevent arrests at needle exchange sites as well as when intervention workers go to people's homes to exchange needles (Andrade et al. 2001). Recognizing the large transgendered sex and sex worker communities that exist in Brazil led to similar intervention efforts with these groups. In dealing with clients of sex workers, their social status and class and their willingness to practice safer sex were incorporated into intervention efforts. There are also interventions directed toward increasing the use of condoms with the steady partners of TGs in Brazil (Grandi et al. 2000).

Brazilian NGOs and CBOs recognize the sex and drug use that occurs among incarcerated people. With a relatively young and economically poor prison population, interventions with this group address the demographic characteristics that exist in this situation (Marins et al. 2000).

Eastern Europe

Eastern European countries also recently established N/SEPs. Since the dissolution of the United Soviet Socialist Republic (USSR), Eastern Europe represents "the fastest [growing] incidence rate of HIV in the world" (Somlai et al. 2002: 295). Having undergone rapid economic, social, political, and sexual changes in the past decade, Eastern Europe has rates of HIV and other STIs that are increasing geometrically, particularly among females (Somlai et al. 2002). While unprotected sexual behavior is the primary route of transmission, IDU is a secondary causal factor. N/SEP programs are relatively new, with about 50–60 percent of IDUs no longer sharing needles (Somlai et al. 2002).

Successful Harm Reduction Programs

There are a number of factors that affect the success of harm reduction models for IDUs. Several programs outside the United States appear to incorporate those variables that increase the chances of success. They include:

developing programs at grassroots, community levels;
using CBOs and NGOs that take advantage of human and local
    resources to implement programs;
working with local law enforcement agencies to establish safe
    zones for needle exchange in areas where needle exchange is
    illegal;
using peer educators and people from the community in education
    and outreach efforts;
establishing programs that meet the linguistic, sexual, and eco-
    nomic needs of the target group;
incorporating safer sex messages into harm reduction models; and
using harm reduction messages that are less judgmental, more
    realistic, developed locally, and less authoritarian.

Adapting some of these successful cross-cultural harm reduction methods in the United States might help to reduce risk.

It is interesting that through NGOs and CBOs, officially Catholic Brazil and Islamic Laos have developed effective safer sex and N/SEP programs. In contrast, the theoretically secular United States presents much legal

---

6.7

Iran is another example of a society that is taking an active position in regards to HIV. Within what is an Islamic, conservative society in some respects, the Iranian government is attempting to maintain its relatively low HIV prevalence rate. Most of the HIV transmission in Iran comes from needle usage. Condoms and clean needles are provided for its prison populations, and condoms are widely distributed and encouraged as a way of preventing transmission in general (Allam 2006).

---

and governmental opposition to both comprehensive safer sex education and needle exchange programs.

While not as prevalent as sexual behavior in the transmission of HIV worldwide, drug usage and needles play a significant role in HIV transmission. They are the second most common form of HIV transmission. Programs to prevent transmission through needle exchange, within medical settings, and through the blood supply are controversial. Intervention and educational harm-reduction programs in the United States and elsewhere tend to be most effective when they are community based, involve peer education, and are nonjudgmental. Despite a lack of official government support of N/SEPs in the United States, Brazil, and Laos, these programs have achieved success in reducing both the incidence and the prevalence of HIV among IDUs.

SUMMARY

Drug and needle usage can either be a direct cause or a cofactor in HIV infection.

The stigma associated with IDU increases the risk for transmission of HIV. It also affects the ability to get tested and receive treatment if infected.

CBOs and NGOs have been effective in reducing needle transmission of HIV through N/SEPs.

Increasingly, drug/needle usage as a risk factor for HIV infection is becoming more common cross-culturally.

The blood supply is statistically safe in the United States and in most industrialized societies.

Thought Questions

What are the sociocultural factors that influence both drug and needle usage and harm-reduction programs in the United States and cross-culturally?

What fears need to be addressed to reduce the concern about HIV transmission from patient to health-care provider and from health-care provider to patient?

Resources

Books

Singer, Merrill. *Something Dangerous: Emergent and Changing Illicit Drug Use and Community Health.* Long Grove, Ill.: Waveland Press, 2005.

Stoller, Nancy E. *Lessons from the Damned: Queers, Whores, and Junkies Respond to AIDS.* New York: Routledge, 1998.

Web Sites

American Red Cross: http://www.redcross.org.

NIAID (National Institute of Allergy and Infectious Diseases): http://www.niaid.nih.gov.

7

AIDS and Women

CHAPTER HIGHLIGHTS INCLUDE

A discussion of women's role as caregivers in the epidemic
A discussion of women's sexuality and sexual risks for HIV
A discussion of women, reproduction, and HIV
A discussion of the roles played by poverty and politics in women's risk
    for and experience with HIV/AIDS
A discussion of ethical issues surrounding women and HIV

Dr. Helene Gayle, an AIDS physician, former researcher for the Bill and Melinda Gates Foundation, and president of the International AIDS Society (IAS), stated at the International Conference on Women and AIDS, "Currently, women make up fifty percent of the people with AIDS worldwide. History will judge us [the United States] by how we deal with women and AIDS" (Gayle 2003).

Women have been infected and affected by HIV since the beginning of the epidemic (Corea 1992; Campbell 1999; O'Leary and Jemmott 1996; Patton 1994). Their experience of HIV differs from that of men. For example, HIV+ women often experience gynecological health problems, and they have issues about pregnancy, childbirth, and breast-feeding that men do not have. While both must deal with a potentially fatal, stigmatized disease and illness, women's roles as caregivers, their sexual and reproductive lives, and their lack of political, social, and economic autonomy in the societies where they live contribute to making HIV in women unique. Furthermore, HIV disease and illness varies among women. Poverty, the lack of formal education women receive in many nonindustrialized societies, and beliefs about women's roles, statuses, and sexuality within and between cultures all impact their risk of infection and their treatment once infected.

Women in industrialized societies who have access to confidential or anonymous testing, safer sex, good medical care, and HAART are in a very different position relative to risks for HIV and the way the disease affects them than are poor women living in industrialized subcultures or in nonindustrialized societies. The difference between the quality of life and resources available to women in industrialized societies versus women in nonindustrialized societies is vast. There are two AIDS epidemics for women living in the twenty-first century: the one affecting women in industrialized countries and the one affecting them in the rest of the world. This chapter explores how HIV/AIDS impacts women around the world.

Women as Caregivers

In most societies, women are the caregivers throughout the life cycle. Women are the ones primarily responsible for socializing children from birth through adolescence. They provide most of the paid and unpaid labor in societies, are the entry points into health-care systems, and provide most of the care for people who are sick and dying. In addition, they tend to take care of their own health last, putting others' needs and health above their own. These behaviors are culturally created and sanctioned (Gender-AIDSeForum 2004; Nyblade et al. 2003; Sargeant and Bretell 1996; Upton 2003; Desgrees du Lou 1999; http://www.aids2004.org).

Women have been involved as caregivers since the beginning of the AIDS epidemic in the United States and cross-culturally. They serve in formal medical contexts such as midwives, *curanderas* (indigenous healers in Mesoamerica), nurses, and doctors to those infected, as well as informally as relatives and friends providing care to those with HIV/AIDS (Shilts 1987; Corea 1992; Schneider and Stoller 1995; Roth and Fuller 1998;

7.1

Men served as the forefront of caregiving in the first wave of the epidemic in the United States. Gay male nurses, doctors, lovers, family, and friends often provided the bulk of care for the largely gay, white, male population who were infected in the epicenters during this time. Groups such as Shanti in San Francisco and the Gay Men's Health Crisis in New York City were early formal sources of care and information for those who were infected as well as their support people.

Anderson 2001; http://www.aids2004.org). Their informal roles comprise the majority of caregiving worldwide; however, their work is less visible and acknowledged. Women provide care to others regardless of their overall health and HIV status (Gender-AIDSeForum 2004; http://www.aids2004.org).

In nonindustrialized societies, women's overall health is worse than men's. Women tend to receive less health care and care that is of poorer quality than do men, regardless of their HIV status (Greenblatt and Hessol 2001; Schneider and Stoller 1995; Sargeant and Bretell 1996; Human Rights Watch 2004). This situation is exacerbated if they are HIV+ themselves; women tend to receive less health care and at a more advanced stage of infection than do men. If there is a choice between HIV+ women or men getting and taking ARVs, generally women will get them less often than men, despite the fact that women access health-care settings more so than do men because of reproductive concerns. In addition, if they are HIV+, they may not have anyone to care for them, and they face rejection from their kin groups and tend to be blamed for having contracted the infection (Human Rights Watch 2004). At the same time, they are expected to fulfill their roles in society as wives, mothers, and laborers. These factors place additional burdens on them as caregivers and as people with HIV/AIDS (Gender-AIDSeForum 2004; http://www.aids2004.org). Caregiving is only one set of the multiple roles women play in society. They are also sexual and reproductive beings. These roles of sex partner/wife and mother comprise the major focus of women's lives in most societies.

Women as Sexual Beings

As discussed in chapter 5, double standards of sexual behavior persist and are culturally widespread (Bankole et al. 2004; Bond 1997; LeClerc-Madlala 2001; McGrath et al. 1993). Generally, women are held to very different sexual mores and behaviors than are men (Whelehan 2001a, 2001b; Hunter and Alexander 1996; Delacoste and Alexander 1987; LeClerc-Madlala 2001). The further women's real or perceived sexual behavior is from a committed, monogamous, heterosexual relationship, the greater the chances are that they will be seen as "bad" girls (Kaschak and Tiefer 2002; Whelehan 2001a). These beliefs and perceptions increase the chances that women will be seen as vectors of transmission in heterosexual sex, will be blamed for spreading HIV/AIDS, and will be set up for societal condemnation and rejection (Upton 2003).

In nonindustrialized societies, it is common for the patrilineage and individual men (brothers, fathers, and husbands) to make the sexual decisions about not only their own sexual behavior but also that of their sisters, daughters, and wives. It is also culturally common that females have sex with older males, and while the females may be monogamous, their male partners often are not, thus increasing the women's risk of HIV infection (Gender-AIDSeForum 2003; Nyblade et al. 2003; Orubuloye et al. 1994; Bankole et al. 2004; McGrath et al. 1993; Heald 2006; Upton 2003) Women may have very little say over the circumstances under which they engage in sex or with whom (Machekano et al. 2000; Saul et al. 2000; Susser 2001; Beyrer 1998; Orubuloye and Orguntimehin 1999; Lyttleton 2000; Yep 1998; Setel 1999).

Biology, Women, and Sexual Risks of HIV Infection

Women who have sex with men bear a disproportionate burden for risk of HIV infection. As discussed in chapter 5, in penetrative sex the receiver is more at risk for infection than is the inserter. The receiver's mucous membranes are more likely to be abraded than the inserter's. Most women are infected with HIV through unprotected penile-vaginal intercourse. In both penile-vaginal and penile-anal intercourse, the surface areas of the vagina and anus and rectum have larger exposure areas to the virus than the penis has. Semen contains a higher concentration of HIV than does vaginal fluid (Tortu et al. 2000). In any given act of unprotected p-v intercourse, healthy women are three to eight times more likely to be infected with HIV than are men (Tortu et al. 2000; Bartlett 2006; Cameron et al. 1989; Hutchinson 2001).

Other biological factors contribute to a woman's risk of HIV infection. These include age, overall state of health, and the presence of other STIs. Youth, malnutrition, diseases such as malaria or tuberculosis, and genital ulcers and sores all become cofactors that put her at increased risk of contracting HIV (Bloom et al. 1997; Eldred and Chiasson 1996; Volberding et al. 1999; Bankole et al. 2004). Females under the age of fifteen do not have mature sexual and reproductive tracts (Bailey 1999). Their vaginal lining is thinner and more porous than that of an adult, and they do not lubricate as much as adult women do (Bailey 1999).

Vaginal lubrication is important for physically comfortable intercourse and to reduce the friction that occurs during intercourse. Vaginal lubrication varies during sexual arousal, over the course of the menstrual cycle, during pregnancy, and after menopause (Bailey 1999; Barbach 1998). A well-lubricated vagina decreases penile-vaginal friction and the risk of vaginal tearing. The presence of other STIs can create tears, lesions, or sores in the external genitalia or in the vaginal walls that can act as portals of entry for HIV (Ferry 1995; Parker and Patterson 1996). In addition, malnutrition and other health problems can impair her immune system, making her more susceptible to infection (Bloom et al. 1997; WHO 2004a, 2004b; UNAIDS 2002; http://www.aids2004.org). All of these biological factors exist and are expressed through culture. They do not exist as pure physiological or anatomical entities removed from a cultural context.

7.2

Cultural practices and beliefs can impact these basic biological factors. Many groups in sub-Saharan Africa and Melanesia, for example, believe that semen and menstrual blood contain their own power. Blocking semen from entering the vagina with the use of condoms could violate deep cultural norms about body integrity, conception, and men's and women's "natural" roles (Butt et al. 2004; Rasing 2003).

Sociocultural Factors in Women's Risk of HIV Infection

There are numerous cultural factors that affect women's risk of contracting HIV sexually. Cultural beliefs and norms about women's sexuality rest on deeply held assumptions about women. As discussed in detail in chapter 5, assumptions relate to how innately sexual or nonsexual women are, their moral worth based on their sexual behavior, and how close to nature they are believed to be. Beliefs based on these assumptions encompass double standards of sexual behavior, women as both seductresses and chaste, and the subjugation of women's sexual needs to those of men (LeClerc-Madlala 2001; Bond 1997; Heald 2006). Based on the beliefs and assumptions made about women's sexuality, cultures define who are acceptable sexual partners, how many sexual partners are acceptable, at what age sex should commence, what kinds of sex are appropriate, and who makes the sexual decisions for and about women.

Women's sexuality generally is defined relative to their male sexual partners. It is not considered as an entity in itself (Aggleton 1994). Therefore, the sexual needs and wants of women tend to be ignored. Two examples illustrate this point. One addresses women who have sex with women. As discussed in chapter 5, both in the United States and elsewhere, women who have sex with women or who identify as lesbian generally are not considered in developing intervention programs, and their risk of contracting HIV sexually is either denied or diminished (Aggleton 1994; Ramos 1997; Raffaelli and Suarez-Al-Adam 1998; Parker and Ehrhardt 2001; Chapkis 1997).

7.3

Obtaining accurate data on how many WSW become infected solely through same-sex behavior is difficult for several reasons. First, the CDC's definition of a lesbian does not fit with lesbians' definitions of themselves. Second, many women who identify as lesbians also have sex with men; this presents a confounding variable in determining whether their exposure to HIV is from men or women. However, WSW do engage in risky sex with other women and do contract other STIs from sex with women, and these can be cofactors for HIV infection. Currently, the best guesstimate for the incidence of HIV among WSW exclusively is that it is "low" (Fethers et al. 2000: 348; Kwakwa and Ghobrial 2003).

The other example involves women who have sex with men. In the United States, we culturally define women's sexuality in comparison with men's, depicting women's sexuality as more passive, less intense, and less driven than a man's and thereby less valid (Parker 1994). In the United States, men are expected, encouraged, and allowed to be sexual from adolescence through old age, to have a number of partners, to be the sexual initiator, and to be more knowledgeable about sex than females are. P-v intercourse remains the standard of acceptable, "normal," adult sexual behavior in this society (Kaschak and Tiefer 2002). These beliefs are deeply entrenched, regardless of the evidence about risk and transmission.

Defining women's sexuality relative to or as a function of men's sexuality leads to biases about women and their risk of AIDS. These biases initially downplayed the risk for contracting HIV among women in the United States and Western Europe by focusing on HIV infection among men who have sex with men and perceiving it as a "gay, white boys' disease" (Shilts 1987; Corea 1992). During the first two waves of the epidemic in the United States, women with HIV/AIDS—particularly ethnic women living in poverty—were underserved relative to prevention efforts, testing, and treatment (Campbell 1999; O'Leary and Jemmott 1996; Patton 1994; Roth and Fuller 1998; Simoni et al. 2000; Basu et al. 1997; Kurth 1993).

Cultural biases about women's sexuality include ambivalence and negativity (Orubuloye et al. 1994; Aggleton 1994; Beyrer 1998; Campbell 1999; Hogan 1998, 2001). In many societies, women are held responsible for transmitting HIV to both sex partners and their fetuses and infants (Noar et al. 2002; Setel 1999; Stine 1997; Anon. 2002; Upton 2003; Heald 2006). Although women can transmit HIV to men, epidemiological and biological data clearly indicate that in heterosexuals, transmission is much more likely from male to female (Tortu et al. 2000; Cohen and Kelly 1995; Bartlett 2006). (Women's transmission of HIV perinatally and during breastfeeding will be discussed later in this chapter.) Seeing women as vectors of sexual transmission of HIV particularly applies to female sex workers.

Female Sex Workers and HIV

A global aspect of female-male sexual relationships is sex work, particularly prostitution. Although sex work covers a wide range of sexual exchange interactions, this section will focus on female prostitution, which is the most common form of sex work worldwide (International Committee for Prostitutes' Rights 1987; Alexander 1996; Kempadoo and Doezema 1998). Female prostitution can put women at risk for HIV infection (Cohen 1999). In discussing female prostitution in a cultural context, one must define what it is and why it occurs, while trying to avoid ethnocentrism.

Prostitution is legally defined in the United States as the exchange of sex (unspecified) for money, goods, or services (Whelehan 2001a). This broad definition leaves room for legal, emic, and etic interpretations of prostitution. For example, the CDC categorizes women who exchange sex for drugs or drug money as prostitutes. However, women who are not substance users but define themselves as prostitutes do not see these substance-using women as prostitutes. Conversely, a woman who exchanges sex for drugs or drug money in the United States may not identify as a prostitute (Whelehan 2001a; Kwiatkowski and Booth 2000; Alexander 1996; Waterston 1997).

Women who are substance users/IDUs are at greater risk of HIV infection than are women who are not (Metsch et al. 2001; Brimlow and Ross 1998; Francis and Cargill 2001; Kwiatkowski and Booth 2000). They are more likely than men to trade sex for drugs or drug money and to practice unsafe sex in doing so. Given the way we structure heterosexuality, sex is a readily available commodity for women to offer men as trade (that is, in the United States, women give sex and men get sex) (Weeks et al. 2004; Koo et al. 2005). Moreover, women who trade sex for drugs or drug money are more likely to contract HIV from their steady sexual partners than from sharing needles. They are also more likely to have a male sex partner who is an IDU than are male IDUs to have a female partner who is an IDU (Francis and Cargill 2001; DesJarlais et al. 1998; see chapter 6). These behaviors increase substance-using women's risk of HIV infection (Francis and Cargill 2001; DesJarlais et al. 1998). Women who are substance users need to have their substance use addressed first and then deal with their sexual behavior, because their drug usage can direct their sexual behavior. Research indicates that safer needle usage is more amenable to change than is sexual behavior (Williams et al. 2001; Brimlow and Ross 1998; Francis and Cargill 2001).

In general, if given a choice, female prostitutes will practice safer sex with clients. This is a business transaction for them; the women do not want to get pregnant or contract an STI, including HIV. Using condoms also provides a physical and psychological way of separating sex at work from sex in their personal life (Whelehan 2001a; Seabrook 2001; Alexander 1996; Cohen 1999). As with prostitutes in industrialized societies, female prostitutes in Southeast Asia, Africa, and India will use condoms with clients if they can but are less likely to do so with steady partners (Campbell 1999; Cohen and Kelly 1995; Cash 1996; Thuy et al. 2000; Newman 2004; Kempadoo and Doezema 1998).

Although female-to-male HIV transmission does occur, female prostitutes generally are not as much the vector of transmission of HIV to their clients as the clients are to them and their other sex partners, including wives (Delacoste and Alexander 1987; Cohen and Kelly 1995; Whelehan 2001a; Padian 1998; Padian et al. 1991). The women are more at risk for contracting HIV from their clients, particularly if they cannot or do not practice safer sex with clients (Seabrook 2001; Alexander 1996). Safer sex intervention efforts with female prostitutes need to be grass roots and peer based and reach their clients as well to be effective (Bolton 1994; Alexander 1996; Rogers et al. 2002; Susser 2001; Campbell 1999; Newman 2004; Renaud 1997).

At the beginning of the twenty-first century, sex work occurs globally. The stigma that accompanies sex work negatively affects adopting safer sex practices (Singer 2003b; Herdt 2001; Auer 1996; Campbell 1999). Cross-culturally, women's choices in sex work differ from those of women in the United States. These differences exist regardless of whether prostitution is a modification of traditional behaviors, as in places such as Thailand and India, or a relatively more recent phenomenon, as in some groups in sub-Saharan Africa.

In much of the world, female prostitution is an economic survival strategy (Setel 1999; Carovano and Schietings 1996; Long and Ankrah 1996; Orubuloye et al. 1994; Seabrook 2001; Bond et al. 1996; Bloom and Mahal 1997; Rogers et al. 2002). If a woman works in a brothel, her ability to practice safer sex may depend on the brothel owner. If she works independently, her income probably will increase if she does not practice safer sex. Generally, male clients will pay more not to use a condom (Setel 1999; Carovano and Schietings 1996; Renaud 1997). If a woman insists on safer sex, she may face violent consequences: beatings, food deprivation, or psychological abuse (Bloem et al. 1999; Wilkinson 1997; Bond et al. 1996; Lau and Tsui 2002; Beyrer 1998; Bloom et al. 1997; Jenkins 1999).

7.4

Activist groups in Thailand and elsewhere have consistently campaigned for safe working conditions for sex workers, which include mandatory condom use in brothels and nonjudgmental health checks for workers to reduce the chances of HIV transmission. In Senegal, for example, sex workers formed collectives to support one another in using condoms with clients. Men who refused to wear a condom did not obtain sex. Collective action in Senegal shows that effective intervention strategies do work (Renaud 1997). However, in many places, sex work has become more dangerous and more stigmatized, and women lost control of their settings and earnings with European contact and globalization in places such as Thailand and sub-Saharan Africa (White 1990; Upton 2003).

Prostitution outside the United States may take on different connotations and not be defined as such. For example, in Haiti and Trinidad, parts of Southeast Asia, and sub-Saharan Africa, casual, nonmarital relationships can involve noncash exchanges of food, shelter, and social support for sex (Furlonge et al. 2000; Kwiatkowski and Booth 2000; Susser 2001;

Amadora-Nolasco et al. 2001; Cleland et al. 1995; Ulin et al. 1996; Farmer et al. 1996). While this may look like prostitution to us, emically these relationships may not be defined as such. It is therefore important to take a culturally relativistic approach so that intervention efforts reflect the reality of these women's lives (Bond 1997; Waterston 1997; Roberts and Cohen 2006; Morof et al. 2004).

International prostitute's rights groups organize and petition to improve working conditions for sex workers in general and prostitutes in particular (International Committee for Prostitutes' Rights 1987; Ninth International Conference on AIDS 1993; Delacoste and Alexander 1987; Alexander 1996). Rather than blaming the victim (that is, the prostitute) for risky sex, the foci are on educating brothel owners and clients about safer sex, providing prostitutes with female condoms to practice safer sex, encouraging safer sex with partners, and discouraging childhood and coerced prostitution (Gender-AIDSeForum 2003, 2004; Lau and Tsui 2002; Patton 1994; Schoepf 1993; Basuki et al. 2002; Newman 2004; Kempadoo and Doezema 1998).

Psycho-emotional Factors and Women's Sexuality

Two aspects associated with women's sexual risk of HIV infection are the ability to consent to sex and emotional involvement with their sex partners. In the United States, the concept of consent is based on individual autonomy to make decisions, free will, and choice. Even within our culture, what constitutes consent is arguable, as in situations of date or acquaintance rape or informed consent for medical procedures (AmFar 2001; Faden et al. 1996; Kendall 1996).

There is considerable research that addresses women's ability to consent in sexual relationships. Forcible rape and intergenerational incest do not connote consent. Other variables such as economic pressures and physical or psychological abuse may affect someone's ability to give sexual consent (Jenkins 1999; Jenkins et al. 2002; Monti-Catania 1997). If women do not have economic independence or a social support system that allows them to leave a relationship or make changes within it or if they fear for their own or their children's health and safety, the meaning of sexual consent differs from that of economically independent and secure, assertive women who have a network of people who will help them (Brimlow and Ross 1998).

Outside of middle-class, Anglo culture, issues of consent can be major factors in whether or not safer sex is practiced. For example, *machismo*, a value in Latino cultures, can incorporate acceptance for male aggression in interpersonal relationships (Saul et al. 2000; Tross 2001; Susser 2001; Campbell 1999). Physical safety may take precedence over safer sex (Wilkinson 1997; Women's Bulletin 2003). Among African Americans and Latinos, women's emotional attachment and respect for cultural values are critical to practicing safer sex (Raffaelli and Suarez-Al-Adam 1998; Margillo and Imahori 1998). For many African American women, loyalty to and support of their male partners is most important (Robinson et al. 2002).

As discussed in other chapters, males and the kin group make the sexual decisions for females in parts of sub-Saharan Africa. Polygyny and the levirate are common practices in much of sub-Saharan Africa (Anon. 2002; Orubuloye et al. 1994; Orubuloye, Caldwell, and Caldwell 1994). While women are expected to be monogamous, men are not. In some places, more than 50 percent of females under the age of eighteen are married to older men, many of whom may carry the virus (Gender-AIDSeForum 2004; Bankole et al. 2004; McGrath et al. 1993; Desgrees du Lou 1999; http://www.aids2004.org). As young, monogamous wives, these women are at risk for contracting HIV from their husbands who have multiple sex partners without practicing safer sex (Gender-AIDSeForum 2004; Bankole et al. 2004; Schoepf 2003b, 2004; http://www.aids2004.org).

Programs that address men's sexual behavior and attitudes are as important in reducing risk as those that try to provide women with sexual, economic, educational, political, or social power (Billowitz 2004; McGrath et al. 1993). When consent rests outside the individual, those people and institutions that grant consent and make decisions need to be incorporated into interventions at a grassroots level to work (Williams et al. 2001; Gielen et al. 2001; Dowsett 1999; Viaud et al. 1997; Byrnes 1996; Preston-Whyte et al. 2000; Gifford et al. 1999).

Emotional and psychological attachment to one's sex partner(s) plays a consistent role in safer sex decisions. Extensive research in the United States and cross-culturally indicates that once emotional involvement and attachment occurs between partners, safer sex practices decrease (Kane 1998; Raffaelli and Suarez-Al-Adam 1998; Margillo and Imahori 1998; Sobo 1995; Pilkington et al. 1994; Klein-Alonso 1996; Helfferich 2000; Desgrees du Lou 1999). Emotional attachment frequently involves trust. In many groups, trust is part of intimate relationships.

How does a person develop trust and still practice safer sex, given that safer sex may imply either noninvolvement or distrust? The challenge is to develop and implement safer sex strategies that reflect emotional involvement and intimacy. These programs need to address couples and their communities, not just individuals. They also need to address women's male sexual partners (Patton 1994; Lau and Tsui 2002; Campbell 1999; Susser 2001; Billowitz 2004).

7.5

"The importance of integrating emotional factors in the AIDS risk is particularly interesting in the family context, where affection for the partner, fear of estrangement, and concern for children far outweigh concerns for self-preservation. . . . [A woman in an African family] must balance the risk of contracting the AIDS virus against that of her husband's rejection if she attempts to negotiate condom use or a halt to family building (which may seem to outweigh the risk of bearing an HIV-infected child)" (Desgrees du Lou 1999:76). Although this quotation is based on research conducted in sub-Saharan Africa, its message has broader applicability.

Focusing only on women's responsibility in safer sex, to the exclusion of the males, reinforces cultural assumptions and biases about heterosexuality and heterosexual relationships (Cash 1996; Billowitz 2004; Schoepf 2003b, 2004; McGrath et al. 1993). Although female condoms have been available since the early 1990s, they are expensive, can be awkward to use, and may be too costly for people in nonindustrialized societies. Accepted by female prostitutes in India and other places as a means of having control over safer sex, their use helps women in the immediate sexual situation but does not address other issues about responsibility for sexual behavior. Female microbicides are being developed. However, currently there are no safe, effective, inexpensive, easily available and reliable, female-controlled safer sex options for women other than abstinence. As discussed in this chapter and in chapter 5, women's desire and ability to be abstinent or monogamous is questionable both in the United States and elsewhere (Saah 1996; Volberding et al. 1999; Marks et al. 2000; Elias and Heise 1996; Gender-AIDSeForum 2003, 2004).

7.6

The development of vaginal and rectal microbicides that women can control generates a great deal of interest among social science and biomedical researchers. There are questions about safety, cultural and individual acceptability, efficacy, and affordability, as well as ethical concerns about how clinical trials are conducted. The implication that women can use microbicides "without their partners' knowledge" also raises issues of trust and potential consequences for the women if their partners discover their use of the microbicides (Weeks et al. 2004; Koo et al. 2005; Feuer 2006; Forbes 2006; Klasse et al. 2006).

Kofi Annan, while secretary general of the United Nations, addressed these issues in his statement recognizing International Women's Day 2004. He reinforced the need for women to be able to exert political, economic, and social autonomy, independence, and control over their own lives. He supported the need for women to have contraceptive and safer sex methods that they can control available to them. He also recognized the need to hold men responsible for their sexual behavior, without that being interpreted as controlling their female partner's contraceptive or safer sex decisions and practices (Annan 2004).

Recently, several programs have been developed that support responsible sexual behavior among adolescent males who have sex with females. Found in Nigeria, Kenya, Brazil, and India, these programs use positive values about male sexuality and gender role to encourage safer sex practices (Billowitz 2004; Schoepf 1993, 2001). If men are not held responsible for their sexual behavior and if effective, comprehensive, culturally sensitive programs are not developed to modify their behavior and attitudes, women will continue to be put at risk for contracting HIV (McGrath et al. 1993; Schoepf 2004; Upton 2003; Heald 2006).

Sexual Practices and Women's Risk of HIV Infection

Indigenous sexual practices other than marital roles can increase the risk of contracting HIV in women. As discussed in chapter 5, numerous sub-Saharan African and Malaysian Islamic groups practice various forms of female genital surgery as a rite of passage. As Hanny Lightfoot-Klein's (1989) and Carla Obermeyer's (2003) research shows, female genital cutting ranges from removal of the clitoral hood (true female circumcision) to infibulation and fulfills a variety of socioeconomic, sexual, and political functions where it occurs (WHO 2004a; Whelehan 2001b; Obermeyer 2003). Since the World Health Organization (WHO) outlawed female genital surgery in the early 1980s, this practice has become more dangerous and covert. Women can experience various infections either from the surgery itself or from the healing process that can increase their risk of contracting HIV (Lightfoot-Klein 1989; Tokars and Martone 1996).

"Dry sex," ritual "widow cleansings," and the belief in the power of ejaculate potentially also put women at risk for HIV infection. These practices are found among some groups in sub-Saharan Africa (Brown et al. 1993). Dry sex entails using various herbal astringents to reduce vaginal lubrication, thus making intercourse tighter (Orubuloye et al. 1994). Lack of lubrication increases the friction and can abrade the vaginal walls, making it easier for the virus to pass through.

Widow cleansings involve ritually purifying widows as part of the levirate. She may have sex with several men in her dead husband's kin group. In some parts of sub-Saharan Africa, this practice currently involves reestablishing older rituals that symbolically instead of behaviorally cleanse the widow, to reduce HIV risk (Setel 1999; Orubuloye et al. 1994). The belief in the power of semen (ejaculate) is widespread cross-culturally. In some sub-Saharan African and Melanesian societies, mixing semen and vaginal fluids and repeated intravaginal ejaculations during pregnancy are seen as necessary for health and proper fetal development (Herdt and Stoller 1990; Butt et al. 2004). Using the concept of symbolic as opposed to behavioral methods of mixing fluids and cleansing widows may prove to be a safer alternative while maintaining traditional beliefs.

Women as Reproductive Beings

Women face a conundrum with safer sex. To get pregnant, they must engage in risky sex. Women in the United States who become pregnant through artificial insemination, however, are safe, since all states now test sperm for HIV (Rochman 2002a, 2002b; CDC 2005a). Eighty-five percent of AIDS in women in the United States alone occurs during their reproductive years (Mitchell et al. 1996: 67). Worldwide, most women become

infected during this stage of the life cycle as well (UNAIDS 2002a; Desgrees du Lou 1999).

Reproduction is essential to perpetuate the species and the group.
There are cultural pressures and expectations on women to reproduce.
Becoming mothers for most women globally is the event that grants them
full adulthood in society. Within patrilineal and bilateral descent groups,
producing a son also serves to continue the kin group and thus raises
women's status. In general, women who do not reproduce and become
mothers risk ostracism, scorn, loss of status, and possible divorce, with
the consequent shame and stigma. These cultural expectations provide a
necessary framework for understanding women with HIV/AIDS or who
are at risk for infection and the realities they face about childbearing and
rearing (Desgrees du Lou 1999).

Reproductively, there are biological and sociocultural variables that
make women's experience of HIV unique. In most societies, fertility and
reproduction are the women's responsibility (Bolin and Whelehan 1999;
Desgrees du Lou 1999). As such, women carry most of the burden of reproduction: pregnancy, birth, and lactation. Because becoming pregnant
can result in infection and mothers can transmit HIV to their fetuses during pregnancy or birth and to their infants through breast-feeding, women
experience HIV reproductively in ways that men do not (Ammann and
Rubenstein 2000; Karim 2000; Fowler 2000; Van de Perre 2000; Anon.
2002; O'Gara and Martin 1996; White 1999; Burke 2004).

As with sex, women in industrialized societies face different risks for
HIV during reproduction than do women in nonindustrialized societies.
First, only about 10 percent of women worldwide know their HIV status
(White 1999: 5; UNAIDS 2006). (In contrast, about 75 percent of **People
Living With HIV/AIDS [PLWH/A]** in the United States know their HIV
status [Klein et al. 2003; CDC 2005b].) Most of those who know their
status live in industrialized societies (Synergy Project 2003). Thus, the
nature of sexual risk and HIV status is an unknown for most women. The
unknown risk of infection is one more risk that occurs in daily life and
does not outweigh the cultural expectation to bear children.

The risk of an HIV+ woman transmitting HIV to her fetus or infant is
variable. It is not 100 percent regardless of where she lives, and that adds
another layer of uncertainty to the situation. Without intervention, the
risk of passing HIV to a fetus during pregnancy or birth (perinatal transmission) ranges between about 16 percent to 25 percent in the United

States and is about 35 percent in nonindustrialized societies (Anderson 2001; Stine 1997; Desgrees du Lou 1999). The risk of perinatal transmission depends on the stage of the mother's infection, including her viral load, and her overall state of health (Anderson 2001; Fawzi 2000; Bulterys et al. 2000). It is important to realize that while women do not want to pass HIV onto their babies, they have internalized the very real and intense cultural pressures and expectations on them to reproduce and continue the kin group.

HIV+ Women and Reproduction

Attitudes about women with HIV who want children have changed in the United States since the first wave of the epidemic, as have the resources that are available to help them. In the first decade of the epidemic, HIV+ women were discouraged from becoming pregnant. There were several reasons for this. First, there were no drugs available then to prevent perinatal transmission. Second, there were few antiretroviral drugs available to treat the women, and there were fears that pregnancy could exacerbate HIV progression. These concerns later proved to be unfounded; pregnancy does not jeopardize an HIV+ woman's health (Anderson 2001; Rochman 2002a, 2002b).

Third, there was a punitive attitude toward HIV+ women who became pregnant: they were blamed for becoming pregnant and potentially infecting "innocent" fetuses. Since most women with HIV are poor and ethnic, this took on racist overtones. There were physicians in the 1980s who refused to care for HIV+ pregnant women (Feldman 1995; Shernoff 1999; Loue 1999). Fourth, those who were pregnant during the 1980s had limited options, because President Ronald Reagan's "gag rule" prohibited health-care workers other than physicians from discussing abortion with women (Rochman 2001b; The Alan Guttmacher Institute 2004). In addition, women were criticized for having babies when there was a high probability that they would not survive to raise the children to adulthood.

7.7

In contrast, women with other, more socially acceptable diseases such as diabetes generally do not receive the same kinds of medical and social censure for becoming pregnant and having children as women who are HIV+ have experienced.

Since 1994 in industrialized societies, the concern about HIV+ women becoming pregnant and passing the virus on to their children has shifted. AZT076 is a drug that dramatically reduces perinatal transmission during pregnancy and birth. Administering the drug from the second trimester of pregnancy through birth reduces the risk of transmission from 15–25 percent to about 3 percent (Fowler 2000; Anderson 2001). Alternatively, a shorter course of treatment may also work. As of 2006, HIV+ women in the United States who have access to and take ARVs during the second and third trimesters of pregnancy and during birth have a "statistically insignificant risk" of transmitting HIV to their fetus/newborn (Bartlett 2006: 50).

When we address the problems of HIV+ women bearing children or of dying and leaving dependent children in the United States, we are not facing the same dilemmas as women and children cross-culturally. For areas heavily impacted by the epidemic, having children holds the promise of continuing the group. For these HIV+ women, their children, even if orphaned, may be the virtual continuation of their culture (Desgrees du Lou 1999).

In nonindustrialized societies with higher rates of perinatal transmission and less ability to pay for a longer course of drugs, there are a couple of options available. Women can take either Nevirapine (a less expensive retroviral that is easier to administer) or a combination of Nevirapine and Combivir, which decreases the chances of later resistance to Nevirapine, to reduce perinatal transmission (Ammann and Rubenstein 2000; Marseille et al. 2000; Mirochnick 2000; WHO/CDC 2004; MEDSCAPE 2004; http://www.aids2004.org). Based on knowledge as of 2004, administering these drugs perinatally reduces transmission. Short-term as opposed to long-term usage of these drugs does not appear to negatively affect the pregnancy, fetus, birth process, or the infant postnatally. This is a dramatic improvement in preventing MTCT (Bulterys et al. 2000; Lindegren et al. 2000; Synergy Project 2003; Center for Health and Gender Equity 2004a; Gender_AIDS@healthdev.net).

Preventing MTCT requires knowing the mother's HIV status. As discussed in chapter 4, there are many ethical issues about whether to make prenatal testing mandatory or voluntary, when to test, and to whom to disclose results. In a study done in 2003 by the Synergy Project, women in Zambia, Kenya, and Tanzania were willing to be tested and disclose their results if they felt secure that they controlled the distribution of test results and if that disclosure did not bring negative consequences such as abandonment, ostracism, loss of economic security, or violence to them or their children (Synergy Project 2003).

In areas of the world where HIV prenatal testing is either unavailable or an HIV+ test result could endanger the women's well-being with her husband or among her kin group, other steps are taken to reduce perinatal transmission during childbirth. Traditional birth attendants (TBAs), or (traditional) midwives, are taught universal precautions. With TBAs, there is a reduction in the number of episiotomies (surgical incisions to open the introitus of the vagina), the number of pelvic exams done during labor, vaginal washings during labor, and caesarian sections (White 1999; Ammann and Rubenstein 2000; Anon. 2002; Karim 2000).

Once the baby is born, the concern for HIV transmission shifts to the risks involved in breast-feeding. This is a complicated issue and a difficult decision for women to make. Just as bearing and rearing children are culturally expected, so too is breast-feeding (O'Gara and Martin 1996). In most nonindustrialized societies, women engage in extended breast-feeding, nursing their children for a period of several months to several years. Breast-feeding is an important nutritional, immunological, and bonding event. Breast milk is nutritionally complete and provides the infant with the mother's antibodies to disease for a number of months (White 1999; WHO/CDC 2004). In areas where clean drinking water is not available, breast milk also protects children from infant diarrhea, a disease that kills eight million children a year (Anon. 2002; Child and Adolescent Health and Development 2003; Kahn et al. 2002; Burke 2004). In many parts of the world, if a woman did not breast-feed, she would be suspected of having HIV or of being a "bad mother" (Solomon et al. 2000; White 1999; Synergy Project 2003; Burke 2004).

If the mother is HIV infected, breast milk contains sufficient concentrations of HIV to be passed on to the infant (White 1999; Child and Adolescent Health and Development 2003). Risk of transmission varies depending on the mother's overall state of health, viral load, and whether she has sore or cracked nipples or her infant has mouth sores. The risk can range from 5 percent to 20 percent (Van de Perre 2000; Semba 2000; WHO/CDC 2004). The decision faced by women in nonindustrialized societies is do I breast-feed and risk transmitting HIV to my infant, or do I bottle feed (if she can afford the formula and supplies) and risk my child dying of infant diarrhea (in some places a much greater risk than HIV transmission)?

The World Health Organization revised its 1998 position on breast-feeding for women with HIV to its current recommendation (Lhotska and Armstrong 2000; WHO/CDC 2004). HIV+ women in industrialized societies who can afford bottle feeding and have access to clean water are encouraged to bottle feed to eliminate postnatal transmission of HIV to their children. For women in nonindustrialized societies, the WHO recommends exclusive breast-feeding for the first six months and then, if possible, to switch to bottle feeding. It strongly discourages **mixed feeding**, which combines breast- and bottle feeding. Mixed feeding increases the risks of infant diarrhea and decreases the health and nutritional benefits of breast-feeding (Child and Adolescent Health and Development 2003; WHO/CDC 2004). The risks that women from nonindustrialized societies face for HIV infection and transmission regarding sex, pregnancy, childbirth, and breast-feeding were eloquently summed up to me by a woman from Tobago who stated, "You white women worry about negotiating safer sex and your rights. We don't know from one week to the next whether we're infected or if we'll be alive" (personal communication at the Ninth International Conference on AIDS, 1993).

Given that having HIV/AIDS is ultimately a death sentence in most parts of the world and that access to HAART slows but does not eliminate HIV/AIDS in those who have access to it, HIV+ women must also face the reality of leaving orphaned children. This applies to women in both industrialized and nonindustrialized societies. Again, there are distinct differences in these women's experiences.

We who live in industrialized societies have become accustomed to losing our parents when we are adults and have lost the cultural memory of orphaned children, largely because of improved standards of health, immunizations, and other public health measures. We also have shifted our kinship structures from large, extended kin groups who took care of family members to smaller, nuclear families, dependent on non-kin-based organizations (for example, day care, friends, social services) to fulfill the needs of the extended kin group. HIV/AIDS has changed that, particularly for the ethnic women living in poverty who make up the vast majority of women with AIDS in the United States.

Most of the AIDS orphans (that is, children with one or both parents who have died of AIDS and who may or may not be HIV+ themselves) are children of African American women or Latinas. While grandparents are accepting responsibility for many of these children, they often are impoverished as well or have their own health problems. There is a pool of AIDS orphans in the United States who are dependent on social services for their care. In states such as California and New York that are heavily impacted by the epidemic, guardianships are being established for children whose parents have died of AIDS (Hudis and Brown 2002; Doran et al. 2002; Campbell 1999; Levine et al. 1996). Depending on the community where these orphans live and the resources available, they can receive various levels of acceptance.

As of 2005, there are an estimated fifteen million AIDS orphans, most of them living in sub-Saharan Africa and India (Solomon et al. 2000; UNAIDS 2002a; CNN 2004; http://www.aids2004.org). Whether or not they are taken in by the extended kin group depends on several factors. First, there have to be enough extended-kin-group members alive to take care of the children. In some villages in these two areas, all the adults are dead from AIDS and the children are left homeless (UNAIDS 2002a; Schoepf 2004; Desgrees du Lou 1999). Second, the stigma of AIDS can extend to the children. If they are shunned because of their mother's illness (AIDS is more stigmatic for women than for men), they may be left without caregivers. Third, AIDS has become a disease of poverty. Extended kin may or may not have the resources to care for another child, regardless of their desire to do so. Fourth, caring for orphans depends on the political and economic infrastructure of the society where they live. If there are resources such as TASO (see chapter 4), orphans may be provided for.

It is in the area of taking care of children orphaned by the effects of the epidemic that **Faith-Based Organizations (FBOs)** have had a dramatic positive impact. FBOs include formal religious organizations and groups that are allied with them. They have provided orphanages, schooling, and medical care to places heavily impacted by HIV/AIDS (UNFPA 2007b; Dilger 2007). A woman's HIV status and risk for HIV affects her, her children, and the larger group. Poverty and politics compound women's risk and HIV status.

Poverty, Politics, HIV/AIDS, and Women

Poverty, the larger economic practices in a society, and politics are inextricably linked to women's risk of HIV infection and their experience with it. Whereas HIV was initially diagnosed in middle-class men in North America, Europe, Brazil, and parts of sub-Saharan Africa, it has become a disease of the poor and dispossessed worldwide. Women are primarily affected by poverty. There are similarities as well as differences in how women in industrialized and nonindustrialized countries experience poverty. Both groups have poorer overall health, fewer resources at hand, and decreased access to resources, and they experience discrimination from formal structures in the larger society regarding receiving help. They face a greater risk of violence, abandonment, and loss of support groups when they have HIV/AIDS than do middle- and upper-class women (Synergy Project 2003; Women's Bulletin 2003; Schoepf 1993, 2003a, 2003b).

There are also differences in how poverty impacts women at risk for or with HIV/AIDS in industrialized and nonindustrialized societies. This section explores how poverty, larger societal economics, and political decisions affect women's risk of HIV infection and their experience of HIV/AIDS.

Women in the United States

Eighty-three percent of the women with AIDS in the United States are either African American or Latina; most of them live in poverty (UNAIDS 2006; Kates 2006; Kaiser Family Foundation 2006; http://www.aids2004.org). A significant number of them are also substance users or the sex partners of substance users (Simoni et al. 2000; Robinson et al. 2002; Raffaelli and Suarez-Al-Adam 1998; Schneider and Stoller 1995; Stoller 1998). This society has ambivalent attitudes about providing health care in general to poor people and to substance users (Bennett 1999; Hutton and Wissow 1991; McCaul et al. 1996; Rothenberg 1996; Acuff 1996; Allen 1996; Faden and Kass 1996). These attitudes are discriminatory because insured people have access to many elective medical procedures such as assisted reproductive technology to help infertile couples have children, drug rehabilitation programs, and care for their dependent children in addition to basic health care (Mayer and Pizer 2000; Aranda-Naranjo and Davis 2001; Singer 2005).

These attitudes are also discriminatory when one contrasts the response to HIV/AIDS with the response to other diseases. Many of our current health problems are lifestyle in origin: high blood pressure, much heart disease, diabetes, and some cancers such as skin cancer or lung cancer from smoking. Each of these has a strong behavioral component in terms of causing the disease. Yet they are accepted, treated, and incorporated into the health-care system with relatively little stigma, rejection, and punishment associated with them or the people who contract them.

Research consistently indicates that well-designed, culturally sensitive prevention programs are more cost-effective and efficient than treatment for HIV/AIDS (Mayer and Pizer 2000). However, the most effective prevention programs involve comprehensive education built around safer sex and safer needle and drug behaviors. The problems with developing and implementing effective programs that stress anything other than abstinence from both sex and drugs are discussed in chapters 5 and 6.

When impoverished ethnic women become infected, they also interact with health-care resources differently than do middle-class women. HAART is expensive, costing US$12,000–15,000 a year, depending on the particular regimen and follow-up care needed (Simoni et al. 2001; Rochman 2001a, 2002a, 2002b; Stine 1997). **AIDS Drug Assistance Programs (ADAP)** are available through individual states to defray the costs of HIV therapies. However, the availability in any given community is dependent on the vagaries of federal funding, the particular political and economic structure of the state receiving funding, the prevalence of AIDS in a community and state, and how disability laws regarding HIV/AIDS are interpreted (Kirkland 1998; Kaiser Family State Health Facts 2006b; NASTAD 2007). Impoverished, primarily ethnic women can easily fall through the bureaucratic cracks in HIV funding and care.

Accessibility to care is another issue facing women. Can they actually get to the health-care facility to receive care, find child care that is affordable while keeping medical and social service appointments, and receive care that is medically and socially appropriate and sensitive for them? Again, research indicates that there are differences in how middle-class and poor women experience this aspect of HIV. Impoverished women receive less care, and it is of poorer quality. They also enter the health-care system at a later stage of disease progression (Allen 1996; Ankrah et al. 1996; Auer 1996; Banks 1996; Bradley 1995).

Larger cultural, political, and social structures as well as values held within ethnic groups also impact women's risk of contracting HIV and their life with HIV/AIDS in the United States. This culture continues to economically and politically discriminate against the poor, with impoverished ethnic women receiving the brunt of the discrimination (Vernon 2001; Robinson et al. 2002; Raffaelli and Suarez-Al-Adam 1998). Political and economic policies that limit reproductive services and options and access to employment, child care, social services, and education all contribute to women's risk of HIV infection by influencing women's choices. If insisting on safer sex means that they face economic or social abandonment by a partner and will not have the economic resources to meet daily needs, then the decision not to practice safer sex is logical, reasonable, and relatively obvious. If the employment options available to them result in less income than receiving aid to dependent children and does not provide health care, then staying on welfare is an economically better decision (Ehrenreich 2002). These issues are discussed in more detail in chapter 8.

The values within various ethnic groups also impact women's risk of HIV infection in the United States. Since most women with AIDS are Latina or African American, looking at cultural beliefs about women and sex and women in relationships can shed light on risk. "Standing by your man" is a value shared by both groups; loyalty and psychosocially and emotionally supporting your man are part of being a good woman in these subcultures. Holding a family together is another value among African Americans and Latinas. These values can supersede any given decision to practice safer sex (Robinson et al. 2002; Kaisernetwork 2004a; Green and Sobo 2000; Margillo and Imahori 1998; Raffaelli and Suarez-Al-Adam 1998).

Being sexual is an important value in African American culture. Women are accepted as sexual beings; the expression of their sexuality may vary depending on their community and socioeconomic status. However, the value exists and is a positive statement about African American women. Interestingly, in the United States and elsewhere, it is women, not men, who are denied their sexuality. It is women who are told to "use condoms," practice safer sex, negotiate sex with their male partners (female-female sex is largely ignored; see chapter 5), and be monogamous. Current research into microbicides is directed toward women; there is not the same kind of energy, time, and resources devoted to having men who have sex with women change their sexual behavior, values, and attitudes or accept responsibility for their sexual behavior (Upton 2003; Gender-AIDSeForum 2003, 2004).

Women in Nonindustrialized Societies

In nonindustrialized societies, the issues plaguing women exist in a more complex cultural setting than in the United States. As discussed in chapters 2, 4, and 5, women in these societies often do not have economic, political, or social autonomy. Decisions about their health, sexuality, and risk of contracting HIV may be made by the kin group or their husbands. Women in these societies are generally in a more precarious economic, political, and social situation in that the larger socioeconomic and politi-

7.8

Since women's primary risk for HIV infection is from having unprotected penetrative sex with infected males, the issue of **sero-discordant couples** arises. Sero-discordance occurs when one partner is HIV- and the other is HIV+. In studies of sero-discordant couples, HIV- women believed that sexuality was denied and removed from the relationship. These women felt that health-care providers, counselors, and others focused on the HIV+ partner. In addition, women felt that it was primarily their responsibility to monitor safer sex and make the relationship "OK" for both themselves and their partners (Van Der Straten et al. 1998: abstract). These views reflect the larger sociocultural attitudes, beliefs, and patterns about gender, women's roles, and sexuality.

The risk of infection lies in the context of the relationship and the balance of power that exists there (Bajos and Marquet 2000; Barker et al. 1998). Two examples illustrate this point. As discussed, African American women carry the additional responsibility of being a buffer and source of support for their partners. Taking on these roles can serve to diminish women's sexuality as an entity of its own and women's right to their own sexual expression and satisfaction. Proportionately, Native Americans comprise the economically poorest sector of the United States. Native women have high rates of HIV, experience sexual violence, and tend to be in poor health overall, which limits their ability to "negotiate" safer sex (Walters and Simoni 2004: 3). As with the other groups of women we have discussed, placing the responsibility for prevention on the woman instead of her partner(s) or seeing prevention as a shared responsibility places further stress on women.

cal structures may be very fragile, compromised, and stressed in and of themselves (Barnett and Whiteside 2002; Schoepf 2004). Poverty is rampant in most of the world. Resources are limited. Warfare between groups and across borders disrupts social and economic life and creates desperate survival situations for people, particularly women (Schoepf 1993, 2003a, 2003b; Synergy Project 2003; Women's Bulletin 2003; Center for Health and Gender Equity 2004a, 2004b). Global Gag Rules imposed by President George W. Bush in 2003 and 2004 that would cut funds from any health-care setting that mentioned abortions put women in nonindustrialized societies at increased risk for both HIV and pregnancy. These centers often are the only place where women can get any health care, information about contraception and HIV, HIV testing, or treatment (Synergy Project 2003; Center for Health and Gender Equity 2004a, 2004b; UNAIDS/UN-FPA/UNIFEM 2004).

The availability and cost of drugs internationally are regulated by **PhRMA**, an international prescription drug group, and other major drug companies within the United States. They determine who gets what drugs, when, and at what price. These decisions are out of the control of the individual who needs the drugs. Providing effective HAART at afford-able costs in a way in which it can be used is the interest of humanitarian efforts such as the Bill and Melinda Gates Foundation and the William J. Clinton Presidential Foundation. It was the goal of the 3×5 initiative of the United Nations. The 3×5 initiative hoped to be able to provide HAART or other antiretrovirals to three million people who would otherwise not receive them by 2005 (Gender-AIDSeForum 2004; http://www.aids2004. org). That goal was not met and has been revised to 10×2010, that is, to have ten million people on ARVs by 2010. Currently, about 17–20 percent of the people who need the drugs receive them (UNAIDS 2006).

Research indicates that women in nonindustrialized societies will prac-tice safer sex, get tested, take HAART, and do what they can to prevent MTCT under the following conditions:

> Their physical safety and security and that of their children are as-sured.
>
> They are in control of getting tested, knowing the results, and de-ciding who has access to those results.
>
> They can practice safer sex, get tested, bottle feed their babies, and receive treatment without being economically or socially ostra-cized and abandoned by their husbands, their families, or their communities.
>
> They can access HAART or other antiretrovirals (Synergy Project 2003; Burke 2004).

Ethics, Women, and HIV/AIDS

The psychological, social, sexual, reproductive, economic, and political factors involved in women's risk of HIV infection and living with HIV/AIDS raise a number of ethical issues. These issues involve safer sex prac-tices, testing and disclosure, treatment options, parenting, and improving women's economic and political status in societies. There appear to be double standards of sexual behavior for safer sex for men and women in this culture and elsewhere: women are held responsible for their own and their male partner's sexual behavior, whereas men who have sex with women are rarely held accountable for their behavior. Programs that focus exclusively on women's practice of safer sex ignore the social, economic, and power differences that exist between men and women. Focusing on women to uphold some cultural sexual norm diminishes the importance of their sexual pleasure and needs and puts them in the position of being blamed if safer sex is not practiced, if they or their partners become infected, or if they transmit HIV to their fetus/child. Because of this focus on women, men are excused from practicing safer sex. Men need to be given correct information, culturally appropriate messages, and support to practice safer sex to protect themselves, their partners, and their families (Billowitz 2004; Bond 1997; LeClerc-Madlala 2001).

Ethical issues involved in mandatory versus voluntary HIV testing and mandatory versus voluntary testing of pregnant women are discussed in chapter 4. Placing the focus on the pregnant woman and not her partner means that she alone is held responsible for the HIV health of herself and her children. Since most women with HIV worldwide live in poverty and are more socially and politically disenfranchised than the middle class in their cultures, programs that establish one set of medical and reproductive standards for impoverished HIV+ women can take on sexist and racist overtones.

Encouraging women to practice safer sex or get tested when the results of doing so could cause them or their children bodily harm, economic loss, social abandonment, and ostracism increases their problems. Ignoring larger, structural economic and political conditions that cause interruptions in women's education and prevent their economic and political autonomy can undermine intervention efforts. HIV/AIDS is a complex phenomenon; it requires holistic, complex responses to reduce incidence and address the needs of those who are infected (Heald 2006).

Women are in a unique position relative to their risk of HIV infection. Biological, sociocultural, sexual, economic, and political factors in our culture and elsewhere put women at greater risk of infection than are men. Once women are infected, the course of HIV can affect not only the women but also their future children. Because women are the center of caregiving in most societies, the state of women's health directly impacts them, their children, and the larger group. The future and course of HIV globally may be measured by how we respond to women and AIDS.

SUMMARY

Women have been infected and affected by HIV/AIDS since the beginning of the epidemic.

Worldwide, women are the caregivers in society, and their health is poorer than men's.

Women's risk for HIV infection is influenced by both biological and sociocultural factors.

Women's sexuality and reproduction are defined and controlled by their culture.

Women's economic and political status affects their risk of infection and the course of the illness if they are infected.

Prevention efforts need to encourage MSW to be responsible for safer sex.

Thought Questions

What biocultural factors make women's risk of HIV infection and experiences with HIV/AIDS unique?

How do larger social, political, and economic structures and beliefs in various societies increase women's risk of contracting HIV?

Resources

Articles

Bajos, N., and J. Marquet. "Research on HIV Sexual Risk: Social Relations Based on Cross-Cultural Perspective." *Social Science and Medicine* 50, no. 11 (June 2000): 1533–46.

Parker, Richard G. 1994 "Sexual Cultures, HIV Transmission and AIDS Prevention." *AIDS* 8:S309–S314.

Van Der Straten, A., K. A. Vernon, K. R. Knight, C. A. Gomez, and Nancy S. Padian. "Managing HIV among Sero-Discordant Couples: Serostatus, Stigma, and Sex." *AIDS Care* 10, no. 5 (October 1998): 533–48.

Books

Corea, Gena. *The Invisible Epidemic: The Story of Women and AIDS.* New York: Harper and Collins, 1992.

Patton, Cindy. *Last Served? Gendering the HIV Epidemic.* Bristol, Penn.: Taylor and Francis, 1994.

Renaud, Michelle Lewis. *Women at the Crossroads: A Prostitute Community's Response to AIDS in Urban Senegal.* The Netherlands: Gordon and Breach Publishers, 1997.

Stoller, Nancy E. *Lessons from the Damned: Queers, Whores and Junkies Respond to AIDS.* New York: Routledge, 1998.

Videos

Bilheimer, Robert. *A Closer Walk.* Santa Monica, Calif.: Direct Cinema Limited, 2003.

Kleiman, V. *My Body's My Business.* Berkeley, Calif.: Cultural and Research Communication, 1992.

Reticker, G., and Amber Hollibaugh. *Heart of the Matter.* New York: First Run/Icarus Films, 1994.

Web Sites

Body, The: http://www.thebody.com.

Guttmacher Institute: http://www.guttmacher.org.

HealthDevelopmentNet: http://www.healthdev.net.

Human Rights Watch: http://www.hrw.org.

NASTAD (National Alliance of State and Territorial AIDS Directories). The ADAP Watch, August 16. http://www.nastad.org/Docs/Public/InFocus/2007816_NASTAD%20ADAP%20Watch%20–%208%2016%2007%20FINAL.pdf, accessed August 16, 2007.

8

The Politics and Economics of AIDS

CHAPTER HIGHLIGHTS INCLUDE

A discussion of how "the face of AIDS" has shifted toward a primarily poor, female, and ethnic profile

A discussion of how biases held by political leaders in the United States and cross-culturally have impacted the course of the epidemic

A discussion of the roles that the pharmaceutical companies and poverty play in prevention, testing, and treatment efforts in the United States and cross-culturally

A discussion of how political and economic policies and decisions about HIV/AIDS disproportionately affect women

A discussion of HIV/AIDS as a human rights issue

We cannot claim that competing challenges are more important, or more urgent. We must keep AIDS at the top of our political and practical agenda.

No progress will be achieved by being timid, refusing to face unpleasant facts, or prejudging our fellow human beings—still less by stigmatizing people living with HIV/AIDS. Let no one imagine that we can protect ourselves by building barriers between "us" and "them." In the ruthless world of AIDS, there is no us and them. And in that world, silence is death. On this World AIDS Day, I urge you to join me in speaking up loud and clear about HIV/AIDS. Join me in tearing down the walls of silence, stigma, and discrimination that surround the epidemic. Join me, because the fight against HIV/AIDS begins with you.

Kofi Annan, statements made on World AIDS Day, December 1, 2003
(United Nations Events and Observances 2003)

Overview of Politics and Economics

As discussed in previous chapters, the risk of contracting HIV and the experience of HIV/AIDS are inextricably linked with poverty and larger economic and political structures in a society. Economic and political variables themselves are interdependent in the roles they play in the AIDS pandemic. **Politics**, the formal decision-making processes found in a group, influence **economics**, the ways in which resources are accessed and distributed within a group. Politics and economics reinforce each other.

Both political and economic factors directly affect resource availability, access, and distribution. These variables have been part of the epidemic since the first diagnosed cases and continue to be major cofactors in risk and intervention efforts. Although HIV/AIDS initially appeared among middle-class or elite populations in North America, Western Europe, Brazil, and parts of Africa during the first wave of the epidemic in the 1980s, it has become a disease of the poor and dispossessed in the twenty-first century. This chapter explores the role that national and international economic and political structures and decisions play in the epidemic.

Political and economic structures are part of all societies. However, indigenous political and economic systems have changed because of the effects of colonization and Westernization over the past several hundred years. In addition, global markets have drastically increased over the past century, further changing these systems. These changes have resulted in qualitative shifts in social structures, loss of traditional subsistence patterns, and a combination of native and Euro-American beliefs and behaviors (Kottak 2000; Parker, Easton, and Klein 2000). These shifts are reflected in the risks for HIV/AIDS among ethnic groups in the United States and elsewhere.

Economics, Politics, and HIV/AIDS in the United States

The changing face of AIDS discussed in chapter 2 is clearly visible in the United States at the beginning of the twenty-first century. The initial appearance of AIDS among middle-class, Anglo, gay men was an economically and politically mixed situation. As a stigmatized group, gay men had few legal rights, and government denial about the seriousness and extent of HIV/AIDS in this population was predominant for much of the first wave of the epidemic (Shilts 1987; O'Leary and Jemmott 1996).

The federal government delayed acting on HIV/AIDS relative to funding research, education, and treatment. It did not initially perceive HIV/ AIDS as a serious health threat. Reinforcing myths and stereotypes about homosexuality, the administrative approach during the early 1980s presented HIV/AIDS as a gay man's disease. Ronald Reagan, president during the first decade of the epidemic, did not speak of AIDS openly until well into his second administration (Shilts 1987; Thomas 2001; Vernon 2001; Mayer and Pizer 2000: part 3). Reagan only officially acknowledged the disease and epidemic after Ryan White, a teenager who had hemophilia and contracted HIV through a blood transfusion, died (Thomas 2001). Ryan White's situation made HIV more "respectable" because it involved an "innocent victim," that is, a teenager who contracted the virus nonsexually through a medical procedure.

Denial also reinforced the perception of AIDS as a "gay disease" (or GRID [gay-related immune deficiency]; see chapter 2) by underplaying its presence in other populations that included IDUs, women, children, and ethnic minorities (Bastos et al. 1998; Simoni et al. 2000). The initial labeling of AIDS as GRID firmly established the perception that this was a disease that affected one population, and one that has been stigmatized at that. This denial resulted in a lack of funding for research, treatment, education, and prevention efforts (Thomas 2001).

However, the fact that AIDS was first diagnosed among an educated, white, middle-class, politically and economically savvy group also helped bring the disease to the country's attention. Gay groups organized to provide social and economic support to those infected, created community-based organizations such as the Gay Men's Health Crisis (the oldest AIDS service organization in the country) in New York, and initiated the safer sex movement. This population had the resources to help themselves (Bastos 1999; Stoller 1998; ACTUP 2003). Had AIDS first been diagnosed within the populations currently seriously affected by the virus (IDUs and

---

8.1

Bathhouses are found in gay-friendly areas. They are sociosexual meeting places for MSM. Public health controversies involving bathhouses as "vectors of infection" led to the closing of several of them around the country in the 1980s. However, in 2006, Gay Men's Health Crisis, the oldest HIV CBO in the United States, found that bathhouses can serve as a venue for eroticizing safer sex, for encouraging safer sex practices, and as an educational medium about HIV/AIDS (Kaiser Daily HIV/AIDS Report 2006h).

Latino/as, African Americans, and Native Americans living in poverty), progress in controlling the epidemic could have been delayed further. These advances included isolating the virus, developing an HIV antibody test and antiretroviral drugs, and implementing safer sex and safer needle-usage campaigns (Institute of Medicine 2001; Anon. 2000b).

By the second wave of the epidemic in the 1990s, the reaction to HIV/AIDS in the United States had become somewhat dualistic. There were the "innocent victims" of the epidemic, including infected children, people who contracted the virus through medical procedures, and the sexual partners of those people who lied about their HIV status. There was a different attitude toward the people who "deserved" to be infected: gays, prostitutes, "promiscuous" people, IDUs. Moralistic judgments have been made about these populations. Groups, not behavior, were seen as being at high risk for infection and responsible for the prevalence of HIV/AIDS in the population (Stoller 1998; Mayer and Pizer 2000; Pott 2000; Institute of Medicine 2001). For example, bisexual men were blamed for bringing the virus into the heterosexual population (Rust 2000). The judgmental attitude toward people in these groups can be contrasted with that exhibited toward people who eat high-fat diets and get no exercise. We do not see them as deserving of having a heart attack. Blaming groups and imposing stigma on behavior tends to create shame and drive that behavior underground, making intervention efforts more difficult.

Economics, Politics, Risks, and Subcultures

The primary means of HIV transmission continues to be unprotected anal and vaginal intercourse. Chapter 5 has a discussion of the difficulties involved in implementing age-, gender-, ethnic-, and sexual-subculture-appropriate comprehensive sex and HIV education programs in the United States. These problems extend to the information on federally funded Web sites such as those of the CDC and the National Institutes of Health (NIH). The Bush administration has altered safer sex information about condom efficacy and has emphasized abstinence as the only appropriate prevention method (TAC 2004a; Planned Parenthood Federation of America 2004; Center for Health and Gender Equity 2004a, 2004b). In addition, three surgeons general—Koop, Elders, and Satcher—who have promoted comprehensive HIV and sex education as prevention strategies since the 1980s all received serious sanction from their respective presidents—Ronald Reagan and William Clinton (Elders 1994; *HIVPlus* 2002a; SIECUS

2003). Elders, in fact, was fired for her statements (see chapter 5). The George W. Bush administration will only support abstinence-only programs in the United States. We will see later in the chapter the problems created by his position on international HIV/AIDS prevention support, which is likewise primarily focused on abstinence.

Injection drug use is second to unprotected sex as a means of transmitting HIV in the United States. As of 2004, most states heavily impacted by HIV/AIDS have needle exchange programs (Editorial Desk *New York Times* 2004). However, their implementation remains controversial, and funding and operation of the programs are subject to local, state, and federal policies. This controversy continues despite recommendations and documented evaluations of their benefits from well-respected organizations such as the Institute of Medicine and the **National Institute of Drug Abuse (NIDA)** (Institute of Medicine 2001; DesJarlais et al. 1998; Anon. 2000b; Buchanan et al. 2004; see also chapter 6).

Substance abuse in this society also results in a high rate of incarceration, particularly if one is ethnic and poor; estimates indicate that 80 percent of the people in prison are there on drug-related charges (Francis and Cargill 2001: 330; Kane and Mason 2001; Waterston 1997). Drug rehabilitation rarely occurs in prison settings, and in many cases there are few options for safer sex in prison.

In prison, the chances of either becoming HIV infected or being reinfected increase. There is variable medical care for HIV+ inmates and few guarantees of confidentiality while incarcerated (see Stimson, DesJarlais, and Ball 1998). While unprotected sex and drug usage are common in prisons, one study of prison guards revealed that only 20 percent of them believed that condoms, bleach to clean injection equipment, or harm-reduction programs should be available to inmates (Abeni et al. 1998; Barrett and Robinson 1996). Confidentiality is difficult to maintain within this population, and that can impact decisions to get tested and receive treatment (Francis and Cargill 2001; Cheever 2001).

In 1993, the CDC redefined what constituted an AIDS diagnosis, which more realistically reflected the situation of infected women. This change not only resulted in a dramatic increase in the number of AIDS cases found among women but also meant that services previously unavailable to women who were HIV positive but did not meet the prior CDC criteria for an AIDS diagnosis could finally be accessed.

The situation regarding women and AIDS in the United States has improved in the third wave of the epidemic. However, women continue to be diagnosed later than men and continue to be seen as the vectors of sexual transmission. Women die sooner from AIDS than do men, and most of the attention is focused on their reproductive role in HIV transmission rather than looking at them as individuals and how gender is socially constructed (Greenblatt and Hessol 2001; *HIVPlus* 2002b; Anderson 2001; Patton 1994). This is due more to gender bias, poverty, and politics than to hormones, pregnancy, and childbirth. Gender-role expectations within ethnic groups and the larger society, violence, and pronatalism interact to increase women's risk for HIV and affect the course of the disease once they are infected (Loue 1999; White 1999; Patton 1994; Banks 1996; Monti-Catania 1997; Treichler 1999; see chapters 5 and 7).

Once women become infected, economics and politics affect women differently than men. Most women with HIV/AIDS are of reproductive age and have children. Therefore, efforts to include them in clinical drug trials and to provide them with HAART and other medical care need to consider not only the women's health but also their child-caring and other obligations. Women without child care or transportation and who are also taking care of other social obligations may need help to adhere to HAART or to keep medical appointments. There are few programs that consider and provide for these other contingencies in their lives (AmFar 2001; Korvick 1996; Lather and Smitheres 1997; Powers 1991). In addition, if the women are substance users and impoverished, they probably will have fewer treatment options available and stand a greater risk of losing their children (Francis and Cargill 2001; Waterston 1997; Kane and Mason 2001; see chapter 7 for a discussion of U.S. and cross-cultural factors in perinatal transmission).

Ethnicity interfaces with sexual, substance use, gender, economic, and political variables (Ramos 1997; Wilkinson 1997; Zierler and Krieger 2000). As discussed in chapter 2, by the late twentieth century, the "face of HIV/AIDS" had shifted to disproportionately affect non-Anglo populations. Most of these people are also impoverished, thereby having worse overall health than middle-class people, and exhibit varying degrees of trust in mainstream health care and political decisions. According to some research, poverty, racism, and access to health care are more fundamental causes of the problems with HIV in the African American community than are indigenous beliefs about family, sex, and women (Loue 1995, 1999; Trotter et al. 1995; SIECUS 2005; Parker, Barbosa, and Aggleton 2000).

For African American men, economic pressures and larger cultural messages about masculinity, including sexual prowess and economic success, reinforce values of virility and heterosexuality as a measure of worth. Poverty, substandard housing, and the relatively easy access to drugs increase the risk of HIV infection. Since HIV/AIDS is still seen as a "gay, white boy's" disease in this community, safer sex practices may be inconsistent (Robinson et al. 2002).

HIV+ African Americans' access to health care and treatment reflects the economic and ethnic discrepancies of health care in the United States (Loue 1999; Anderson 2001; Zierler and Krieger 2000). There are fewer clinical trials that include African Americans and other ethnic groups (*HIV-Plus* 2002a). HAART is expensive. The cost can range from US$12,000 to US$15,000 a year, depending on the regimen (*HIVPlus* 2002a). African Americans are less well insured than Anglos. Medicare programs that include HIV care are susceptible to federal government budget fluctuations (McGuire 2000; Kaiser Family State Health Facts 2006b).

There are differences in the ways in which African American and Anglo substance users are treated legally and medically. Among middle-class Anglo communities, drug dependency is more often considered a disease, with detox and rehabilitation programs and facilities available. Health insurance may also pay at least a part of their cost. Drug dependency within the African American community is more often seen as a crime by the larger society. There are higher rates of incarceration and removal of children from families, particularly for female substance users, in African American communities than in Anglo ones (Schneider and Stoller 1995; Perrone et al. 1989). The combination of social, economic, and political factors in the African American community contributes to the risk for HIV infection, the higher incidence and prevalence rates found, and lower survival rates among this group. As discussed in chapter 6, racism and sex phobia exists within and between subcultures as well.

The Economics and Politics of HIV Testing

The development of an HIV antibody test in 1985 raised numerous political and economic concerns. With the availability of the test, some conservative groups called for mandatory HIV testing of people in "high-risk groups" or for "immoral behavior," with quarantines for those who tested HIV+ during the first decade of the epidemic (Shilts 1987). The states of Illinois and Louisiana even required HIV premarital testing for a brief time but abandoned this requirement because it was economically unfeasible and people could circumvent the test by going to a neighboring state to get married (Bayer 2000; McGuire 2000; Farmer et al. 2000; Owens 1998; AIDS Action Committee 2005). Fortunately, the calls for quarantines have ended. The incidences of overt discrimination in housing, employment, education, and medical care have diminished greatly since the first wave of the epidemic (Kirkland 1998; Stine 1997; ACTUP 2003; Bastos 1999; Americans with Disabilities Act 2004).

Generally, HIV testing in the United States is voluntary (see chapter 4). The debate over mandatory versus voluntary testing primarily resides with pregnant women (Bennett and Erin 1999; Faden et al. 1991; Stoto et al. 1999; Hutton and Wissow 1991). Although HIV testing is recommended for pregnant women, in 2002 about 50 percent of pregnant women received information about and requested an HIV test (Rochman 2002a, 2002b). As discussed in chapter 4, as of 2003, the CDC recommends opt-out testing for pregnant women, whereby they receive an HIV antibody test unless they sign a waiver declining one. Since most pregnant women with HIV are ethnic and poor, opt-out testing has the potential for being discriminatory because of language or literacy barriers (see chapters 4 and 7).

The CDC exerts political and economic pressure on states that have confidential HIV test sites. As a major provider of HIV-test funding to states, the CDC requires states to adopt mandatory name reporting at confidential test sites. States such as New York, which has the highest incidence of HIV/AIDS in the country, then must choose to either comply with the HIV mandate or lose several million dollars worth of funding. New York State chose to comply (Office of the Medical Director 2000).

The decision to get tested has political and economic ramifications for the individual as well. Before HAART was available, some people decided not to get tested and to practice safer sex instead, since knowing that one was HIV+ without having effective treatments meant dealing with an almost-certain death sentence (Bartlett 2002; Owens 1998; Loue 1999). HIV antibody tests are not free, though alternative test sites often offer the test on a sliding scale. Reporting an HIV test to one's insurance company or asking the insurance company to cover the cost of an HIV test can result in higher premiums or dropped coverage, particularly if one is HIV+ (Bartlett 2002). As of 2003, an estimated 25 percent of the people who are HIV+ do not know their status, and an estimated 40 percent of people

---

8.2

On September 22, 2006, the CDC issued a statement endorsing routine, opt-out HIV testing with assent (but not written informed consent) and with a minimum of pre- and posttest counseling. This is an attempt to address the 25 percent of the HIV+ people in the United States who do not know their status. The response to this proposal has varied. A recent survey conducted by the Kaiser Family Foundation concerning attitudes toward HIV testing in the United States revealed the following:

- More African Americans and Latinos than Anglos have been tested in the past year.
- Sixty-two percent of those surveyed in general believe that there would be no stigma if friends or family found out that they had had a HIV test (this is for having the test only; not for learning that they were HIV+ if that were the case). Twenty-one percent of the people surveyed believe that people would think less of them for having a test.
- Sixty-seven percent of those surveyed believe that the test should be routine, while about twenty-five percent believe that written consent and other "special procedures" should be followed before having a HIV test (Kaiser Public Opinion Spotlight 2006; MMWR 2006b).

---

with HIV do not know their status until they develop AIDS-like symptoms (Klein et al. 2003; CDC 2003a).

The Economics and Politics of Vaccine and Drug Development and Treatment

Economics and politics also factor into vaccine development and HIV treatment. The first decade of the epidemic was fraught with medical frustration and discovery, economic roadblocks and funding opportunities, medical avoidance of people with HIV/AIDS, heroic medical efforts, and career building (Bayer and Oppenheimer 2000; Daniels 1995; Epstein 1996; Shilts 1987; Feldman 1995). Once the virus was discovered and an antibody test developed and made available, funding for HIV/AIDS vaccine and treatment research became more acceptable and available (Shilts 1987; Thomas 2001). In the third decade of the epidemic, with neither a

---

8.3

The controversies surrounding access to and distribution and cost of ARVs both within the United States and cross-culturally continue. In the fall of 2006, Senator Edward Kennedy and Representative Henry Waxman asked for an investigation of U.S. trade agreements and international health (Kennedy and Waxman 2006).

---

vaccine nor a cure available, controversies about funding research, financing prevention efforts versus developing a vaccine, and finding a cure continue. Most of the ARVs are financially out of reach for the vast majority of the people worldwide who are HIV+ or have AIDS. The drug companies such as Merck that make many of the ARVs believe that the high costs of the drugs allow for research. However, only about 14 percent of drug-company income actually goes toward research (Moynihan and Cassels 2005).

Within biomedicine, there is a split between academic and institute researchers ("pure scientists") and applied scientists (practicing physicians) (Thomas 2001). Pure scientists tend to want to understand the mechanism of the virus; applied scientists tend to want to create a vaccine that can prevent infection or slow the progression of the virus in infected people.

According to Patricia Thomas, a medical journalist, this division applies to HIV vaccine development. In her book, *Big Shot: Passion, Politics, and the Struggle for an AIDS Vaccine,* Thomas details the struggle at places such as the NIH and CDC as well as at private laboratories and research facilities in developing an effective HIV vaccine. Research funding is finite; HIV/AIDS research must compete for money with other medical projects that are less controversial and more acceptable, such as diabetes and heart disease. Her book describes national and international efforts to not only develop a vaccine but also work collaboratively if one becomes available. Thailand, for example, is working with the U.S. Army on creating a vaccine. Thailand has also stipulated that it is willing to conduct clinical trials among its population as long as Thai people are not abandoned once a vaccine becomes available (Thomas 2001). As of 2008, there is no preventive vaccine for HIV.

Part of the problem in developing a vaccine rests with a bias in biomedical research and practice. The bias is to treat the disease first. This means that money that might be put into vaccine research is spent on treatment.

People who are ill want help now; vaccines are less likely to help them than drugs to ease symptoms, treat infections, or slow the progression of the virus. Researchers and medical people are sensitive and sympathetic to this need (ACTUP 2003; Shilts 1987; Thomas 2001; Grady 1995).

ACTUP (discussed in chapter 2) was one of the first community-based organizations to actively and aggressively protest the cost of antiretrovirals, the length of time required to make drugs available to people, and research protocols. Their efforts in the first two waves of the epidemic, before they came to support Duesberg, pressured major pharmaceutical companies to reduce prices and push new treatments through the approval process (ACTUP 2003; Thomas 2001; Shilts 1987). These changes included greater sensitivity to what constitutes informed consent, and more patient involvement in health-care decisions, resulting in a less authoritarian doctor-patient relationship. These changes also laid the groundwork for women to be included in clinical trials of anti-HIV drugs (Bastos 1999; Thomas 2001; Loue 1999; Epstein 1996).

Activism also challenged medical ethics concerning whether physicians and other health-care workers could refuse to treat people living with HIV/AIDS (PLWH/A). Those doctors who did treat PLWH/As during the first wave of the epidemic have come to be seen as heroes in parts of the AIDS community (Feldman 1995; Bastos 1999; Bayer and Oppenheimer 2000; Daniels 1995; Epstein 1996). They treated patients and conducted research when fears about transmission and lack of institutional or peer support were common. Ironically, these activist efforts also factored into slowing interest in an HIV vaccine, as funds were directed into drugs (Thomas 2001).

There are challenges that face the pharmaceutical industry as well. They include developing, testing, marketing, and making available anti-HIV drugs that are safe, effective, tolerable, and affordable (Anon. 2000b; Bloom et al. 1997; Innocenti and Pilling 2001; Palmedo 2002). A significant part of this process involves clinical trials. Clinical trials are the three-part research and development efforts required by the FDA before a drug can be made available. Who is involved in these clinical trials and who receives the drugs after they have gained FDA approval are additional aspects of the economics and politics of AIDS.

Until the mid-1990s, middle-class Anglo males were the primary subjects involved in clinical trials for antiretrovirals. Women and people from various ethnic groups were largely omitted from the trials but were then prescribed the same drugs after their approval. The sexism and racism inherent in this approach are apparent; the concern that these drugs could affect women and ethnic minorities differently than middle-class white men is a related consideration (Thomas 2001; Korvick 1996).

Including women in clinical trials is important. If there are aspects of the drugs that specifically affect women gynecologically, reproductively, or sexually, it is important to know this before drugs are approved (Long 1996; Tavris 1992). Many drug trials also provide health care during the trial and/or provide a stipend for being part of the study. Since most women infected with HIV are also ethnic and poor, excluding them from clinical trials meant that they lost an avenue for health care and for HIV treatment (Powers 1991; Korvick 1996). The inclusion of women in drug trials more recently has also needed to incorporate cultural sensitivity regarding confidentiality, community and kin-group norms, child care, and transportation requirements to keep the women involved (AmFar 2001; Lather and Smitheres 1997; Loue 1999).

The safety and efficacy of HAART are major considerations for anyone taking it. HAART is analogous to being on chemotherapy for the rest of one's life. These drugs have toxic side effects. There needs to be careful monitoring of liver, kidney, and heart functioning as well as bone integrity while on them (Schooley 1996; Wormser and Horowitz 1996; Volberding et al. 1999). HAART can involve specific food restrictions and proscriptions against alcohol usage as well as time adherence for dosage. Until the advent in 2004 of **Fixed Dosage Combination (FDC)** drugs that require fewer pills taken less often, people developed a life around adherence to their anti-HIV drug regimens. Adherence to HIV therapy can be a major issue for some people.

Having to deal with the safety and efficacy of HAART presumes that people can afford the drugs. As stated, HAART is expensive. Specific drugs, such as T-20 (used by people who are resistant to other drug combinations), can cost US$15,000–20,000 a year for just the one drug (Palmedo 2002; Holtgrave 1998; Anon. 2000a, 2000b). How are people going to pay for HAART, particularly given that most PLWH/As are poor?

People with private insurance may be able to defray some costs; Medicaid and Medicare pay for some for those who economically qualify. ADAP operates in states to offset the cost of HAART (Anon. 2000b). However, with the exception of private insurance, these other programs are subject to the vagaries of federal funding. Politically conservative administrations tend to cut or reduce funding for these programs; liberal ones tend to maintain them.

Drug companies also bear responsibility for drug costs. While it is expensive to develop, test, market, and receive approval for drugs, most of the costs do not go toward developing new drugs. Most of the costs go toward making similar drugs and toward drug companies' profits (ABC News 2004; Moynihan and Cassels 2005). Activists since the late 1980s have protested the cost of anti-HIV drugs here and cross-culturally (ACTUP 2003; Thomas 2001). The current revolt against large pharmaceutical companies' fees for HAART is a major topic in the discussion of politics and economics outside the United States later in this chapter.

People on HAART live longer and are able to resume work and other activities. The reintegration of HIV-infected people and PLWH/As into the workforce involves the **Americans with Disabilities Act (ADA)**. PLWAs have been protected by the ADA since the 1980s. In 1998, being HIV+ was included and protected (Americans with Disabilities Act 2004).

There are direct economic, political, and confidentiality issues involved with covering HIV+ people under ADA. Workplaces may need to provide accommodations for people with HIV/AIDS relative to areas where they can take or store medications, or disability-accessible work environments for people returning to work. Who is going to pay for this: the employer, the government, grants? If people at work or children in school need to take HAART during the workday or school day, how is this done while maintaining confidentiality? If AIDS becomes a chronic but manageable disease similar to other diseases such as arthritis or diabetes, will it remain a disability, and will it still protected by ADA? These are very difficult and complicated issues. There have been lawsuits over what must or may be covered in these situations (*HIVPlus* 2002b).

Politics and economics play important roles in every aspect of HIV, from prevention efforts involving education and testing to treatment. They also impact risk. If people are not given correct HIV prevention information, because of political and economic pressure to provide abstinence-only programs, that affects risk. If people are judged as immoral, sinful, or dirty based on either their behavior or their membership in a group that is heavily impacted by the epidemic, this affects their risk by creating shame, driving behavior underground, and encouraging people not to seek help. Providing or recommending condoms to "high-risk groups" stigmatizes people in those communities and implies that the rest of the population is not at risk (Parker and Aggleton 1999).

If HIV testing is prejudicially used for or against certain groups or if community norms about confidentiality are not respected, that discourages people from getting tested. If HAART is unaffordable, then people will not get the drugs they need, escalating health care costs, loss, and trauma (Barnett and Whiteside 2002; McGuire 2000; Farmer et al. 2000). Research consistently indicates that effective prevention is more cost-effective than treatment (Barnett and Whiteside 2002; Mayer and Pizer 2000).

There are community-based and nongovernmental programs that have been successful in reducing risk. The California Prostitutes/Prevention Education Program (CALPEP) is one such agency. It has been in existence for more than twenty years and currently is located in Oakland, California. I have been actively involved with CALPEP since 1994 and have known its director, Ms. Gloria Lockett, since 1987. This program, originally created to reduce the risk of HIV infection among street prostitutes in San Francisco, has expanded to include other populations such as the homeless, substance users, and adolescents. CALPEP has engaged in a variety of HIV prevention efforts, including HIV testing and safer sex street outreach, and now is working on reducing the risk of transmission for people who are HIV+. The survival of a community-based organization such as CALPEP, however, often depends on receiving grants that may be subject to governmental approval or funding. CALPEP has managed to weather local, state, and national economic and political challenges by adapting and being flexible to the changing needs of the community it serves and to redefinitions of what is fundable by the state and national agencies.

Successful programs in the United States that survive budget cuts and changing political atmospheres appear to embody the following characteristics:

> They are adaptable and flexible.
> They accommodate the changing face of AIDS.
> They are aware of and respond to larger political and economic shifts and seek out multiple sources of funding.
> They hire and involve people from the community, incorporate community values, and are grounded in a grassroots approach.
> They are holistic and relativistic and follow harm-reduction models appropriate to their population (Office of the Surgeon General 2001; Institute of Medicine 2001; Waterston 1997).

These characteristics can serve as a model for developing and implementing programs.

Politics, Economics, and HIV/AIDS Cross-Culturally

"AIDS . . . is more than a health issue. This is a social issue, this is a political issue, this is an economic issue, this is an issue of poverty. It is an issue of the destruction of a society" (Colin Powell, former U.S. secretary of state, commenting about the AIDS epidemic in Africa during a four-nation tour of Africa in 2001 quoted in Quist-Arcton 2001).

The economic and political gulf between the experience of HIV/AIDS in the United States and other industrialized countries and the experience in nonindustrialized ones is qualitative (Greenblatt and Hessol 2001; Anon. 2000a). As controversial as the politics and economics of HIV/AIDS are in industrialized countries, they become even more so when dealing with those countries that are not. There are numerous reasons for these differences.

People in industrialized countries tend to have better overall health, nutrition, and education and higher socioeconomic status with concomitant access to goods and services than do people living elsewhere (Wolffers and Josie 1999). The availability of AZT076 since 1994 for pregnant women and of HAART since 1996 in the United States are two examples that illustrate the gap between AIDS here and elsewhere.

In much of the nonindustrialized world, daily life involves struggle for economic survival at the most basic level relative to procuring food, clothing, and shelter. Living at what is considered this most basic level of existence creates its own risk for infection. For example, poverty sets the foundation for a thriving sex-work industry as an economic survival strategy that pays better than other available work and in which decisions about safer sex are tied to economics (see chapters 5 and 7) (Pitayanon et al. 1997; Seabrook 2001; Beyrer 1998; Rogers et al. 2002; Steffan and Kraus 2000; Wolffers and Bevers 1997).

In societies such as Haiti and much of sub-Saharan Africa, where tuberculosis (TB), malaria, and malnutrition are immediate and daily health threats, the risk of HIV infection appears to be more remote. Feeding and taking care of one's children, one's self, and the extended kin group require one's first and primary attention (Greenblatt and Hessol 2001; Basu et al. 2000; Farmer 1992, 1999; Farmer et al. 1996, 2000). South Africa's President Mbeki's position that poverty rather than HIV is the cause of AIDS, while incorrect, takes on a different connotation in this context

---

8.4

Most people in sub-Saharan Africa live on less than one U.S. dollar per day. With the cheapest ARVs costing several hundred dollars a year, this means that based on affordability alone, treatment is beyond the means of most PLWH/As. In addition, for those who do have access to drugs and live longer as result, there is a good chance that these people will become resistant to the first-tier ARVs they were originally prescribed and will need to move to second-tier drugs, which are even more expensive. With HIV+ people who receive the drugs living longer, there also needs to be sustained prevention intervention support to reduce the transmission of HIV to their sex and needle-sharing partners. Although people are less infectious once they are on an effective ARV regimen, there is still a risk for infection. The complexities of HIV infection, prevention, and treatment are pervasive and require a holistic response.

(Cherry 2000a, 2000b; TAC 2004a; see chapter 2). Poverty is a significant cofactor in both the risk of infection and the progression of the virus once infected.

The effects of cultural change over the past several hundred years also impact the risk of HIV infection. Anthropologically, **syncretism** is the emergent behaviors, beliefs, and norms that result from culture contact and change. We have seen evidence of syncretism in examples of sexual practices in subcultures in the United States, Brazil, and sub-Saharan Africa, as discussed in chapters 5 and 7. Syncretism is also reflected in economic and political practices.

Increasing Westernization over the past several hundred years and twentieth-century globalization altered traditional economic, political, and social patterns in much of sub-Saharan Africa, India, Southeast Asia, and Native North America. Women lost their traditional economic base and their autonomy (Vernon 2001; Pitayanon et al. 1997; Bloom et al. 1997; Orubuloye and Orguntimehin 1999; Wolffers and Josie 1999; Wolffers and Bevers 1997). For example, they lost control over goods and services they provided. Women in Africa and India living under British colonization became subject to British inheritance and property rights, which turned their property over to their husbands and fathers (White 1990; Setel 1999; Orubuloye et al. 1994). Both indigenous and Euro-American expectations of women as caregivers, good wives, and mothers reinforced putting the needs and welfare of others before their own (Hogan 2001; Carovano and Schietings 1996). Christian views of sexuality changed traditional marriage and sexual practices, driving some of them, including previously accepted same-sex sexual behavior, underground (Susser 2001; Teunis 2001; Setel 1999; Orubuloye et al. 1994; AFROL 2003). These changes provided a socioeconomic and political backdrop for HIV and AIDS (Mufune 2003; Rasing 2003; Stanley 1999).

Fear and HIV/AIDS

People outside industrialized societies clearly experience the devastation of HIV/AIDS and do not want to get infected. However, their fear of infection occurs in the context of the realities of daily life. Immediate concerns for economic survival and pressing health issues take precedence. They also have a love-hate relationship with Euro-American economic, political, and medical policies and practices. On the one hand, antibiotics, immunizations, and HAART save lives; on the other hand, unethical research and imposition of Euro-American economic and political structures have hurt numerous groups and individuals (Bastos 1999; Grady 1995; Moatti and Spire 2000; Adams and Pigg 2005; De la Gorgendière 2005; LeClerc-Madlala 2005; see chapter 2). Fear fuels conspiracy theories about the origins of HIV/AIDS (as discussed in chapter 2) and the skepticism behind being used as test cases for vaccine development or drug trials (Thomas 2001; Lather and Smitheres 1997; Burhansstipanov et al. 1997;http://www.aids2004.org).

Fear and ignorance are behind the belief within some groups that having p-v intercourse with a virgin will prevent HIV/AIDS. This behavior puts the female at risk from the men who are choosing perceived or known virgins as sex partners and brings in the question of whether the sex is coerced or consensual (Setel 1999; Orubuloye et al. 1994; LeClerc-Madlala 2001). Fear can reinforce denial, thus increasing the risk of infection. Countering the fear requires not only accurate information and respect for local norms about confidentiality but also dissemination of information through respected leaders and access to resources (Thornton 2002; Dilger 2007).

Developing culturally sensitive, safe environments with language and behaviors that are meaningful to the target audience are important strategies (Vollmer 2000; Orubuloye et al. 1994; Setel 1999). Examples of successful strategies have occurred in include areas of India, Africa, and

China. Truck drivers who have sex along their trade routes in India and areas of sub-Saharan Africa are finding HIV information along the truck routes. In India, the information is provided in the form of tea parties (Marck 1999). In Tanzania, Zimbabwe, and Kenya, there are road-stop informational centers (Setel 1999; Bujra 2000). Providing safer sex information and condoms to men who have sex with women is a way of reducing heterosexual transmission of HIV and having men assume responsibility for their sexual behavior (South African Development Commission 2006).

In the twenty-first century, China is working to counteract the stigma and fear around HIV/AIDS that dominated much of its policy decisions during the 1980s and 1990s. Recent efforts in China include developing its own antiretrovirals to distribute among its HIV+ population and vaccine research, increasing education among the populace and health-care workers, and efforts to reduce the stigma about HIV through awareness and through providing correct prevention information (Anon. 2004b; Cohen 2004a, 2004b; Hepeng 2004).

Using local leaders and incorporating traditional customs are also effective parts of treatment efforts (Vollmer 2000; Thornton 2002). For example, in India, anti-HIV drugs are dispensed by indigenous healers as well as at clinics. India uses a combination of biomedical and traditional practices and treatments (AmFar Treatment Insider 2002b, 2002c; d'Adesky 2002a).

Politics, Economics, and HIV Decision Making

From data presented in chapters 4 and 7, we know that people outside the United States will have an HIV test if they feel safe, can test and get results in the same visit, and control the dissemination of the test results. However, other factors also enter into the decision to get an HIV test. The major variables are getting accurate information about testing, having access to a test site, and having access to antiretrovirals if people test positive. In most places of the world, people who receive an HIV+ test result do not have access to drugs. It is roughly analogous to decisions to get tested in the 1980s in the United States, when there was a lack of drugs to maintain T-cells and suppress viral load.

Politics and economics exert a direct influence on the dissemination of HIV information. While most people worldwide have heard about or witnessed the effects of HIV/AIDS within their communities, access to

---

8.5

Lesotho and Botswana are two countries in South Africa with a high prevalence of HIV/AIDS. They are also countries that have or are implementing universal, voluntary HIV testing. While the intentions are to identify and treat people who are HIV+ and to prevent HIV transmission to sex partners and perinatally, there are concerns about confidentiality and how voluntary these policies are. Human rights groups have urged caution and oversight of the universal HIV testing policies for these two countries (Kaiser Daily HIV/AIDS Report 2005, 2006d).

---

accurate information about the disease is lacking. Casual-contact fears abound, and access to safer sex and needle-usage information and supplies do not match the awareness about the illness (Bankole et al. 2004; Human Rights Watch 2004). The most accurate and available information about HIV/AIDS cross-culturally is found where NGOs and CBOs exist. NGOs and CBOs are found more often in urban areas. Brazil, India, Thailand, Uganda, and Indonesia are some examples of countries that have or have had effective HIV/AIDS intervention programs in some of their urban areas (Hogan 2001; Preston-Whyte 1999; Orubuloye et al. 1994; Setel 1999). These programs work around governmental and religious opposition, tend to focus on literate populations, and work with charitable and international organizations to obtain and keep funding.

8.6

President George W. Bush's multiyear and multibillion-dollar AIDS relief program, the **President's Emergency Plan for AIDS Relief (PEPFAR)**, and his reimposition of the Global Gag Rule regarding sex workers, needle exchange, and comprehensive reproductive health care have generated much controversy. PEPFAR only recently allowed generic drugs to be distributed to the fifteen countries in the program. Thirty percent of all prevention funds must be allocated to abstinence-only programs, which is posited as one possible factor in the recent increase of HIV in Uganda (Kaiser Daily HIV/AIDS Report 2006e, 2006f).

Safer sex programs must address the behaviors and values within their targeted groups. Uganda's ABC model has been discussed as a controversial safer sex program (Allen 2002; see chapter 5). However, in the spring of 2004, Yoweri Kaguta Musveni, president of Uganda, potentially bowed to the economic pressure exerted by the Bush administration's AIDS relief plan to focus on abstinence-only programs (TAC 2004a; http://www. aids2004.org). This is an example of external, international political and economic influence on program implementation. As of 2006, Musveni is increasingly supporting abstinence-only programs (Kaiser Daily HIV/ AIDS Reports 2006e).

The internal economic realities and external economic pressures on nonindustrialized societies affected by HIV/AIDS are startling. Given that 80 percent of AIDS worldwide exists in sub-Saharan Africa alone and that most PLWH/As currently are poor and politically disenfranchised, it is reasonable to see poverty as a primary cofactor in HIV infection (see chapter 2; Bastos 1999; Barnett and Whiteside 2002; Basu et al. 2000; Lyttleton 2000).

Economic stability and viability provide an infrastructure for intervention efforts, including prevention, production of and availability of treatments, and provision of medical care. Without either a stable economic infrastructure or individual and group resources to provide outreach and medical facilities and buy the drugs, most PLWH/As face a death sentence. Some societies (such as in India, Thailand, and Brazil) are manufacturing their own generic versions of HAART in response to the cost of brand-name drugs, and PhRMA, an international group of drug companies, sets the prices of and access to prescription drugs (Bastos 1999; d'Adesky 2002a, 2002c; TAC 2004a; Center for Health and Gender Equity 2004b; Okie 2006).

The cost of HAART, however, is only one of the economic aspects of the epidemic. The loss of productive labor due to illness and death exacts another toll from societies heavily impacted by AIDS. As of 2002, 25 percent of South African females between the ages of twenty and twenty-nine are HIV+. More than 40 percent of South Africa's teachers have died of AIDS. Economic projections indicate that by 2010, South Africa's national economy will be reduced by US$22 billion (Anon. 2002).

In Zimbabwe and Zambia, a child born in 2000 was more likely than not to die of AIDS (Anon. 2000a: 1). The life expectancy for people in countries for whom greater than 5 percent of the population has HIV/AIDS, which includes most of sub-Saharan Africa, has decreased from sixty-four years to forty-seven years over the course of the pandemic (Anon. 2000a: 1). Much of sub-Saharan Africa remains agrarian; the urban areas are more industrialized. With HIV/AIDS prevalence and incidence rates this high, the economic, social, and political futures of many of these societies are bleak.

In India, the economic impact of adults who are dying of AIDS creates household poverty. The loss of adult wage earners burdens extended kin groups. Economic responsibilities can shift to these groups (Basu et al. 1997). Members of upper-caste households are left without an income, since many of the women do not work outside the home. Overall, the economic losses in India due to AIDS exceed ten times its per capita income (Bloom and Mahal 1997: 10). India is predicted to have the largest number of AIDS cases in the future. With a population exceeding one billion (1,000,000,000), India will have a proportionately large number of people with HIV/AIDS (Bloom and Mahal 1997; UNAIDS 2006).

Unlike the United States, Brazil, and some parts of Africa, HIV/AIDS first occurred among the poorest people in Thailand. This left that population with few resources and contributed to young females in particular entering sex work as a survival strategy (Seabrook 2001; Lyttleton 2000; Pitayanon et al. 1997). Programs that were effective to reduce HIV transmission in the 1980s and 1990s need continued support to suppress the currently increasing rates of HIV in Thailand (Altman 2004).

After the dissolution of the Soviet Union, rapid social and economic changes occurred within the former Soviet republics (Somlai et al. 2002). Changes included intra- and intergroup conflict, an increased illegal drug trade, and adult and child prostitution within and across borders (Rosenbrock and Wright 2000; Steffan and Kraus 2000; Somlai et al. 2002). Coerced work also involves sweatshops and child and slave labor. In Eastern Europe, drugs and prostitution are cofactors in susceptibility to the virus (Steffan and Kraus 2000). Women who are forced into these forms of work across Eastern Europe tend to be young, have few marketable skills, and have little ability to negotiate safer sex with their clients. Many of these women are unable to establish their own businesses and work for managers in brothels who control their working conditions, including safer sex practices (Amnesty International 2002). Intervention efforts need to address safer sex practices for the clients; viable economic options for the women who want to avoid entering sex work and for those who want to leave it; and overall reduction in the stigma associated with these women.

HIV/AIDS generally infects people in their most productive and re-productive years. By reducing the adult labor force, HIV/AIDS affects a group's gross national product, interrupts the socialization of the young, and compromises the overall quality of life of the group (Anon. 2000a, 2001). Thus, it can directly affect the survival of individuals and their group.

8.7

An additional depletion of the workforce in sub-Saharan Africa is "**brain drain**." Brain drain refers to the practice of industrialized countries, particularly the United States and Great Britain, hiring professionals from nonindustrialized societies to fill positions in health care and engineering. These professionals leave their native countries for better pay, benefits, and safer and more comfortable working conditions, and the hiring countries gain professionals who will work for lower pay and benefits. This practice results in fewer qualified professionals in areas of the world already overstretched on resources, leaving serious shortages in the health-care and industrial sectors in their home countries. There have been international calls to end brain drain by improving the infrastructure of the sending nations and of sending interns from industrialized countries to help train workers and provide services to underserved areas (Kaiser Daily HIV/AIDS Report 2006a; Adams and Pigg 2005; Bond 1997; Jooma 2006; IOM/HDN Project Team 2005).

These economic considerations particularly affect women in nonindustrialized societies. They are the ones whose education is most often interrupted when adult caregivers die. Women are the ones encouraged to be monogamous and held responsible if they or their partners or their infants become infected. They are the ones with the fewest social, political, and economic resources, and they are most severely stigmatized for having the disease (Synergy Project 2003; Center for Health and Gender Equity 2004a, 2004b; Human Rights Watch 2004).

Women need economic opportunities that are under their control and offer them viable means of supporting themselves and their families. This can take the form of small businesses, restoration of earlier economic trade networks that existed in various parts of sub-Saharan Africa, education, and the ability to access and control the distribution of their income (Basu et al. 1997; Kurth 1993; Outwater 1996; Patton 1994; Steffan and Kraus 2000; Setel 1999; Bond 1997; Schoepf 2004).

Politics is inseparable from this discussion of economics and AIDS outside the United States. The situation in Thailand regarding the development of an HIV vaccine is an example of this connection. There are vaccine trials occurring in Thailand, Brazil, parts of sub-Saharan Africa, and the United States. Thailand agreed to participate in these trials with the United States (and the U.S. Army) as long as any effective vaccine that was developed stayed in Thailand. Thailand stipulated that pharmaceutical companies cannot test the vaccine on Thais and then take the rights to it out of the country and sell it back to Thailand. The agreement also stated that informed consent had to meet Thai standards and be implemented before vaccine trials could begin. Finally, Thailand insisted that some form of compensation was to be agreed upon in case adverse reactions to the vaccine occurred. In making these conditions, Thailand showed that it could take steps to protect its population and still be able to take advantage of biomedical technology (Thomas 2001).

Perhaps the most dramatic example of the power that external political and economic forces have on the AIDS pandemic concerns the availability of, access to, and distribution of HAART and other antiretrovirals. PhRMA, which includes a number of United States–based drug companies, limits and sets prices for HAART and other retrovirals. The United States has been sued for its attempts to block the use of generic drugs in sub-Saharan Africa and has repeatedly backed out of international trade agreements that would make cheaper but effective drugs available. Most

---

8.8

The debate over the cost of, access to, and use of generic ARVs rather than brand-name drugs is often framed as a discussion over intellectual property rights and how they apply in an international context. The Doha Declaration of 2001 stated that public health takes priority over the protection of patents. The controversy centers on what constitutes the "threat" to public health and for how long. Brazil is one country that broke patent rights to provide ARVs to its HIV+ population. This debate is ongoing and far from resolved (Westerhaus and Castro 2006).

recently, President Bush's opposition to the World Health Organization's recommendation of using Fixed Dosage Combinations (FDCs) for people without access to them in nonindustrialized societies has engendered additional criticism of our government's international AIDS policies. FDCs are combined antiretroviral drugs that need to be taken only twice a day, with fewer pills, and at less expense. (TAC 2004a; Love 2003; Palmedo 2002; http://www.aids2004.org).

President Bush also reinstituted the Global Gag Rule and put forward his US$15 billion AIDS intervention plan. The Global Gag Rule withdraws United States funds from any international agency that mentions or provides abortions as part of its services, similar to Reagan's "gag rule" in this country in 1980s. Most of these organizations are NGOs and CBOs, and the only place where people, women in particular, can receive health care, contraceptives, and HIV information and services (Center for Health and Gender Equity 2004a, 2004b). The Global Gag Rule also extends to N/SEPs and to agencies that work with sex workers (Ditmore 2005; http://www.pepfarwatch.org).

In fact, to receive PEPFAR funds, agencies that work with sex workers must sign an oath, commonly referred to as the "Anti-Prostitution Pledge," which states that they openly oppose sex trafficking and prostitution. What constitutes "sex trafficking" and "prostitution" is left undefined. Frequently, NGOs and CBOs are the only place sex workers/prostitutes can go for condoms, health check-ups, and contraceptive and HIV prevention information. Having to publicly denounce the people for whom groups are trying to provide services is counterproductive. This funding criterion has generated international debate and a lawsuit against the U.S. government on First Amendment grounds. The legal decisions and appeals are still in process (Masenior and Beyrer 2007).

President Bush's AIDS relief plan to places such as Haiti and countries in sub-Saharan Africa would provide US$5 billion per year to countries heavily impacted by AIDS. However, one-third of that money must go toward abstinence-only programs. Condoms would only be available to "high-risk groups"—prostitutes, drug users, and MSM. This not only stigmatizes condom use but also ignores the reality of people's sexual behaviors. As of 2006, only some of the money pledged has been encumbered for AIDS relief. The stipulations about who can receive how much money and for what is helping some people but stifling prevention and treatment efforts for others (TAC 2004a; SIECUS 2005; South African Development Commission 2006). Interestingly, 56 percent of the U.S. public surveyed believe that the federal government is not doing enough to address the AIDS epidemic domestically or internationally; 36 percent believe that HIV/AIDS is the second most serious health problem in the United States after cancer; and 34 percent believe that it is the greatest health threat in the world (Kaiser Public Opinion Spotlight 2006).

More hopefully, both the Bill and Melinda Gates Foundation and the William Jefferson Clinton Foundation continue to provide AIDS relief, primarily in the form of treatments, to nonindustrialized societies. Smaller corporations such as MAC Cosmetics also contribute to HIV/AIDS relief (U.S. Philanthropic Commitments for HIV/AIDS 2006). In addition, the **Treatment Action Campaign (TAC)** poses a challenge to President Mbeki and South Africa's Health Ministry's position on HIV and AIDS (TAC 2004a, 2004b; see chapter 2). TAC is an activist group working to provide HIV/AIDS education, prevention, and treatment to people in South Africa. TAC has the support of both WHO and UNAIDS. In 2003, TAC filed a lawsuit against the Health Ministry of South Africa. The lawsuit "demands" that governments provide standard, medically accepted, prevention and treatment resources to PLWAs, including AZT076 and Nevirapine to pregnant women to reduce MTCT (TAC 2004a, 2004b). These struggles continue.

Successful interventions outside the United States incorporate a number of strategies. Brooke Schoepf is an anthropologist who has worked in Africa since the 1980s to establish programs that reduce transmission. Highly critical of the U.S. government's international AIDS efforts, she and many others have recommendations about what works to reduce transmission. General recommendations by her and others include the following:

Involve the communities in program development and implementation.

Know local sexual norms and behaviors and develop programs that consider them.

Provide safer sex options that not only reflect community norms but also are available without discrimination, stigma, and judgmental attitudes.

Create programs that are holistic and address other pressing economic issues as well.

Provide viable alternatives to breast-feeding and drugs that are accessible and affordable.

Work with kin groups and communities to foster tolerance and accurate HIV information.

Use traditional values and beliefs that support safer sex practices, value women and men, and emphasize kin group and community cooperation.

Provide educational and economic opportunities for women (Schoepf 1993, 2001, 2003a, 2003b, 2004; Teunis 2001; Gifford et al. 1999; Sobo 1995; Susser 2001; Basuki et al. 2002).

HIV/AIDS and Human Rights

The HIV/AIDS pandemic can be seen as a human rights issue, particularly as it impacts disenfranchised groups, the poor, and women. Chapters 2, 4, 5, 6, and 7 discuss various aspects of human rights relative to HIV/AIDS. These aspects—stigma, discrimination, sexual exploitation, testing, and the role of women—all exist within political and economic contexts. Ethical concerns about research, testing, and treatment discussed in the current and previous chapters include a human rights component.

Kofi Annan's statement about HIV/AIDS as a human rights concern opened this chapter. There are a number of steps that need to occur to protect human rights, including

developing and implementing comprehensive, holistic, culturally relativistic and sensitive prevention efforts;

strengthening political and economic infrastructures in areas heavily impacted by AIDS to reduce cofactors of poverty, malnutrition, and other diseases that impair the immune system, disrupt people's lives, and increase their risks for infection;

increasing educational and economic autonomy for women;

providing education and support for engaging in safer sex practices for MSW (South African Development Commission 2006);

correcting casual contact fears;

reducing stigma; and

consulting with local leaders and incorporating indigenous health measures into intervention efforts (Dowsett 1999; Gifford et al. 1999; Bhutani and Khanna 2001; Susser 2001; Grady 1995; Geller and Kass 1991; Human Rights Watch 2004).

The political and economic aspects of HIV/AIDS cross international boundaries, span the life cycle, and include gender and ethnic considerations. Political and economic variables have the potential either to be significant cofactors in the risk of infection and the course of the disease or to provide the resources that can help to reduce risk, alleviate suffering, and control the spread of infection. Understanding the intricate roles that political and economic factors play in the epidemic requires community, local, regional, and global awareness, sensitivity to cultural differences, and collaboration to effectively reduce the risk of infection.

SUMMARY

Politics and economics are interdependent and have been inextricably connected to the AIDS pandemic since the beginning of the epidemic.

Conservative politics in both the United States and elsewhere increase the risk for HIV infection and impede research efforts, resource availability, and resource allocation.

Intrasocietal and intersocietal political and economic decisions affect risk, intervention efforts, program availability, and success.

Political and economic decisions can disproportionately negatively affect women and the poor.

Successful programs are holistic, nonjudgmental, interdisciplinary, and geared toward the specific needs of the target population.

Thought Questions

What are the economic and political variables that affect both risk for HIV infection and the course of the disease among different populations?

How have culture change, Euro-American colonization, and global economic and political policies impacted the risk of infection and the response to HIV/AIDS in nonindustrialized societies?

Resources

Articles

Stanley, Laura D. "Transforming AIDS: The Moral Management of Stigmatized Identity." *Anthropology and Medicine* 6, no. 1 (April 1999): 103–20.

Books

Alexander, Priscilla. *Totem and Taboo: AIDS and Prostitution.* London: Taylor and Francis, 1995.

Farmer, Paul. *AIDS and Accusation: Haiti and the Geography of Blame.* Comparative Studies of Health Systems and Medical Care 33. Berkeley: University of California Press, 1992.

Gostlin, Lawrence O., and Zita Lazzarini. *Human Rights and Public Health in the AIDS Pandemic.* New York: Oxford University Press, 1997.

Seabrook, Jeremy. *Travels in the Skin Trade: Tourism and the Sex Industry.* 2nd ed. Sterling, Va.: Pluto Press, 2001.

Setel, Philip. *A Plague of Paradoxes: AIDS, Culture, and Demography in Northern Tanzania.* Chicago: University of Chicago Press, 1999.

Shilts, Randy. *And the Band Played On: Politics, People, and the AIDS Epidemic.* New York: St. Martin's Press, 1987.

Thomas, Patricia. *Big Shot: Passion, Politics, and the Struggle for an AIDS Vaccine.* New York: Public Affairs Books, 2001.

Video

Bilheimer, Robert. *A Closer Walk.* Santa Monica, Calif.: Direct Cinema Limited, 2003.

Web Sites

ADA (Americans with Disabilities Act): http://www.usdoj.gov/crt/ada/adahom1.htm.

Global Fund: http://www.theglobalfund.org.

Henry J. Kaiser Family Foundation (Kaisernetwork and Kaiser Daily AIDS/HIV Report): http://www.kff.org.

Masenior, Nicole Franck, and Chris Beyrer. "The U.S. Anti-Prostitution Pledge: First Amendment Challenges and Public Health Priorities." *PLoS Med* 4, no. 7 (2007): e207. http://medicine.plosjournals.org/perlserv/?request=get-documents&doi=10.1371/journal.pmed.0040207, accessed July 24, 2007.

South African Development Commission: http://www.sadc.int/attachments/news/SADCPrevReport.pdf.

Treatment Action Campaign (TAC): http://www.tac.org.za.

UNAIDS: http://www.UNAIDS.com.

World Bank: http://www.worldbank.org/.

9

The Sociopsychological Aspects
of HIV/AIDS

CHAPTER HIGHLIGHTS INCLUDE

A discussion of how stigma affects the sociopsychological aspects of HIV/AIDS for people with the virus and their communities

A discussion of the sociopsychological issues facing people with HIV/AIDS in the United States and cross-culturally

A discussion of the sociopsychological dimensions facing the caregivers, family, and friends of people with HIV/AIDS in the United States and cross-culturally

> If it [HIV test] is positive it will be difficult for me to the extent that I will die; I will kill myself. There would be quarrels in my family. There would be no peace of mind. My husband would leave the house. Keeping the children, I would suffer, wondering whether I would live or die.
>
> Statement from a pregnant HIV+ woman in India (Van Hollen 2007: 8)

The Sociopsychological Aspects of Stigma

The associations among stigma, fear, and AIDS are almost universal (Green and Sobo 2000; Alexander 1996; Stoller 1998; ICRW 2005; Kruger and Richter 2003; Lyttleton 2004; Moore et al. 2006). The specific sociopsychological aspects of stigma vary by gender, ethnicity, risk factors, and modes of transmission and whether one lives in an industrialized or nonindustrialized society (Lyttleton 2004; ICRW 2005). While shame, fear, and grief are human emotions all associated with stigma, their triggers and expression are culturally constructed.

In nonindustrialized societies, stigma and fear take on survival characteristics. AIDS-related stigma can become a death sentence when it results in the inability to obtain food, clothing, and shelter and leads to rejection by your kin group, and where there are no social services to provide these necessities. In some parts of India, Thailand, and sub-Saharan Africa, stigma and ostracism may accompany HIV testing, safer sex practices, or bottle feeding. Denial, fear, and lack of or inconsistent prevention efforts can take precedence in these areas to avoid AIDS-associated stigma (Anon. 2000a; Solomon et al. 2000; Orubuloye et al. 1994; Beyrer 1998; Burhansstipanov et al. 1997; Lather and Smitheres 1997; ICRW 2005).

HIV/AIDS differs from other diseases of the twentieth and twenty-first centuries in the degree and kind of stigma associated with it (Herdt 2001; Solomon et al. 2000; Beyrer 1998; Hedge 1999; Green and Sobo 2000; Patton 1994; Singer 2003b). Factors that contribute to this include the modes of transmission (primarily unprotected sex and drug/needle usage), the fatal nature of the disease, and the disfigurement that is caused by some OIs. As discussed in chapters 5, 7 and 8, specific gender, socioeconomic, and ethnic variables can impact the effect of stigma as well.

Stigma, Sex, Gender, Orientation, and Drugs

As a primarily sexually transmitted disease, HIV evokes strong cultural responses about appropriate sexual behavior. HIV/AIDS exposes generally private behavior and sexual experiences to public scrutiny. Sex education in many cultures traditionally is seen as private or as occurring intergenerationally within the kin group, not in public settings (Orubuloye et al. 1994; Setel 1999; Rasing 2003: 4). The influence of Christianity and of Euro-American attitudes about sexuality cross-culturally contributes to the sexual stigma associated with HIV/AIDS as well (Orubuloye et al. 1994; White 1990; Setel 1999; ICRW 2005; Dilger 2007; Pfeiffer 2004). In societies that view sex as primarily for reproduction and assign negative religious judgments to sex outside of that context, discussions about safer sex other than abstinence and monogamy can evoke social censure for the people involved (Dolcini and Catania 2000; Bonivento 2001). The censure extends to discussions of gender and sexual orientations (Diaz 1998). As discussed in chapter 8, President Bush's international AIDS program that emphasizes monogamy and abstinence with condoms available only for "high-risk groups"—that is, prostitutes, gay men, drug users, and "those who cannot be abstinent or monogamous"—reinforces the stigma around sexual behaviors, safer sex messages, and condom usage (Feuer 2004a; ICRW 2005).

HIV-infected IDUs experience dual stigmas from their drug use and HIV status. Female IDUs tend to disclose their status to their male sexual partners more often than male IDUs disclose to their female sexual partners. These women, therefore, potentially face a greater chance of rejection by their male partners than do males by their female partners. Intervention and treatment programs need to address the dual stigmas. Treatment programs that address these issues have greater chances of success (Metsch et al. 2001; Anderson 2001; Roth and Fuller 1998).

Women collectively experience AIDS stigma. While WSW are generally ignored in the epidemic, WSM are held responsible for not only their own but also their male partner's behavior (Alexander 1996; Orubuloye et al. 1994; Patton 1994). WSM are seen as horizontal and vertical "vectors of transmission" to their sex partners and children. They are blamed for heterosexual transmission of HIV, for lapses in safer sex practices with men, and for infecting "innocent fetuses and children" (Patton 1994; Murrain 1997; Lyttleton 2004; Kruger and Richter 2003; see chapters 5 and 7).

Associating sexuality negatively with either proscribed behavior or membership in disenfranchised groups impedes comprehensive prevention efforts and increases stigma. For example, the association of condoms with drug users, with people in sexual communities, and with "promiscuity" creates the perception that if people practice safer sex, then they are drug addicts, gay, sexually immoral, or untrustworthy. Concomitantly, if one is a member of these groups, then one often is perceived as having HIV or AIDS. Practicing safer sex thus increases suspicions about people's behavior and moral worth with sex partners, family, and the community. It may also provide a false sense of security: if I am married, am not a drug user, and do not identify as "gay," then I am "protected" from HIV and do not need to practice safer sex.

9.1

Ironically, the life-saving drugs people take can also affect people's body image. Lipodystrophy, a condition where body fat is redistributed, is one side effect of taking some ARVs.

Stigma, Illness, and Death

HIV stigma occurs relative to the disfiguration that can accompany OIs and the high AIDS mortality rates. Full-blown AIDS can create highly visible physical changes in the person. There can be large, purplish lesions from Kaposi's sarcoma, an OI common among MSM. Wasting syndrome, called "The Slims" in many parts of sub-Saharan Africa, depletes body mass, leaving people looking skeletal. The physical signs of AIDS are very noticeable, making PLWH/As stand out from the rest of the group.

The high mortality rates of AIDS in the United States during the first two waves of the epidemic and in nonindustrialized countries since the 1980s contribute to AIDS stigma. Death is a physical, symbolic, and subjectively viewed part of life. Cultural responses to death vary, but most societies recognize death as a serious loss to the group. Losing large numbers of one's group, particularly those who are young and productive members, places burdens on the society as a whole. These include immediate and direct economic and social losses such as loss of labor and income and a lack of people to carry out daily nonwage work (Basu et al. 1997; Lyttleton 2004; http://www.aids2004.org). Without an income or laborers, households and kin groups cannot be maintained. The illness dimensions of HIV/AIDS relate to the symbolic aspects of death.

Attitudes about disease causation and process and the afterlife become part of AIDS stigma. These attitudes include misinformation, casual-contact fears about transmission, and religious explanations about the morality of disease and death. Among some Christian groups in the United States and elsewhere, AIDS is seen as retribution for an "immoral" lifestyle (Synergy Project 2003; TAC 2004a; Mayer and Pizer 2000). HIV/AIDS often is associated with violations of social norms and rules (ICRW 2005). Rarely do communities perceive HIV neutrally as a virus that infects people, causing disease and death.

Beliefs about the afterlife influence the degree of stigma associated with AIDS. If HIV/AIDS violates social norms, then an afterlife that is structured as punitive or exclusionary or part of witchcraft becomes associated with HIV. One is a bad or evil person for having HIV and will be punished in the afterlife for being bad.

Fatalism is another symbolic and religious belief that affects HIV risk and stigma. Research indicates that people who are fatalistic are less likely to practice safer sex and feel that they have little control over whether they become infected or over the course of the disease if infected (Ramirez et

---

9.2

Faith-based organizations (FBOs) such as the African American church in the United States and Pentecostal and Islamic groups in sub-Saharan Africa are a core element of many groups (Dilger 2007; Pfeiffer 2004; Howell 2007). Strategies need to be developed to work with these organizations and their leaders about prevention methods. The primary means of transmission worldwide—unprotected sex and needle usage—involve behaviors that are often private, censured, and have a number of taboos associated with them. FBOs and their affiliates may hold moralistic views about sexuality and drug usage (Bonivento 2001; UNFPA 2007b; Pfeiffer 2004; Dilger 2007). To reduce risk and respect individuals' and groups' religious views, intervention efforts with FBOs need to take a "bottom-up" approach by working with leaders in FBOs to mitigate stigma and negativity associated with HIV/AIDS (Howell 2007; Dilger 2007).

---

al. 2002; Orubuloye and Orguntimehin 1999; Awusabo-Asare et al. 1999). This is shown by the attitudes of some adolescent males in Tanzania, in a study of men in Nigeria, and in studies of groups of sex workers in Southeast Asia (Bujra 2000; Amadora-Nolasco et al. 2001; Basuki et al. 2002; Bond et al. 1996; Orubuloye and Orguntimehin 1999).

Because HIV/AIDS is primarily a disease of the poor worldwide, the stigma of poverty and the stigma of HIV/AIDS reinforce each other (Basu et al. 2000; Setel 1999; Seabrook 2001; Feuer 2004b). HIV/AIDS highlights all that the poor lack: overall health, resources, status, and access to prevention and treatment. Poverty combined with drug usage and marginalization not only increases the chances of infection but also contributes to the lack of care and to ostracism once infected. Stigma itself almost acts as a cofactor for infection and for the ability to receive treatment (Basu et al. 2000; Moore et al. 2006; ICRW 2005).

In Thailand, AIDS stigma persists and can extend to the entire family. If younger members of the Thai kin group die from AIDS, then the elderly are left without a basis of socioeconomic support. One response to counteract the stigma has been to develop work collectives for women whose husbands have died of AIDS. Work collectives provide income for the immediate and extended kin group and a potential source of sociopsychological support for the widows (Beyrer 1998; Pitayanon et al. 1997). Social support groups for people with HIV/AIDS have appeared in northern Thailand over the past several years. Largely comprised of women, they serve to re-establish a Buddhist sense of order and balance in those who are infected and have helped to destigmatize the disease (Lyttleton 2004).

Stigma and Grief

HIV/AIDS stigma affects the grieving process. Grief is culturally defined and expressed. It is a way of accepting and surviving loss individually and societally. Because HIV/AIDS is stigmatized, expressing grief over AIDS deaths often is hidden or denied. Socially created support mechanisms may not apply to AIDS deaths if the deceased is shunned and survivors are ostracized, thus creating no outlet for individual or group grief.

Survivors may also experience guilt by association for knowing or being family members of the person who died from AIDS. They may not experience whatever healing processes exist in the culture because they, too, are stigmatized for knowing the person with AIDS. Additionally, the sheer quantity of AIDS deaths within a group can be overwhelming. There may not be extended kin left to bury the body and perform funeral rituals, take care of dependent children, or help surviving members cope financially, psychologically, or emotionally (Schoofs 1999).

The enormity of multiple AIDS deaths affects the grieving process. The loss of one's entire support group, one's entire kin group, or one's entire community to the virus impacts coping mechanisms and the ability to grieve. AIDS isolates individuals, groups, and communities. If one has HIV, then the death of others from the virus is a symbolic precursor of one's own future. For both the infected and uninfected survivors, it is another marker of all who have been lost and the increasing narrowing of one's world. For example, a friend of mine was a graphic designer with AIDS. Several months before his death, he stated, "In three months, I lost fifteen people in my support group to AIDS. They were all gone. I had a meltdown."

Using the group's spiritual and symbolic structures to ease the death and dying process helps people cope with grief. It can help the survivors function. Ongoing educational campaigns that address misinformation about transmission and address casual-contact fears may eventually reduce the stigma associated with AIDS (Hogan 2001; Catalan 1999; ICRW

2005). Positive messages about treatment of people with HIV/AIDS may also reduce stigma, making it easier for people to get tested and to cope with the disease. To be effective, these efforts need to be continuous, widespread, and nonjudgmental and should originate from within the group.

Peer education can be more effective in providing psychosocial support than that which derives from authority figures. Research on adolescents in both South Africa and the United States indicates that peer socialization and support can positively impact safer sex practices and reduce the degree of stigma associated with HIV/AIDS (Kruger and Richter 2003). Use of traditional values and beliefs to educate and provide support presents information in a familiar context. Efforts to establish trust and respect for Euro-American research and pharmaceutical groups are important steps in promoting drug adherence. Societally, shoring up the ecological, political, and economic infrastructure among groups heavily impacted by AIDS will help to reduce cofactors in HIV transmission. Once again, a holistic, integrated approach is called for.

Sociopsychological Issues for People with HIV/AIDS

There are multiple sociopsychological issues for people with HIV/AIDS. They vary by culture and over the course of the disease and include facing one's own illness and mortality as well as managing social and sexual relationships with others. One of the initial issues is whether to have an HIV test (see chapter 4). If treatments are not available for people who test positive or to prevent MTCT, are the risks of getting testing worth the potential social disruption if others learn the test results (Solomon et al. 2000; Synergy Project 2003)? Testing positive raises immediate issues about confidentiality, sexual behavior, children, illness, and mortality (Green and Sobo 2000; Johnston 1995; Kanuha 2000; ICRW 2005). There are also concerns about one's psychological state upon receiving an HIV+ test result. Although the risk of committing suicide is highest upon first finding out one's HIV+ status, few people actually attempt suicide (Mitchell 1999). Well-developed pre- and posttest counseling can help to mitigate this risk (see chapter 4).

Receiving an AIDS diagnosis is much different from receiving HIV+ test results. AIDS is medically more serious. Most people outside the United States do not know they are HIV+ until they receive an AIDS diagnosis (Campbell 1999; Beyrer 1998). Even in the United States, people can learn their HIV status at a relatively advanced stage of the disease. At one HIV/

AIDS service clinic in the San Francisco Bay area, 45 percent of the people did not know they were HIV+ until they became symptomatic (Klein et al. 2003). An AIDS diagnosis can compress one's sense of time, increase one's sense of mortality, and immediately raise the issues of economic and social survival or rejection.

The more depressed, isolated, and stressed the PLWH/A is, the greater the chances are that this will affect disease progression in several ways. Unresolved stress may impair the immune system. Depression, lack of social support, and stress can impact adherence to HAART. These factors may affect sexual and drug risk-taking (Golin et al. 2002). Increasingly, research indicates that those people who have good social support systems live longer and cope better with crises than those who do not have them (Catalan 1999; Moatti and Spire 2000; *HIVPlus* 2001; Lyttleton 2004).

An AIDS diagnosis can also upset the individual's and group's sense of "the natural order of things" (Campbell 1999: 144). As AIDS is primarily a younger person's disease, there is not only the sense of losing someone young but also the knowledge of the effect that this will have on one's family and group (Luna 1997; Odets 1995; Basu et al. 1997). This sense of loss becomes part of individual and group grief and stress, and it can reinforce fatalistic beliefs (Orubuloye and Orguntimehin 1999; Meursing 1999; Awusabo-Asare et al. 1999).

In sub-Saharan Africa, where entire villages have been lost to AIDS and more than 20 percent of the adult population is infected in some areas, the threat of loss of the group and its culture is a reality. Anglo gay men in industrialized societies faced a similar situation in the 1980s. Ethnic groups in the United States could potentially experience something similar in the twenty-first century (Odets 1995; Tielman 1991; Shilts 1987; CDC 2001a, 2001b).

For those people on HAART, death may not be an immediate issue, but the side effects of the drugs can be. HAART has serious side effects, including heart, liver, kidney, and bone damage (Wormser and Horowitz 1996; *HIVPlus* 2002a, 2002b). HAART is effective for about 50 percent of the people who take it; for others, their bodies may "wear out." Another friend of mine died of AIDS in January 2003. His doctor, a respected AIDS physician, told him, "Even without an OI, most of my patients in your situation live only two to three years. Their bodies just can't take any more." While taking daily medications is common for many people living in the United States, taking HAART poses unique challenges. It requires strict adherence to the regimen, the side effects of the drugs can be toxic, the drugs are expensive, and there is the possibility of eventual drug resistance or intolerance. These effects pose a constant reminder of one's vulnerability.

Taking HAART requires people to be both medically and psychologically ready to do so. Psychological readiness includes

Acceptance of disease progression, often without symptoms for people in the United States. (This contrasts with those nonindustrialized societies where HAART is available, and often is given after symptoms develop.)

Acceptance of one's HIV status and health.

A willingness to adhere to the dosing regimen and make whatever lifestyle adjustments are necessary.

A willingness to deal with side effects of the drugs.

A willingness to meet with both medical people and various social service agencies to address the medical, social, and economic aspects of HAART.

A decision about confidentiality and disclosure, particularly if one is working or in school.

A willingness to deal with the unknown since HAART is relatively recent, new treatments are being developed, and the long-term efficacy or side effects of the drugs are not known.

For those people in nonindustrialized societies who have access to HAART, there are concerns about confidentiality, volition, and informed consent. There are concerns about who is selected for drug trials and for treatment. In response to these concerns, Thailand, Brazil, and India have developed generic forms of antiretrovirals, making these available to their own infected populations and to people in sub-Saharan Africa (Thomas 2001; Cleland et al. 1995). Concerns raised in industrialized societies

---

9.3

While FDCs simplify the number and frequency of drugs taken, their availability and accessibility are recent and variable. A friend of mine who is a long-term survivor spoke to my Anthropology of AIDS class in September 2006. While he is currently on a twice a day regimen, he spoke about having to take twenty or more pills a day on a highly regimented time and food-adherence schedule up until about a year ago.

about adherence to HAART in nonindustrialized societies are unfounded. People with AIDS generally adhere to the regimen if they can get the drugs (TAC 2004a; Center for Health and Gender Equity 2004b; Synergy Project 2003; Feuer 2004b).

Sexuality and PLWH/As in the United States

The sociopsychological aspects of sexuality change for those with HIV/ AIDS. Most HIV prevention efforts focus on those who are not HIV+ and adopt a **Knowledge, Attitudes, and Behavior (KAB)** model. These models are useful in providing quantitative data and analysis for large numbers of people. However, emotions and the psychological aspects of sexuality tend to be absent from these models. They also tend not to incorporate cultural variables or psycho-behavioral strategies for addressing the sexuality of people with HIV/AIDS.

In most societies, sexual behavior, particularly with steady partners such as spouses and lovers, entails a psycho-emotional component. As discussed in chapter 5, the more emotionally involved that sexual partners are, the less likely they are to practice safer sex (Afifi 1999; Cleland et al. 1995; Sobo 1995; Cummings et al. 1999; Pilkington et al. 1994; Margillo and Imahori 1998). This holds true regardless of age, gender, sexual orientation, ethnicity, socioeconomic status, education, or self-esteem. The emotional aspects of sexual relationships can influence people to behave differently than what they know they "should" do. For example, it is common for prostitutes to practice safer sex with their clients when they have that option, but not with their primary sex partners (SIECUS 2005; Morof et al. 2004; Weeks et al. 2004). Etically defined risky sex is not necessarily experienced or perceived as risky for most people who engage in it. Unprotected sex is an act of love, commitment, and support (Moore et al. 2006). Unprotected sex can also symbolize trust, respect, and support for one's partner in Anglo, African American, and Latino communities (Pilkington et al. 1994; Diaz 1998; Raffaelli and Suarez-Al-Adam 1998; Robinson et al. 2002; Margillo and Imahori 1998).

The redefinitions of what constitutes safer sex, monogamy, and main partners within gay male communities in the United States and Australia during the second and third waves of the epidemic also support the role of emotions in risk taking. These decisions include whether or not to disclose one's HIV status, what kinds of sexual behavior are acceptable,

---

9.4

In many societies, structural norms and values that support women's deference to men's sexual preferences also play a role in the practice of safer sex (see chapters 5 and 7). These norms and values can be framed in terms of "being a good wife/woman," being "there" for their men, and being "chaste."

---

what constitutes an identity as a gay man, and crossover behavior. Crossover behavior involves MSM having penetrative sex with women without disclosing that they also have it with men. This behavior also occurs with Latino and African American men, referred to as "on the down low" in African American communities (Clay 2002; Diaz 1998; Campbell 1999).

For people taking HAART and living longer, practicing safer sex becomes a long-term, lifelong behavior to avoid both "superinfection" (that is, becoming infected with another strain of the virus) and transmitting the virus. Consistently maintaining safer sex behaviors over extended periods of time can be difficult, particularly when one is emotionally involved with one's partners. The difficulty in consistently practicing safer sex for extended periods of time is currently reflected among MSM between eighteen and twenty-four years old in the United States. Since the late 1990s, data suggest that not practicing safer sex is increasingly common for this population (CDC 1999, 2001b, 2003a; Anon. 2003a, 2003b; Anon. 1998). The reasons for this are not well understood. There may be several factors involved.

The first of these is that with the development of HAART, deaths from AIDS have decreased and the visible physical signs of AIDS are much less common. Second, HAART is marketed as allowing people to resume their usual lifestyles and live longer, without signs or symptoms of HIV. Third, HAART can successfully suppress viral loads to undetectable levels and increases T-cell counts. These factors may foster a sense that one is no longer infectious or really has a disease. Fourth, if HAART successfully transforms HIV/AIDS into a chronic but manageable disease, the seriousness of becoming infected may diminish for some people. Fifth, with new drugs appearing that may result in taking fewer pills and less often (FDCs; see chapter 8), drug adherence may increase. The effect of all of these variables may make HIV/AIDS appear to be a less serious disease than in previous decades and may as a result impact risk taking (*San Francisco Chronicle* 2003a, 2003b; Bingman et al. 2001; Chng et al. 2003; Clatts and Sotheran 2000; McFarland et al. 2004; O'Donnell et al. 2002).

However, data from research conducted in the late 1980s indicate that safer sex among sero-discordant couples does prevent HIV transmission. Sero-discordant couples are those in which one person is HIV+ and the other is HIV-. Safer sex practices among gay men in the United States resulted in a decline in HIV for that population during the later 1980s.

Nancy Padian, a researcher at the University of California–San Francisco (UCSF), conducted studies on sero-discordant heterosexual couples. Those who consistently practiced safer sex for vaginal and anal intercourse remained sero-discordant. The HIV-negative partner did not become infected. Her research also provided twenty-four-hour hotlines for couples to call with safer sex questions and to be able to receive psychological support to maintain safer sex practices (CDC 2001b, 2003a; Padian et al. 1991).

Cross-Cultural Sociopsychological Factors

As discussed in chapters 5 and 7, the sexual risks of contracting HIV outside industrialized societies, including the United States, have their own characteristics. This extends to the sociopsychological aspects of sexuality as well. The following examples illustrate this point. Among the Chagga in Tanzania, romantic love is a factor in partner selection and safer sex decisions, just as it is in industrialized societies (Setel 1999). In many parts of sub-Saharan Africa, women used to be able to follow cultural sexual taboos around menstruation, pregnancy, and breast-feeding to withhold sex from their male partners. European contact, colonization, and the resultant culture change altered these taboos and women's ability to make their own sexual decisions. Women lost a lot of their negotiating power about the circumstances under which they would have sex (Orubuloye et al. 1994; Setel 1999; Rasing 2003: 16).

In response to these cultural changes, Uganda established recommendations about sexual behavior to reduce the incidence of HIV/AIDS. Their (admittedly controversial) ABC model, presented in chapter 5, encourages an older age for having intercourse, a reduction in the number of partners and marital monogamy, referred to as "zero grazing," and condom usage (Schoepf 2001, 2003a, 2003b; Green 2003; Hogle et al. 2002). Increased education for women, restoration of their legal rights, and economic opportunities for them have also been part of Uganda's successful efforts to prevent infection and reduce incidence, strategies that some researchers believe were as effective in reducing seroprevalence as the controversial ABC model was (Schoepf 2003b).

In nonindustrialized societies, the social survival of the group and the culture are intrinsically related to the economic and political aspects of the disease, as discussed in the previous chapter. The enormity of the loss of individuals to AIDS impacts local economies in rural areas and villages (Solomon et al. 2000; Moore et al. 2006). In India, middle-class wives are not expected to work outside the home. When their husbands die of AIDS, the widows do not have the marketable skills to provide for their family, nor do they have the social support to obtain the skills to help them find work. When their extended kin group will not help them because of stigma and ignorance about transmission, they and their children face a survival crisis (Solomon et al. 2000).

In sub-Saharan Africa, Thailand, and areas of rural China, the impact that AIDS has on the local economies stimulates survival prostitution (see chapters 5 and 7). The stigma associated with both AIDS and prostitution further isolates people from traditional means of social support (Lyttleton 2004).

Sociopsychological Factors for the Caregivers and Survivors

Survivor Guilt and Fatalism

HIV/AIDS entails major changes for individuals, groups, and societies. The illness affects not only those who are infected but also those who take care of them in a variety of ways and those who are not HIV+. There are concerns about risks for infection and survivor guilt.

Survivor guilt is a common phenomenon. It often occurs among people who do not physically succumb to catastrophes, such as the Holocaust in World War II or the AIDS pandemic (Odets 1995; Shilts 1987; Johnston 1995). Survivor guilt can manifest as questions about why the individual was spared when others such as family and friends were not. Depending on the circumstances and the social support available to the survivors, survivor guilt may be expressed positively or self-destructively.

Survivor guilt relative to the AIDS epidemic may lead to safer sex and safer drug practices, taking good care of oneself, community involvement in prevention or treatment efforts, and formation of new social networks.

However, survivor guilt may express itself in fatalistic ways in both industrialized and nonindustrialized societies.

Fatalism can take the form of a sense of invulnerability to the virus—which may be playing out among some younger people in the third wave of the epidemic—or as a sense of inevitability for risk of infection. It may also be expressed as depression, which may lead to risky behaviors (Odets 1995; Mitchell 1999; Green and Sobo 2000). Cross-culturally, the feeling of inevitability has been documented. Younger males in parts of sub-Saharan Africa and some female prostitutes in parts of Southeast Asia have expressed a fatalistic attitude toward infection (Orubuloye and Orguntimehin 1999; Amadora-Nolasco et al. 2001; Basuki et al. 2002; Bond et al. 1996). The belief that preventing HIV infection is beyond one's control and belief in the inevitability of death can lead to risky sexual behaviors.

Caregivers

The caregivers of people with HIV/AIDS include a wide range of people. In both industrialized and nonindustrialized societies, they are family members and friends, as well as biomedical and traditional health-care providers. The illness aspects of AIDS particularly affect the caregivers.

Caregivers face **burnout** as part of dealing with PLWH/A. Burnout is a sociopsychological phenomenon that may include physical symptoms such as sleep disturbances and irritability or emotional distancing from the people under their care. These caregivers may engage in overwork and focus exclusively on their caregiver roles until they can no longer effectively meet their other responsibilities. If this happens, their own personal relationships may suffer, and their patients' well-being may be negatively affected (Odets 1995; Bennett et al. 1995).

Burnout among HIV caregivers is common and occurs for several reasons. There is the frustration of dealing with a disease that is often fatal. AIDS is primarily a younger person's disease. Losing large numbers of people who are in their thirties and forties is a different kind of loss than that incurred with caring for the elderly. Younger people are at the beginning of their contributions to society; older people have lived what many cultures see as the "normal" life cycle.

As HIV/AIDS becomes more of a chronic disease and illness, the sense of dealing with something incurable and eventually debilitating may develop. During the first two waves of the epidemic, caregivers could also be affected by AIDS stigma. This could manifest itself as a lack of compassion and support for the caregivers themselves. Lastly, gender is a factor in caregiver burnout. Worldwide, most of the AIDS caregivers are women who take care of PLWH/As in addition to other economic, social, and familial responsibilities they have. The culturally widespread gender-role expectations of women as caregivers increase the pressure to provide care, regardless of one's own needs (Bennett et al. 1995; Moore et al. 2006; Lyttleton 2004).

Health-care workers in the United States such as physicians, nurses, and mental health professionals face specific sociopsychological issues about AIDS beyond their own risks for burnout and the accompanying sense of loss and grief for their patients and clients who have died. Medical technology raises ethical questions about pain relief and how and when death occurs.

HIV/AIDS-related pain can occur as a side effect of OIs, as one of the effects of disease progression, or as a side effect of HAART (Nedeljkovic 2002). The medical profession has a conflicted view about pain relief that is related to larger cultural values about stoicism and strength and fears about addiction. There is a specific fear about treating pain in substance users, as many prescription pain relievers contain narcotics. There is concern that providing adequate pain relief may create or contribute to drug dependence (Sottile et al. 2002; Bader 2002). These fears are more a function of cultural attitudes than they are founded in drug physiology. Pain receptors in people experiencing severe, chronic pain, particularly as a result of terminal disease progression, operate differently and respond to drugs differently. Physicians who are experienced in dealing with PLWH/As realize the necessity of adequate pain management (Nedeljkovic 2002).

9.5

One of the ongoing and more controversial aspects of pain and other symptom relief is the use of marijuana. Despite recommendations from the Institute of Medicine and other respected medical authorities, the use of marijuana to stimulate appetite and to alleviate pain and nausea brought on by both the progression of AIDS-related symptoms and the drugs remains illegal in most parts of the United States. Medical marijuana usage continues to be a political rather than a medical issue (Institute of Medicine 2001).

End-of-life concerns are another ethical and social issue for medical caregivers. Industrial societies have the technology available to extend life that other societies do not have. Technology allows people to live when they would not otherwise. Who makes these decisions and how are they carried out (Nedeljkovic 2002; Stumpf 1996)? People in the United States who have written health-care proxies can stipulate that life support be withheld and no extraordinary measures taken. Hospice provides this kind of care as well as pain relief. However, as a society, we do not legally or socially accept active euthanasia, in which drugs are given to hasten death. There is a medical, legal, and ethical irony involved in being able to keep someone alive beyond that which would occur naturally but not allowing them to die (van den Boom et al. 1999).

These particular end-of-life concerns are primarily an issue in industrialized societies. In societies that do not have this technology, death does occur sooner. For example, among middle-class Latinos in Peru, much of the health care for seriously ill people takes place at home. Visiting nurses, physicians, and the extended kin group provide home care. Resources generally are not available to prolong life through extraordinary measures. When my Peruvian husband became seriously ill with advanced AIDS, he decided to leave the United States and return to Peru. He did not want to make or have the family make "end-of-life decisions." He died at home with pain relief and without medical interventions to prolong his life.

AIDS deaths in nonindustrialized societies usually occur soon after an AIDS diagnosis. Effective pain relief is variable, and high-tech life support is rarely available. The sociopsychological issues about pain relief and death and dying focus on how to make the person comfortable and how the caregivers will survive after the person's death.

Without access to HAART, people with AIDS live about two to four years (Stine 1997; CDC 2001b). This period may include repeated bouts of OIs, loss of work and income, changes in one's physical appearance, increasing dependence on others to meet daily needs, and eventual death. Loss of functioning and dependence on others not only impacts the sick person but also increases the responsibilities and stresses on the caregivers and others involved with the PLWH/AS. In most societies, these increased responsibilities fall upon members of the kin group, particularly women.

Women primarily fill these caregiving roles in both industrialized and nonindustrialized societies (Moore et al. 2006). The use of resources from social service agencies such as home health aides, social workers, and visiting nurses in industrialized societies to manage daily needs supplements the help from family and friends. Most of the people in these social service or personal situations who provide care are women.

Women provide caregiving to PLWH/As in addition to their other responsibilities and regardless of their own health status (chapter 7). The sociopsychological experiences of women include economic concerns about loss of income to households and the redirection of their own energies away from resource acquisition and toward caregiving. They must cope with additional workloads, ongoing child care responsibilities, and their own sense of grief. If women caregivers are also HIV+, they worry about leaving dependent children (Cummings et al. 1999; Wissow et al. 1996; Bennett et al. 1995; Campbell 1999; Moore et al. 2006).

AIDS Orphans

The impact of AIDS on kin groups is very apparent when addressing the topic of AIDS orphans. Etically, AIDS orphans are the minor children whose parents have died of AIDS. These children may or may not be HIV+. The numbers of AIDS orphans vary worldwide and are increasing in nonindustrialized societies that do not have access to HAART. There are an estimated 15 million AIDS orphans worldwide as of 2004, with an estimated 125,000 in the United States as of 2000 (Simpson and Williams 1996; CNN 2004). The fate of AIDS orphans depends on where they live.

In the United States, which has the fewest AIDS orphans proportionately relative to PLWH/As here and elsewhere, there are various options available to parents. Generally, if there is an active, functioning social support system for the children, they can psychologically cope with the loss of their parent(s) (Sherr 1999; Wissow et al. 1996). Many middle-class, Anglo parents make arrangements for their surviving children well before the parents die (Hutton 1996). Generally, these children go to live with family or adult friends.

Depending on a given ethnic group's views, children may or may not be aware of their mother's AIDS diagnosis. Ethnic orphans living in poverty may come under the aegis of social service agencies and be placed in foster care, depending on their age and circumstances. Some social service agencies are encouraging the use of expanded definitions of family to take care of these children (Sherr 1999; Simpson and Williams 1996; Mellins et al. 1996). Both foster and adoptive parents in the United States legally can know a child's HIV status before the child is taken in.

Extended kin fill active, important roles in African American, Latino, and Native American families. Extended kin among these groups are similar in composition to those in nonindustrialized societies and incur similar obligations. Two examples illustrate this point. Grandmothers in many African American families are raising AIDS orphans (Doran et al. 2002; Joslin 2002; Pointdexter 2002). Native American female caregivers often incorporate spirituality in their roles as surrogate parents to their orphaned nieces and nephews and grandchildren (Burhansstipanov et al. 1997). All of these families need socioeconomic and psychological support to raise their children and to grieve their losses (Hedge 1999; Kimoto 1998; Hogan 2001; Bradley 1995; Doran et al. 2002). Fortunately, with the availability of HAART in the United States, there are fewer AIDS orphans in the twenty-first century than there were here in the 1980s and 1990s.

The situation of AIDS orphans outside the United States is different. Traditionally, extended kin would raise the children. This practice continues when there are surviving extended kin available. FBOs and organizations such as TASO (chapter 8) also provide some relief for AIDS orphans (UNFPA 2007b; Dilger 2007). Those who are left without family are homeless and increasingly are becoming the majority in parts of sub-Saharan Africa. Elderly family members assume responsibility for AIDS orphans in Thailand (Beyrer 1998; Pitayanon et al. 1997). In India, extended kin take care of these children, who also face being stigmatized because their parents died of AIDS (Basu et al. 1997; O'Leary et al. 2007). Their futures as adults remain unknown. They carry not only the burden of being an orphan and having reduced economic resources available to them but also the stigma of AIDS.

This chapter illustrates how HIV/AIDS affects people socially and psychologically as well as sexually, economically, and politically. The sociopsychological aspects of the epidemic reflect the illness of HIV/AIDS as it impacts individuals who are infected, their families, and communities. These aspects need to be addressed as much as do the modes of transmission, cofactors in risk, and the larger economic and political factors that contribute to the spread of the virus. Reducing stigma through education and social support, addressing the needs of PLWH/As holistically, and providing resources for those who care for PLWH/As will contribute to ameliorating the psychosocial stresses that accompany this disease.

SUMMARY

The stigma associated with HIV/AIDS is universal and expressed through individual cultural beliefs and norms.

Stigma affects not only those infected with the virus but also their families, friends, and caregivers.

The sociopsychological dimension of HIV/AIDS is an expression of the illness of HIV/AIDS.

Sociopsychological issues for PLWH/As involve concerns about their own health and mortality, acceptance or rejection by their families and communities, and economic and relationship fears.

Sociopsychological issues for caregivers of PLWH/As relate to fears about social and economic survival, loss, grief, and the stresses involved in caring for PLWH/As.

The number of AIDS orphans is increasing because of the deaths of adults in nonindustrialized societies.

Thought Questions

How does stigma affect intervention efforts for PWLH/As and their communities, caregivers, families, and friends?

What culture-specific strategies are necessary to address the sociopsychological concerns of PWLH/As and their communities, caregivers, families, and friends?

Resources

Books

Campbell, Carole A. *Women, Families, and HIV/AIDS: A Sociological Perspective on the Epidemic in America.* Cambridge: Cambridge University Press, 1999.

Catalan, Jose, ed. *Mental Health and HIV Infection: Psychological and Psychiatric Aspects.* London: UCL Press, 1999.

Herek, Gregory M., and Beverly Greene, eds. *AIDS, Identity, and Community,* vol. 2, *The HIV Epidemic and Lesbians and Gay Men.* Psychological Perspectives on Lesbian and Gay Issues. Thousand Oaks: Sage Publications, 1995.

Joslin, Daphne, ed. *Invisible Caregivers: Older Adults Raising Children in the Wake of HIV/AIDS.* New York: Columbia University Press, 2002.

Sontag, Susan. *Illness as Metaphor and AIDS and Its Metaphors.* London: Peter Smith Publishers, 1995.

Videos

Kleiser, Randall (director). *It's My Party.* Santa Monica, Calif.: MGM/UA Studios, 1998.

Web Sites

The Body, The: http://www.thebody.com.
HIVPlus. 1997–present. http://www.hivplusmag.com.
POZ. 1994–present. http://www.poz.com.

10

Conclusion

AIDS in the Twenty-First Century

CHAPTER HIGHLIGHTS INCLUDE

A discussion of the need for a holistic, integrated, and interdisciplinary
approach to the pandemic

An overview of the pandemic at the beginning of the twenty-first
century

A review of successful intervention efforts

Discussion of anthropology's contributions to intervention efforts

> Let us change the world. . . . We live in a world threatened by unlimited
> destructive force, yet we share a vision of creative potential. . . . AIDS
> shows us once again that silence, exclusion, and isolation—of individuals,
> groups, or nations—creates a danger for us all.
>
> Jonathan Mann, quoted in memorial service to him, 1998 (FXB Foundation
> 2005)

Overview of the Pandemic

HIV/AIDS has the potential to be one of the most devastating health phenomena in human history. It poses a global biomedical, social, political,
and economic crisis. HIV/AIDS illustrates the interdependency of biology
and culture. The response to it, therefore, needs to be comprehensive,
collaborative, and continuous. A holistic, integrated, and interdisciplinary approach is necessary to address the pandemic. The response to this
pandemic requires efforts from the basic medical and biological sciences
and epidemiology, from the social sciences, and from humanistic and human rights groups.

Jonathan Mann, an epidemiologist and human rights activist, was the founder and head of the World Health Organization's AIDS campaign. As early as 1987, Mann encouraged interdisciplinary and international cooperation in responding to the pandemic. He advocated for anthropological contributions to elucidate the cultural variables involved in risk, prevention, and treatment (Armelagos et al. 1990: 253). Mann approached the AIDS epidemic holistically. He saw it as both a disease and an illness that is expressed within the context of specific social, political, and economic systems.

There are universal aspects of AIDS. AIDS is caused by infection with a virus. However, infection is not viewed neutrally wherever it occurs but is placed within a context that has included fear, ignorance, shame, and blame. Without medical intervention, HIV/AIDS is fatal, affecting individuals, communities, and societies from conception through death. There are social, political, and economic consequences of AIDS in the communities where it exists. Given the global nature of HIV/AIDS, the responses to it require cultural sensitivity and specificity.

HIV/AIDS in the United States in the Twenty-First Century

There are two worlds of the AIDS pandemic: the one in what is sometimes referred to as "northern" (that is, north of the equator) industrialized societies that have access to education, testing, and HAART/ARVs, and the one in what has been referred to as "southern" (that is, south of the equator), nonindustrialized societies that have limited resources and access to these preventive and treatment strategies. While both worlds share the health threat that the virus poses, the effect and course of the disease on those infected and their societies are very different. As such, there are epidemics within the pandemic that are functions of gender, ethnicity, and socioeconomic status.

Since the first identified outbreak of HIV/AIDS in 1981, industrialized societies (specifically, the United States) have shown both the problems that surround addressing intervention efforts and the progress that has been made in slowing the spread of AIDS. During the first wave of the epidemic in the United States, the fear and stigma associated with sexually transmitted diseases and with sexual communities slowed medical progress and prevention efforts. The fear and stigma extended to social, legal, economic, and political sectors of our society as casual-contact fears proliferated. Discrimination occurred toward people with HIV/AIDS. Biases affected research about the virus (exemplified by initially referring to AIDS as GRID), prevention efforts, HIV testing efforts, and treatments. All of these variables faced political roadblocks.

The second wave of the epidemic in the United States saw epidemiological, medical, legal, social, economic, and political changes. These included the development of HAART and other antiretrovirals, as well as resistance to holistic prevention efforts and treatments for PLWH/As. The face of AIDS increasingly shifted toward a poorer, more ethnic, and female population. HIV test centers proliferated, and AIDS Drug Assistance Programs (ADAP) were created to financially assist People Living With HIV/AIDS (PLWH/As). ADAP was expanded to include PLWH/As, and various NGOs, CBOs, and social service agencies instituted intensive intervention efforts. At the same time, prevention efforts such as N/SEPs and comprehensive safer sex programs experienced criticism and censorship from local and national conservative groups.

In the third wave of the epidemic, which includes the beginning of the twenty-first century, the epidemiological, medical, social, economic, and political dimensions of HIV/AIDS are mixed. There is still neither a vaccine nor a cure for HIV/AIDS. Recent calls for routine, universal testing are admirable in intent but need careful oversight so that testing remains voluntary, particularly for groups already discriminated against, such as people living in poverty, women, and ethnic minorities (Kaiser Daily HIV/AIDS Report 2006g).

While there has been a dramatic reduction in MTCT, HIV infections are increasing, particularly among young adult MSM, African Americans, Native Americans, and Asian/Pacific Islanders. Impoverished ethnic women continue to constitute about 83 percent of the women with HIV/AIDS in the United States (UNAIDS 2006; Kaiser Family Foundation 2006; http://www.aids2004.org). Most of the PLWH/As are poor, and programs developed in the 1980s and 1990s to help them, including ADAP and ADA, are threatened with economic cuts (*Nation* 2004; State Health Facts 2006b). HAART dramatically improves people's health and increases longevity but has serious side effects, only works for about 50 percent of the people who take it, and is not available to all who need it.

Social programs and research that emphasize comprehensive sexual approaches to prevention are under attack by conservative political and religious groups. Safer sex programs that include methods other than abstinence-only and lifelong monogamy face budget cuts and censorship. Concurrently, activists work to reduce stigma, provide new prevention approaches to reflect the changing demographic patterns of the epidemic, and provide culturally sensitive and aware intervention efforts regarding sexual and needle/IDU transmission of the virus.

Social programs exist based on economic and political decisions. The first decade of the epidemic saw delays in funding and delays in federal acknowledgement of the situation (Shilts 1987). After the isolation of the virus, the development of an HIV antibody test, and intense political activity by groups such as ACTUP, funding for prevention, treatment, and testing increased during the second wave of the epidemic. Research and implementation of comprehensive safer sex, IDU, and N/SEP programs received economic and political support locally or federally. Conservative religious and political groups continued to press for abstinence-only programs and reduced federal support of CBOs.

During the third wave of the epidemic, federal support for HIV intervention efforts has become restricted. ADAP assistance has been cut, resulting in several states having no or reduced ADAP funding. This includes West Virginia and Kentucky as of 2004, South Carolina in 2006 and 2007, and Alaska in 2007 (NASTAD 2007). Federally funded organizations such as the CDC and NIH have had safer sex information changed on their Web sites and in their printed material. NIH researchers seeking grants to conduct sexuality research are under federal scrutiny, and peer-approved proposals are not being funded (*Nation* 2004; Kaiser 2003).

The response to federal cuts and censorship means that CBOs and researchers adapt to federal mandates to maintain their programs. CBOs may increase their range of services and seek sources of nonfederal funding, as CALPEP has done. There is a group of AIDS researchers and various organizations that are protesting censorship of sexuality-based research, including the Global Gag Rule, which would cut funds to international programs that support N/SEPs, provide services to sex workers, and offer comprehensive reproductive health care. To survive political and economic challenges during the third wave of the epidemic, groups and individuals are looking for alternatives to continue their work.

HIV/AIDS in the Nonindustrialized World in the Twenty-First Century

HIV/AIDS continues to wreak havoc in most of the world. In 2006, it was the leading cause of death among people between fifteen and fifty-nine years old worldwide (WHO 2004a; UNAIDS 2006). While there have been dramatic successes in either the reduction or the stabilization of HIV/AIDS in Uganda, Zambia, Senegal, and Sierra Leone, there are disturbing situations in other countries (UNAIDS 2006; Green 2003; Hogle et al. 2002). Current predictions are that the emerging epidemiological pictures in Southeast Asia, including India and China, portray an epidemic that could be worse than what is found in sub-Saharan Africa (Russell 2004; UNAIDS 2006).

The state of the pandemic in nonindustrialized societies clearly illustrates the interdependence of ecological variables, the virus, and social, political, and economic cofactors in the spread of the disease. Correcting ecological conditions that promote malaria, tuberculosis, or diarrhea from contaminated water reduces the risk of HIV infection posed by these cofactors. Building up the agrarian infrastructure to ensure crop production provides resources that can help counter malnutrition and supply HIV+ people with food (Armelagos et al. 1990; Parker, Easton, and Klein 2000; http://www.aids2004.org).

Social, political, and economic factors that perpetuate poverty, violence, gender inequality, and suppression of information and access to HAART or other antiretrovirals contribute to the spread of HIV. International political and economic decisions that restrict access to health-care services, censor information about safer sex other than abstinence and monogamy, and block access to WHO-approved generic drugs and FDCs contribute to the dichotomy between survival with AIDS in industrialized societies and survival elsewhere.

Ignorance, shame, and stigma about HIV deter people from receiving accurate information about prevention, testing, and treatment. Lack of viable economic resources increases the prevalence of risky safer sex decisions being made out of economic survival. Blaming women for HIV transmission places an inordinate amount of responsibility on them for prevention and leads to condemnation if they become infected or transmit the virus to their fetuses or children. The cofactors for HIV infection in areas heavily impacted by the epidemic involve both emic and etic factors.

The effects of culture change on sexual and marital practices can increase risks for women, while leaving them with few economic skills and options. Social, political, and economic interventions that are generated from Euro-American models of sexuality, gender, kinship, choice, and bureaucracy have a decreased chance of success over those that are derived from local community norms. Without a holistic approach to prevention, testing, and treatment that addresses individual, community, and societal beliefs and behaviors as well as steps to change infrastructure problems of poverty, war, and malnutrition, the virus will continue to proliferate.

Successful programs in Brazil, Thailand, and Uganda integrated industrialized approaches to intervention and treatment with their own cultural beliefs. In these societies, the epidemic was recognized early, and sustained intervention and treatment efforts since the 1980s have reduced the incidence and prevalence rates. To maintain their lower incidence and prevalence efforts, there needs to be greater economic, political, and social autonomy for women, and prevention strategies need to address adolescents and young adults (Altman 2004; Schoepf 2003a, 2003b; Parker, Barbosa, and Aggleton 2000; Waterston 1997).

The development and availability of generic drugs in India, Thailand, and Brazil that have received WHO approval for efficacy pose a challenge to PhRMA and other pharmaceutical corporations. The controversy over cost and delivery of drugs to PLWH/As in nonindustrialized societies continues.

Successful Intervention Efforts

Despite much international concern about the devastation of the AIDS epidemic, there have been successful interventions. As discussed in chapter 8, prevention is more cost-effective than treatment is. Successful intervention efforts worldwide share several characteristics. First, they are adaptable and find ways to work with and around official policies. This includes NGOs that developed safer sex programs in Indonesia, governmental policies about condoms in prisons in Iran, and N/SEPs in Brazil and the United States. The Islamic countries Indonesia and Iran recognized that Islamic views on sexuality and legal restrictions on needle exchange programs, respectively, could negatively impact their efforts. Groups in these areas sought nongovernmental funding and support to establish and maintain their programs.

Second, successful programs tend to be grassroots based, culture specific, and culturally sensitive; use peer educators; speak in the language and mores of their target groups; and encourage involvement from local leaders and support from national leaders. They are not top-down programs but are derived from local needs. Third, successful programs are ongoing. They are not one-time intervention efforts but become established as part of their target communities.

Fourth, programs that succeed are neither moralistic nor judgmental in their philosophy, implementation, or options that are offered to their target populations. They incorporate community norms about privacy, confidentiality, and dissemination of information. These programs are inclusive and holistic in approach. For example, if researchers want women to participate in clinical trials, then they need to recognize and incorporate the women's needs. This can include provision of transportation and child care accommodations.

Fifth, successful programs are holistic. They recognize not only the direct and immediate risks for HIV but also the cofactors. They incorporate recommendations or policies that address the social, political, and economic stressors that increase the risks for infection, deter testing efforts, and impede access to drugs. A successful program will not only discuss safer needle options, for example, but will also try to get people into rehabilitation programs. Programs to prevent heterosexual transmission will incorporate culturally sensitive efforts for both men and women.

Sixth, ethical research, testing, and treatment methodologies are important to program success. Programs that succeed do not discriminate or have double standards regarding gender, ethnicity, or socioeconomic status as part of their development and implementation. Overall, successful programs incorporate numerous anthropological principles and perspectives (Bond 1997; Heald 2006).

The Value of an Anthropological Approach in HIV Interventions

This book began with a discussion of anthropology and the value of an anthropological perspective in confronting the challenge of AIDS. Anthropology has theoretical, methodological, and applied contributions to make in intervening in this epidemic.

Jonathan Mann emphasized the importance of an ecological approach to this pandemic, of including local environmental factors that can increase the risk of infection, affect the course of the virus, and expose people to various OIs once infected (Armelagos et al. 1990). Applied, critical medical anthropology as articulated by the physician and anthropologist Paul Farmer (1992) is a significant theoretical component of anthropological work in HIV. This approach explores how globalization affects local economic and social structures that can increase the risk for infection or difficulty in accessing services. It removes analysis from the realm of the individual to that of the group, looking for holistic solutions that integrate behavior with beliefs.

The risk of contracting the virus varies. Risk is based on individual, community, and larger socioeconomic and political factors. Individuals exist within social groups. Their behavior is shaped and influenced by the group and the larger society. Critical medical anthropology focuses on the larger socioeconomic and political factors within cultures and internationally that affect risk. This includes malnutrition, poverty, and diseases such as malaria and tuberculosis that impair the immune system. In addition, development efforts that limit economic opportunities for indigenous populations and governmental policies that inhibit prevention strategies or limit access to drugs exacerbate the problem.

Critical medical anthropology offers holistic responses to the epidemic that address the infrastructure of societies and the effects of culture change on traditional beliefs and practices, as well as approaches that present alternatives that incorporate community norms. For example, a critical medical anthropology approach would educate local healers about transmission and risk to have them serve as resource people. Indigenous healing methods such as acupuncture that can ease symptoms of the disease or side effects of medication can provide a familiar form of relief to people with HIV/AIDS.

The crux of anthropological methodology, participant-observation, is an invaluable tool in obtaining data about sexual mores and behaviors, the context in which behaviors occur, and observations on daily life over time. Through participant-observation, people's daily needs are articulated such that they can provide information about how to establish effective interventions regarding prevention, testing, and treatment. Work by anthropologists such as Brooke Schoepf in Africa in the 1980s and 1990s, and Merrill Singer in the northeastern United States with substance users illustrate how taking an emic approach is useful in developing prevention efforts that reflect the needs of the population being served (Schoepf 1993, 2001, 2003a, 2003b; Singer 2005; Singer et al. 2005).

Anthropologists have been studying sexuality since the nineteenth century. We have a wealth of data about traditional and current sexual practices and beliefs that can be used to establish safer sex programs, can incorporate symbolic ritual beliefs that can replace risky behaviors, and can be framed in the context of larger norms and values. We can act as brokers between the biomedical, epidemiological, and Euro-American etic approaches to present a group's needs.

Anthropologists also have contributions to make regarding implementing programs. We know how to access local leaders and healers who are the spokespeople for their groups. We know how to enter communities to assess people's needs and can advocate for groups, enabling them to speak for themselves. Our theoretical and methodological perspectives allow us to gather the "thick data" discussed in chapter 1 that is necessary in implementing programs.

HIV/AIDS is a complex phenomenon. It requires complex responses across disciplines. To begin to reduce the incidence and prevalence of this pandemic requires cooperation, flexibility, concerted effort, and commitment to programs that work. We have the opportunity to express the best of what is human in responding to the HIV/AIDS challenge.

SUMMARY

HIV/AIDS is potentially the most devastating disease to occur in human history.

Biological (malnutrition, age, other STIs, tuberculosis, and malaria), socioeconomic, and political cofactors significantly increase the risk of HIV infection.

HIV antibody tests and HAART are examples of significant progress in responding to the pandemic.

Judgmental and punitive cultural responses and international profiteering impede intervention efforts.

Successful intervention programs are characterized by early responses to the epidemic, comprehensive prevention strategies, and culturally sensitive and specific programs, including use of local leaders, cultural relativism, holism, and adaptability.

Anthropological theoretical and methodological approaches are useful in developing interventions.

Thought Questions

What kinds of problems prevent successful intervention programs from being developed, being implemented, and succeeding?

What specific anthropological perspectives contribute to successful interventions?

Resources

Articles

Parker, Richard G., Delia Easton, and Charles H. Klein. "Structural Barriers and Facilitators in HIV Prevention: A Review of International Research." *AIDS* 14, suppl. 1 (2000): S22–S32.

Books

Barnett, Theodore, and Alan Whiteside. *AIDS in the Twenty-first Century: Disease and Globalization.* New York: Palgrave MacMillan, 2002.

Mayer, Kenneth H., and H. F. Pizer, eds. *The Emergence of AIDS: The Impact on Immunology, Microbiology, and Public Health.* Washington, D.C.: American Public Health Association, 2000.

Web Sites

Columbia University Mailman School of Public Health: http://www.mailman.hs.columbia.edu/.

Global Fund to Fight AIDS, Tuberculosis and Malaria: http://www.theglobalfund.org/en/.

Medscape HIV/AIDS: http://www.medscape.com/hivaidshome.

Menstuff: http://www.menstuff.org/issues/byissue/worldaidsday.html.

Nation, The: http://www.thenation.com/directory/hiv_aids.

Glossary

ACTUP—AIDS Coalition to Unleash Power. An AIDS activist group whose positions on the causes of AIDS and the drugs to treat it have changed over the course of the epidemic.

Acute disease/illness—Disease or illness that usually has a sudden onset, short course of infection, and relatively quick resolution through either a return to health or death.

AIDS—Acquired Immune Deficiency Syndrome— The end result of HIV infection, is characterized by the presence of antibodies to the virus, compromised immune system, and/or the presence of one or more opportunistic infections.

AIDS Drug Assistance Programs (ADAP)—State programs heavily funded by the federal government that provide financial assistance to buy HAART for people who cannot afford the drugs.

The AIDS Support Organization— *See* TASO

Alternative test site/anonymous test site—An HIV test site where the person's identity is kept anonymous for counseling and reporting of test results.

Americans with Disabilities Act (ADA)—A federal law that protects people with disabilities from discrimination.

Antibodies—Substances produced by the body in response to the presence of a foreign entity.

Antiretroviral drugs (ARVs)—Those drugs that attempt to slow the progression of HIV through a variety of mechanisms.

AZT076—An antiretroviral given to pregnant women to reduce the risk of perinatal transmission of HIV.

Bilateral descent—Tracing one's family through both the father's and mother's sides for purposes of receiving a name, membership in a kin group, inheritance, and/or socialization into the society.

Bisexual (bi)—Sexually and romantically attracted to people of one's own and the other sex. This is a culture-bound term generally applying to and used by Euro-American people.

Brain drain—The practice of industrialized countries, particularly the United States and Great Britain, hiring professionals from nonindustrialized societies to fill positions in health care and engineering. These professionals leave their native countries for better pay, benefits, and safer and more comfortable working conditions, and the hiring companies gain professionals who will work for lower pay and benefits. This practice results in areas of the world already overstretched on resources having serious shortages in their health-care and industrial sectors.

Burnout—A physical and psycho-social response to overinvolvement and overextension with work that can negatively impact the person's ability to function effectively.

Centers for Disease Control and Prevention (CDC) —A federally funded interdisciplinary organization that sets standards and definitions of diseases, sets standards and protocols for diseases, and makes recommendations and policies about health issues and diseases in the United States.

Changing face of AIDS—Demographic changes in terms of who is infected with HIV over the course of the epidemic.

Chronic disease/illness—Disease or illness that has no cure, may be treatable, and impairs but does not stop a person's functioning.

Cofactor—A variable that increases the risk of HIV infection but does not directly cause infection.

Community-based organizations (CBOs)—Organizations that do not stem from local, state, or federal government budgets and supervision.

Confidential test site—An HIV test site where identifying information is recorded for people having an HIV test.

Critical medical anthropology—An activist branch of anthropology that examines current health practices and decision making to create awareness about political, social, and economic influences in health care.

Cross-cultural, cross-cultural comparison—The examination of behaviors and beliefs outside mainstream U.S. culture.

Cultural relativism—The practice of not imposing one's beliefs upon another culture or judging another culture by one's own cultural standards.

Culture—The learned, patterned system of shared values, symbols, and beliefs within a group.

Cunnilingus—Oral stimulation of the vulva, the female genitalia.

Deductive approach—A way of analyzing data based on testing theories through hypotheses.

"Down low"—A term used within the African American community to refer to MSW who also have sex with men.

Economics—The ways in which resources are distributed within a group or society.

ELISA test—Enzyme-Linked Immunosorbent Assay test. The standard blood test to detect antibodies to HIV.

Emic—The approach to data from the insider's or the research subject's perspective.

Endemic—Widespread presence of a disease within a society.

Envelope—The outer layer of a virus.

Epicenter—A geographic area that has a high incidence and prevalence of a disease.

Epidemic—The rather sudden, rapid appearance of a disease or pathogen within a population.

Epidemiology—The study of the patterns of disease within and between societies.

Erotophobia—The fear of sexuality.

Ethnicity—The common identity that individuals share within a group, based on beliefs, values, language, and a possibly similar gene pool.

Ethnocentrism—The belief that one's society and individual beliefs, values, and behaviors are better than another's.

Etic—The approach to data from the outsider's or researcher's perspective.

Evolution—An irreversible process of qualitative change from one form to another.

Faith-Based Organizations (FBOs)—Formal religious organizations and the groups affiliated with them.

Fellatio—Oral stimulation of male genitalia.

Fixed Dosage Combination (FDC)—An antiretroviral regimen that requires fewer pills taken once or twice a day.

Food and Drug Administration (FDA)—A federal agency that regulates food and (legal) drug availability in the United States.

FTMs/F2Ms—Female-to-male transsexuals.

Gay—A male who is sexually and romantically attracted to other males and is open about it. This is a culture-bound term generally applying to Anglo males or those who have assimilated those values.

Gender—The designation of an individual as male, female, or another gender.

Gender identity—The sense people have of themselves as male, female, or another gender.

Gender role—The culturally defined expectations of how individuals are supposed to think, feel, and behave based on their gender.

GRID—Gay-Related Immune Deficiency. An early term for AIDS.

HAART—Highly Active Antiretroviral Therapy. A combination of drugs to reduce viral load, increase the number of T-cells, and reduce the risk for OIs.

Harm-reduction model—A process of behavior change in which people reduce their risks or problematic behavior to achieve an end.

Heterosexual—Sexual attraction to people of the "other" sex.

Histocompatible—Cells that are not foreign to each other.

HIV—Human immunodeficiency virus. The virus widely believed to cause AIDS.

HIV indeterminate—HIV test results that are neither clearly HIV negative nor HIV positive.

HIV negative (HIV-)—An HIV test result that shows no antibodies to the virus.

HIV positive (HIV+)—An HIV test result that indicates the presence of antibodies to the virus.

HIV test—A test, usually a blood test, that detects the presence of antibodies to HIV.

Holism, holistic—The approach to data that looks at numerous variables and their interrelationship.

Homophobia—The irrational fear of people perceived or known to be homosexual.

Homosexual—Someone who is sexually and romantically attracted to members of his or her own sex.

Human T-cell lymphotrophic viruses (HTLV)—Viruses implicated in the cause of some leukemias.

Immune system—That part of the body that helps to respond to pathogens and disease.

Incidence rate—The number of new cases of a disease.

Inductive approach—A way of looking at and analyzing information by gathering data and finding patterns within the data from which generalizations may be made.

Injection drug use (IDU)—The use of needles in intravenous, intramuscular, or subcutaneous injections. Generally, in reference to the risk for

HIV infection, injection drug use refers to recreational, often illegal, intravenous drug usage.

Injection drug user (IDUs)—In the context of risk for HIV infection, someone who injects drugs intravenously, often recreationally and illegally.

Integrase—A protein produced by a virus that helps the virus to integrate into the DNA of the cell.

Kaposi's Sarcoma (KS)—A cancerous OI that expresses itself as blotchy purple lesions in and on people's bodies.

Key informants—Those people in a society or group who appear to well represent the ethos of the group.

Knowledge, Attitudes, and Behavior (KAB)—A HIV prevention interventional model based on the assumption that behavior change will follow changes in knowledge and beliefs.

Lesbian—A female who is sexually and romantically attracted to other females. This is a culture-bound term generally applying to Anglo females or those who have assimilated those values.

Levirate—The practice in polygynous societies of widows marrying their dead husband's brother(s).

Long-term survivors—Those people with HIV/AIDS who have lived with the virus for more than fifteen years and remain healthy.

Major histocompatibility complex (MHC)—A cluster of genes that maintain the immune system.

Male circumcision (MC)—Removal of the foreskin from the penis.

Male-to-female transmission—In unprotected sex, the transmission of HIV from the male to the female. Semen contains higher concentrations of HIV than do vaginal fluids, and in p-v intercourse, the vagina has a larger exposed surface area than does the penis.

Mandatory contact tracing—The practice of notifying sex and needle-sharing partners of someone who tests HIV+.

Mandatory HIV testing—HIV testing that is ordered by courts, the military, or in some parts of the federal government by employers, with or without the individual's consent.

Mandatory name reporting—The practice of reporting an individual's name, date of birth, gender, ethnicity, and address to the Center for Disease Control and Prevention if the person tests HIV+.

Matrilineal descent—Tracing one's family members through the mother's side of the family.

Men Who Have Sex With Men (MSM)—Epidemiologically, *MSM* is a commonly accepted term/acronym. While there is ongoing controversy over risk-exposure categorization and terminology (see Diaz 1998), *MSM* generally is preferred over *gay* or *homosexual*. The term *MSM* covers a broader range of behavior and takes on fewer political connotations in terms of identity in the United States than does either *gay* or *homosexual*. It is also more applicable cross-culturally and within subcultures in the United States (Carrier 2001; Tielman 1991).

Mixed feeding—Combining both breastfeeding and formula as sources of foods for infants.

Modes of transmission—The ways in which HIV can be transmitted through blood, semen, vaginal fluids, and breast milk and from mother to child during pregnancy or birth

Monogamy—The practice of having one sexual partner for life.

Mother-to-child transmission (MTCT)—Transmission of HIV from mother to fetus during pregnancy or birth or to the child after birth through breast-feeding.

MTFs/M2Fs—Male-to-female transsexuals.

National Institute of Drug Abuse (NIDA)—A federally funded organization that conducts research, investigates, and sets standards about the use of various drugs.

National Institutes of Health (NIH)—A federally funded organization that conducts research and sets health policy for health and disease concerns.

National Institute of Mental Health (NIMH)—A federally funded organization that conducts research and sets health policy regarding mental health issues.

Needle/Syringe exchange programs (N/SEPs)—Programs established to reduce HIV transmission through dirty needles. People exchange used needles for clean ones at specified locations and at specific dates and times.

Nevirapine—An antiretroviral drug that is effective in reducing MTCT of HIV during pregnancy, birth, and breast-feeding.

Nongovernmental organizations (NGOs)—Organizations that often are funded by grant money. Relative to HIV, these organizations develop and implement prevention, testing, and treatment programs.

Nonprogressors—Those individuals infected with HIV who do not become ill or develop OIs or AIDS.

Opportunistic infections (OIs)—Those diseases that generally only affect people with compromised immune systems.

Opt-in/opt-out—An informed-consent decision to either specifically agree to a medical procedure (opt-in) or to refuse the procedure (opt-out).

OraQuick®—An HIV antibody test that can give initial results in twenty minutes.

Pandemic—The presence of a disease globally.

Participant-observation—An important methodological technique in anthropology, in which the researcher spends extended periods of time living with the group being studied.

P-a sex—Penile-anal intercourse.

Patrilineal descent—The practice of tracing one's family for purposes of belonging to a kin group, receiving a name, inheriting property or goods, and/or being socialized by the father's side of the family.

Pattern I, II, or III countries—During the first decade of the HIV/AIDS epidemic, a way of following incidence and prevalence rates around the world, largely by modes of transmission.

People Living With HIV/AIDS (PLWH/As)—A term used for people living with HIV or diagnosed with AIDS.

PEPFAR—President's Emergency Plan for AIDS Relief

Perinatal transmission—The transmission of HIV from a pregnant woman to her fetus during pregnancy and/or birth.

PhRMA—An international pharmaceutical trade group that blocks access to generic antiretrovirals.

PLWH/As—*See* People Living With HIV/AIDS

P-NAP—Partner Notification Assistance Program.—

Pneumocystis Carinii Pneumonia (PCP)—A common OI and virulent form of Pneumonia

Politics—The formal decision-making process within a group or society.

Polyandry—The practice of a woman having more than one husband at a time.

Polygamy—The practice of having more than one spouse or culturally recognized sex partner at a time.

Polygyny—The practice of a man having more than one wife at a time.

Postexposure prophylaxis (PEP)—A thirty-day treatment of antiretrovirals taken to prevent HIV infection in health-care workers who have had needle-stick exposures.

Posttest counseling—HIV test counseling that occurs when results of the HIV antibody test are given.

Prevalence—How widespread a given disease or pathogen is in a population.

Pretest counseling—HIV test counseling that is given prior to having an HIV test.

Pronatalism—Concern for the woman as a reproductive being and for her fetus(es) rather than for her own health and safety.

Protease—An enzyme involved in a late stage of HIV replication.

Protease inhibitor (PI)—A class of anti-HIV drugs that blocks the replication of protease.

Provirus—A virus chromosome integrated into the DNA of the host cell.

P-v sex—Penile-vaginal intercourse.

Rapid Immuno-Assay Test—A new HIV test that can give preliminary results in twenty to thirty minutes.

Reservoirs of infection—Pockets of HIV infection that may be undetectable.

Retrovirus—A class of viruses that contain DNA and reverse transcriptase.

Reverse transcriptase (RT)—An enzyme used by retroviruses to transcribe genetic information from RNA to DNA.

Safer sex—Sexual behaviors in which the risk of transmitting HIV or other STIs is reduced by the use of latex or polyurethane barriers such as male or female condoms, vaginal dams, finger cots, and gloves.

Safe sex—Sexual behaviors in which there is no risk for transmitting HIV or other STIs.

Serial monogamy—The practice of having one sexual partner after another.

Seroconversion/Seroconvert—The process of developing antibodies to HIV, which are eventually detectable.

Sero-discordant—A situation where one partner is HIV- and the other partner is HIV+.

Seronegative —No antibodies to HIV present or detectable.

Seropositive —Antibodies to HIV present and detected.

Sero-status—The HIV status of an individual, described as HIV negative (HIV-), HIV positive (HIV+), or indeterminate

Sexual cleansing of widows—Ritualized symbolic or behavioral intercourse between a widow and her dead husband's male relatives (also referred to as widow cleansings).

Sexuality—A holistic term used to refer to gender identity, sexual orientation, and gender-role expression across the life cycle. Sexuality incorporates behaviors, beliefs and values that are culturally defined and expressed.

Sexually Transmitted Infections/Diseases (STIs/STDs)—Sexually transmitted infections involve those infections by organisms that are contracted through various forms of sexual behavior. Sexually transmitted diseases are the bodily changes that result from having a sexually transmitted infection.

Sexual orientation—The sex of the person that someone is sexually and romantically attracted to.

Sexual risk continuum—The risk for contracting HIV sexually, measured from the riskiest sexual behavior to the least risky.

Society—The learned, patterned, and shared rules, norms, and behaviors that exist within a group.

Straight—Colloquial term for heterosexual.

Survivor guilt—Feelings experienced by some people who have physically outlived a disaster.

Syncretism—Sociocultural beliefs, values, and norms that result from culture contact and change.

Systems/ecological approach—A holistic, theoretical model in which a feedback interaction occurs between the individual, culture, and environment.

TASO—The AIDS Support Organization. TASO, located in Uganda, provides various services for people with HIV/AIDS.

T-cell—One component of the immune system that helps the body to ward off and respond to pathogens and infections.

Terminal disease/illness—Referring to diseases and illnesses whose outcomes are death.

Thick data—Qualitative data obtained from participant-observation that provide context and depth.

Third and fourth genders—Gender identities that are something other than male or female.

Transsexuals/transgenders (TSs/TGs)—People in industrialized societies whose gender identities are other than male or female, most often biological men who perceive themselves to be women and biological women who perceive themselves to be men.

Transvestites (TVs)—An etic designation generally applied to men who dress in women's clothes.

Treatment Action Campaign (TAC)—An NGO in South Africa that challenges President Mbeki's views on HIV/AIDS and provides information about prevention, testing, and treatment.

"Two Spirits"—Among southwestern Native American groups, specifically the Zuni, this term is applied to men whose gender identity is something other than as a male and who may fulfill the gender roles of females in these societies.

Universal precautions/standards—Medical practices designed to reduce the transmission of pathogens found in bodily fluids and tissues.

Vectors of transmission—Those people who transmit HIV to others.

Viral load—The number of HIV particles detectable in the blood.

Virons—Viral particles.

Virus—A cellular organism that replicates inside host cells.

Western Blot test—The test that confirms a positive ELISA HIV antibody test by looking for specific antibodies to HIV.

Widow cleansings—The practice in some patrilineal descent societies, in which a widow engages in symbolic or actual ritual intercourse with her dead husband's male relatives (also referred to as sexual cleansings of widows).

"Window period"—The time before someone who has been exposed to HIV has built up sufficient antibodies to the virus for the antibodies to be detectable.

Women Who Have Sex With Women (WSW)—A generic term applied to women who may or may not identify as lesbian but who have sex with other women.

World Health Organization (WHO)—An international group that addresses a variety of health issues globally.

"Worried well"—Individuals who are at low risk for contracting HIV but experience anxiety over the possibility of becoming infected.

Zoonotic—Organisms that can transfer from one species to another.

Bibliography

AARG
  2003 Electronic document, http://puffin.creighton.edu/aarg,accessed April 7, 2006.
  2001 Electronic document, http://puffin.creighton.edu/aarg, accessed December 22, 2005.

abcNews.com
  2004 "Bitter Medicine: Pills, Profit, and the Public Health." Electronic document, http://abcnews.go.com/onair/ABCNEWSSpecials/pharmaceuticals_020529_pjr_feature.html, accessed June 24, 2004.

Abel, Laurent
  2002 "Human Genetic Variability and Susceptibility to Infectious Disease." In *Chemokine Receptors and AIDS*. Thomas O'Brien, ed. Pp. 105–6. New York: Marcel Dekker.

Abeni, Damian, Carlo A. Perucci, Kate Dolan and Massimo Sengalli
  1998 "Prison and HIV-1 Infection among Drug Injectors." In *Drug Injecting and HIV Infection*. Global Dimensions and Local Responses. Gerry Stimson, Don DesJarlais, and Andrew Ball, eds. Pp. 168–82. Bristol, U.K.: UCL Press.

Abrams, Donald
  1996 "Alternative Therapies." In *A Clinical Guide to HIV and AIDS*. Gary P. Wormser, ed. Pp. 379–96. Philadelphia: Lippincott-Raven.

ACTUP. *AIDS*
  2003 Electronic document, http://www.actupsf.com/nav/aids/aids.htm, accessed February 7, 2006.

Acuff, Katherine L.
  1996 "Perinatal Drug Use: State Interventions and the Implications of HIV-Infected Women." In *HIV, AIDS and Childbearing. Public Policy, Private Lives*. Ruth R. Faden and Nancy E. Kass, eds. Pp. 214–53. New York: Oxford University Press.
  2005 "AIDS Optimism, Condom Fatigue or Self-Esteem? Explaining Unsafe Sex among Gay and Bisexual Men." *Journal of Sex Research*. 42(3)(August): 224–37.

Adams, B.
  2002 "A Fortune Retold." *HIV Plus* 5(3): 12–20.

Adams, Jad
  1989 *AIDS: The HIV Myth*. New York: St. Martin's Press.

Adams, Vincanne, and Stacy Pigg, eds.
  2005 *Sex in Development: Science, Sexuality and Morality in Global Perspective*. Durham, N.C.: Duke University Press.

Adimora, Adaora A., and Victor J. Schoenbach
    2005   Social Context, Sexual Networks, and Racial Disparities in Rates of Sexually
            Transmitted Infections. Journal of Infectious Diseases 191:S-115–S122.
Adjuik, Martin, Tom Smith, Sam Clark, Jim Todd, Anu Garrib, Yohannes Kinfu, Kathy
Kahn, Mitiki Mola, Ali Ashraf, Honorati Masanja, Ubaje Adazu, Jahit Sacarlal, Nurul
Alam, Adama Marra, Adjima Gbangou, Eleuther Mwageni, and Fred Binka
    2006   "Cause-specific mortality rates in Sub-Saharan Africa and Bangladesh."
            Bulletin of the World Health Organization. March. 84(3):181–92.
AF-AIDSeForum
    2004   "AF-AIDSeForum2004." Electronic document, af- aidseforums.health.dev.
            org, accessed December 15, 2005.
Afifi, Walid A.
    1999   "Harming the Ones We Love: Relational Attachment and Perceived Conse-
            quences as Predictors of Safe-Sex Behavior." The Journal of Sex Research 36
            (2): 198–207.
AFROL
    2005   "Legal Status of Homosexuality in Africa." Electronic document, http://
            www.afrol/com/Categories/Gay/backgr_legalstatus.htm, accessed April 13,
            2005.
Aggleton, Peter
    2007   Roundtable. "'Just a Snip?' A Social History of Male Circumcision." Repro-
            ductive Health Matters 15(29): 15–21.
Aggleton, Peter, ed.
    1994   Learning About AIDS: Scientific and Social Issues. 2nd edition. New York:
            Churchill Livingstone.
Aggleton, Peter, Peter Davies, and Graham Hart, eds.
    1994   Learning about AIDS: Scientific and Social Issues (2nd edition). Philadel-
            phia: W. B. Saunders.
Ahlemeyer, Heinrich W.
    2000   "AIDS Prevention as a Social System interaction Risk-Taking in the Context
            of Different Types of Heterosexual Partnerships." In Partnership and Prag-
            matism: The German Response to AIDS Prevention and Care (Social Aspects
            of AIDS). Rolf Rosenbrock and Michael T. Wright, eds. Pp. 106–18. New
            York: Routledge.
AIDS Action Committee of Massachusetts
    2005   Electronic document, http://www.aac.org/site/PageServer?pagename=
            action_testimonySen647, accessed November 6, 2006.
AIDS and Anthropology Research Group (AARG)
    2003   Electronic document, http://www.groups.creighton.edu/aarg, accessed
            April 7, 2006.
AIDS and Anthropology Research Group (AARG) Newsletter
    1988   v.1 (1)(July-Sept):1–4.
AIDS_Asia@yahoogroups.com
    2006   "Regular, Routine HIV Tests for All Between 13 and 64, cdc. Monday Sep-
            tember 25, 2006." Electronic document, http://www.groups.yahoo.com.
            groups/AIDS_Asia, accessed September 25, 2006.

AIDS Community Resource Newsletter
    2006   "25 Years of AIDS Timeline." (May 2006): 2.
AIDS Support Organization (TASO)
    2002/2004 Electronic document, http://www.tasouganda.org, accessed April 13,
            2008.
AIDS TREATMENT NOW
    2003   Issues #40, 41, 44. Electronic document, info/newsletter.htm, accessed De-
            cember 15, 2004.
Aing, Tade A.
    1991   "Patterns of Bisexuality in Sub-Saharan Africa." In *Bisexuality and HIV/
            AIDS: A Global Perspective*. Rob Tielman, Manuel Carballo and Aart Hen-
            driks, eds. Pp. 81–90. Buffalo, N.Y.: Prometheus.
Ajzen, Icek, and Martin Fishbein
    1980   *Understanding Attitudes and Predicting Social Behavior*. Englewood Cliffs,
            N.J.: Prentice Hall.
Alan Guttmacher Institute (AGI)
    2004   Electronic document, http://www.agi-usa.org, accessed April 9, 2006.
    2003   "A, B, and C in Uganda: Roles of Abstinence, Monogamy and Condom Use
            in HIV Decline." New York: AGI.
Alcamo, I. Edward
    2003   *AIDS The Biological Basis*. 3rd edition. Sudbury: Jones and Bartlett.
Alexander, Priscilla
    1996   "Women Who Go Out." In *Women's Experiences with HIV/AIDS: An Inter-
            national Perspective*. In D. Long Lynellen and E. Maxine Ankrah, eds. Pp.
            75–90. New York: Columbia University Press.
Allam, Hannah
    2006   "Iran Leads Mideast in Fighting AIDS." Electronic document, http://www.
            kansascity.com/mld/kansascity/news/world/14352264.htm,   accessed
            May 5, 2006.
Allen, Anita
    1996   "Moral Multiculturalism, Childbearing and AIDS." In *HIV, AIDS and Child-
            bearing. Public Policy, Private Lives*. Ruth R. Faden and Nancy E. Kass, eds.
            Pp. 367–407. New York: Oxford University Press.
Allen, Arthur
    2002   "Sex Change: Uganda v. Condoms." *New Republic* May 27: 14–15.
Altman, Lawrence
    2004   "Former Model of Success, Thailand's AIDS Effort Falters," *U.N. Re-
            ports*. Electronic document, http://www.nytimes.com/2004/07/09/
            international/asia/09Aids.html?th, accessed July 9, 2004.
Amadora-Nolasco, Fiscalina, Rene E. Alburo, Judy T. Aguilar Elmira, and Wenda R.
            Trevathan
    2001   "Knowledge, Perception of Risk for HIV and Condom Use: A Comparison
            of Registered and Freelance Female Sex Workers in Cebu City, Philippines."
            AIDS and Behavior 5(4): 319–30.
American Anthropological Association
    1997   "National Institutes of Health Consensus Development Conference on

Interventions to Prevent HIV Risk Behaviors. Statement of the American Anthropological Association on AIDS Research and Education January 24, 1997." Electronic document, http://www.aaanet.org/stmts/nih.htm, accessed February 20, 2006.

American Red Cross
2003   Electronic document, http://www.redcross.org, accessed April 30, 2004.

Americans with Disabilities Act (ADA)
2004   Electronic document, http://www.usdoj.gov/crt/ada/adahom1.htm, accessed June 30, 2006.

American Social Health Association (ASHA)
2003   *FAQS-STD*. Electronic document, http://www.ashastd.org/nah/faqs.html, accessed August 5, 2006.

AmFar
2001   *AIDS/HIV Treatment Directory*. New York: The Foundation.

"The AmFar Treatment Insider"
2002a   2(6). In *HIV Plus*. 5(1): 2–6.
2002b.   3(1). In *HIV Plus*. 5(2):1–8.
2002c.   3(2). In *HIV Plus*. 5(3):1–8.
2001.   1(4). In *HIV Plus*. 4(5):1–8.

Amirkanian, Yuri A., Jeffrey A. Kelly, Elena Kabakchieva, Timothy L. McAuliffe and Sylvia Vassileva
2003   "Evaluation of a Social Network HIV Prevention Intervention Program for Young Men Who Have Sex with Men in Russia and Bulgaria." *AIDS Education and Prevention* 15(3): 205–20.

Ammann, Arthur J.
2000   "Introduction to the Second Conference on Global Strategies for the Prevention of HIV Transmission from Mothers to Infants." *Prevention and Treatment of HIV Infection in Infants and Children* 918: 1–2.

Ammann, A.J., and A. Rubenstein eds.
2000   *Prevention and Treatment of HIV Infection in Infants and Children*. v. 918. New York: New York Academy of Sciences.

Amnesty International
2002   *World AIDS Day: Human Rights Central to Battle against AIDS*. Electronic document, http://web.manesty.org/library/index/ENGPOL300082002, accessed June 25, 2004.

Anastos, Kathryn, Risa Deneberg, and L. Solomon
1996   "Clinical Management of HIV-Infected Women." In *A Clinical Guide to HIV and AIDS*. Gary Wormser, ed. Pp. 69–83. Philadelphia: Lippincott-Raven.

Anderson, Gregory
1996   "The Older Gay Man." In *HIV/AIDS and the Older Adult*. Kathleen Nokes, ed. Pp. 63–79. Washington, D.C.: Taylor Francis.

Anderson, Jean
1996   "Gynecologic and Obstetric Issues for HIV-Infected Women." In *HIV, AIDS and Childbearing: Public Policy, Private Lives*. Ruth R. Faden and Nancy Kass, eds. Pp. 31–62. New York: Oxford University Press.

Anderson, Jean, ed.
    2001   *A Guide to the Clinical Care of Women with HIV.* 2001 Edition. Rockville: Womencare.

Anderson, John R. and Robert L. Barrett, eds.
    2001   *Ethics in HIV-Related Psychotherapy: Clinical Decision-Making in Complex Cases.* 1st edition. Washington, D.C.: American Psychological Association.

Andrade, Tarcisio, P. Lurie, M.G. Medina, K. Anderson, and I. Dourado
    2001   The Opening of South America's First Needle Exchange Program and Epidemic of Crack Use in Salvador, Bahai-Brazil." *AIDS and Behavior* (1): 51–64.

Ankrah, E. Maxine, Martin Schwartz, and Jaclyn Miller
    1996   "Care and Support Systems." In *Women's Experiences with HIV/AIDS: An International Perspective.* Lynellen Long and E. Maxine Ankrah, eds. Pp. 264–93. New York: Columbia University Press.

Annan, Kofi
    2004   "Secretary-General's Remarks on 2004 International Women's Day." Electronic document, http://www.un.org/apps/sg/sgstats.asp?nid=806, accessed April 24, 2008.

Anonymous
    2004a   "HIV Diagnoses Increased in More Than Half of the United States. Infectious Disease News." Electronic document, http://www.infectiousdisease-news.com/200401/frameset.asp?article=hiv.asp, accessed January 22, 2004.

    2004b   "Tackling AIDS in China." SciDevNet, accessed May 18, 2004.

    2003a   "AIDS Cases up in U.S.—First time since {ap}93." *San Francisco Chronicle,* February 12, 2003: A4.

    2003b   "Chiron's Global Operation." Electronic document, http://www/chiron.com/investor/annual/2001/pdf/Chiron_2001_Pipeline.pdf, accessed May 15, 2004.

    2003c   "South African President Pressured to eliminate discourse on HIV and AIDS." *Health Education AIDS Liason,* Toronto. Electronic document, http://www.healtoronto.com/mbeki.html, accessed December 15, 2004.

    2003d   "Talking Teen Sex." *San Francisco Chronicle,* July 6, 2003: E4, E5.

    2002   "Love life and Independent Newspapers Join South African Fight against HIV/AIDS." *SIECUS Report* 30(5): 24.

    2001   AIDS Epidemic Turns Twenty: A Timeline. North CountryAIDS Outreach Summer 2001: 1.

    2000a   *Intensifying Action against HIV/AIDS in Africa: Responding to a Development Crisis.* Washington, D.C.: World Bank, 2000.

    2000b   "The NIDA Community-Based Outreach Model: A Manual to Reduce the Risk of HIV and Other Blood-Borne Infections in Drug Users." In *National Institutes of Health, Center on AIDS and Other Medical Consequences of Drug abuse.* NIH Publication Number 00–4812.

    1998a   "Mayor's Summit on AIDS & HIV San Francisco: Final Report." San Francisco: Office of the Mayor.

1998b "Natural Resistance to HIV/AIDS. AIDS SA-Update on HIV and the Health Care Worker" 6(3). Electronic document, http://www.cig.salk.edu/extra_html/etc_natural_resistance.htm, accessed April 6, 2004.

Aranda-Naranjo, Barbara, and Rachel Davis
2001 "Psychosocial and Cultural Considerations." In *A Guide to the Clinical Care of HIV in Women*. Jean Anderson, ed. Pp. 275–88. Rockville: Women Care.

Aries, Philippe
1989 *Centuries of Childhood: A Social History of Family. Life*. London: Vintage.

Armelagos, George J., Alan H Goodman, and Kenneth Jacobs
1978 "The Ecological Perspective in Disease." In *Health and the Human Condition: Perspectives on Medical Anthropology*. Michael H. Logan and Edward E. Hunt Jr., eds. Pp. 71–84. North Scituate, R.I.: Duxbury Press.

Armelagos, George J., Mary Ryan, and Thomas Leatherman
1990 "Evolution of Infectious Disease: A Biocultural Analysis of AIDS." *American Journal of Human Biology* 2: 353–63.

Arya, O., and C. Hart, eds.
1998 *Sexually Transmitted Infections and AIDS in the Tropics*. New York: CABI.

Auer, Carrie
1996 "Women, Children and HIV/AIDS." In *Women's Experiences with HIV/AIDS: An International Perspective*. Lynellen Long and E. Maxine Ankrah, eds. Pp. 236–63. New York: Columbia University Press.

Awusabo-Asare, Kofi, Albert M. Abane, Delali M. Bedasu, and John K. Anarfi
1999 "'All Die Be Die': Obstacles to Change in the Face of HIV Infection in Ghana." In *Resistances to Behavioural Change to Reduce HIV/AIDS Infection in Predominantly Heterosexual Epidemics in Third World Countries*. John C. Caldwell, Pat Caldwell, John Anarfi, Kofi Awusabo-Asare, James Ntozi, I. O. Orubuloye, Jeff Marck, Wendy Cosford, Rachel Colombo, and Elaine Hollings, eds. Pp. 125–32. Canberra: Health Transition Centre, National Centre for Epidermiology and Population Health, Australian National University.

Bader, A.
2002 "Preoperative Evaluation of the HIV-Infected Patient." In *Pain Management of HIV/AIDS Patients*. Srdjan S. Nedeljkovic, ed. Pp. 195–99. Boston: Butterworth-Heinemann.

Bailes, Elizabeth, Feng Gao, Frederic Bibillet-Ruche, Valerie Courgnaud, Martine Peeters, Preston A. Marx, Beatrice H. Hahn, and Paul M. Sharp
2003 "Hybrid Origin of SIV in Chimpanzees." *Science 300*(5626):1713–15.

Bailey, M.
1999 "Young Women and HIV: The Role of Biology in Vulnerability." In *Mental Health and HIV Infection: Psychological and Psychiatric Aspects*. Jose Catalan, ed. Pp. 159–69. London: UCL Press.

Bailey, Robert C., and Daniel T. Halperin
2000 "Male Circumcision and HIV Infection." *Lancet* 355 (9216): 926–27.

Bailey, Robert C., S. Neema, and R. Othieno
1999 "Sexual behaviors and other HIV risk factors in circumcised and uncircumcised men in Uganda." *Journal of Acquired Immune Deficiency Syndromes* 22(3) (November 1): 294–302.

Bailey, Robert C., Francis A. Plummer, and Stephen Moses

    2001   "Male Circumcision and HIV Prevention: Current Knowledge and Future Research Directions." *The Lancet. Infectious Diseases.* 1 (November): 223–31.

Bailey, William A.

    1995   "The Importance of HIV Prevention Programming to the Lesbian and Gay Community." In *AIDS, Identity and Community. The HIV Epidemic and Lesbian and Gay Men.* Gregory M. Herek and Beverly Greene, eds. Pp. 210–25. Thousand Oaks, Calif.: Sage Publications.

Bajos, N., and J. Marquet

    2000   Research on HIV Sexual Risk: Social Relations Based on Cross-Cultural Perspective. *Social Science and Medicine* 50(11)(June): 1533–46.

Bakari, J.P., S. McKenna, A. Myrick, K. Mwinga, G.J. Bhat, and S. Allen

    2000   "Rapid Voluntary Testing and Counseling for HIV. Acceptability and Feasibility in Zambian Antenatal Care Clinics." *Prevention and Treatment of HIV Infection in Infants and Children* 918: 57–63.

Ball, Andrew L.

    1998   "Overview: Policies and Interventions to Stem HIV-1 Epidemic Associated with Injected Drug Use." In *Drug Injecting and HIV Infection. Global Dimensions and Local Responses.* Gary Stimson, Don DesJarlais and Andrew L. Ball, eds. Pp. 201–32. Bristol, U.K.: UCL Press.

Balmer, Donald, Olga A. Grinstead, Francis Kihuho, Steven E. Gregorich, Michael D. Sweat, Claudes M. Kamenga, Frank A. Plummer, Kevin R. O'Reilly, Samuel Kalibala, Eric van Praag, and Thomas A. Coates

    2000   "Characteristics of Individuals and Couples Seeking HIV-1 Prevention Services in Nairobi, Kenya: The Voluntary HIV-1 Counseling and Testing Efficacy Study." AIDS and Behavior 4(1): 15–23.

Bandura, Albert

    1986   *Social Foundations of Thought and Action: A Social Cognitive Theory.* Englewood Cliffs, N.J.: Prentice Hall.

Bankole, Akinrinola, Susheeha Singh, Vanessa Woog, and Deidre Wulf

    2004   *Risk and Protection. Youth and HIV/AIDS in Sub-Saharan Africa.* New York: Alan Guttmacher Institute. Electronic document, http://www.guttmacher.org/pubs/riskandprotection.pdf, accessed August 3, 2006.

Banks, Taunya L.

    1996   "Legal Challenges: State Intervention, Reproduction and HIV-Infected Women." In *HIV, AIDS and Childbearing. Public Policy, Private Lives.* Ruth R. Faden and Nancy Kass, eds. Pp. 143–77. New York: Oxford University Press.

Barbach, Lonnie

    1998   *The Pause: Positive Approaches to Menopause.* Collingdale, Del.: Diane Book Publishing.

Barker, Judith C., Robynn S. Battle, Gayle L. Cummings, and Katherine N. Bancroft

    1998   Condoms and Consequences: HIV/AIDS education and African-American Women. *Human Organization* 57(3):273–83.

Barnett, Theodore, and Alan Whiteside
    2002   *AIDS in the Twenty-First Century. Disease and Globalization.* New York: Palgrave MacMillan.
Barrett, Robert L., and Adam Robinson
    1996   "Red Clay and Red Necks: HIV Prevention in Rural Southern Communities." In *AIDS Education: Reaching Diverse Populations.* Melinda K. Moore and Martin Forst, eds. Pp. 171–81. Westport, Conn.: Praeger.
Barth, Frederik
    1998   *Ethnic Groups and Boundaries.* 2nd edition. Prospect Heights: Waveland Press.
Bartlett, John G.
    2006   "Pocket Guide. Adult HIV/AIDS Treatment." January 2006. The Johns Hopkins AIDS Service. Electronic document, http://www.hopkins-aids.org and http://hopkins- aids.edu/publications/ Pocketguide/pocketgd0106.pdf, accessed April 7, 2006.
    2002   *The Johns Hopkins Hospital 2002 Guide to Medical Care of Patients with HIV Infection.* 10th edition. Philadelphia: Lippincott Williams and Wilkins.
Bartlett, John G., and Ann K. Finkbeiner
    1998   *The Guide to Living with HIV Infection.* 4th edition. Baltimore: Johns Hopkins University Press.
Bastos, Cristiana
    1999   *Global Responses to AIDS: Science in Emergency.* Bloomington: Indiana University Press, 1999.
Bastos, Francisco I., Gary Stimson, Paulo R. Telles, and Christovam Barcellos
    1998   "Cities Responding to HIV-1 Epidemics among Injecting Drug Users." In *Drug Injecting and HIV Infection. Global Dimensions and Local Responses.* Gary Stimson, Don DesJarlais, and Alan Ball, eds. Pp. 149–67. Bristol, U.K.: UCL Press.
Basu, Alaka M., Devandra B. Gupta, and Geetanjali Krishna
    1997   "The Household Impact of Adult Morbidity and Mortality: Some Implications of the Potential Epidemic of AIDS in India." In *The Economics of HIV and AIDS: The Case of South and Southeast Asia.* David E. Blooman and Peter Godwin, eds. Pp. 102–54. New York: Oxford University Press.
Basu, Sanjay, Kedar Mate, and Paul Farmer
    2000   "Debt and Poverty Turn a Disease into an Epidemic." *Nature* 407(6800): 14.
Basuki, Endang, Ivan Wolffers, Walter Deville, Noni Erlaini,Dorang Luhpuri, Rachmat Hargono, Nuning Maskuri, Nayoman Suesen, and Nel van Beelen
    2002   "Reasons for Not Using Condoms among Female Sex Workers in Indonesia." *AIDS Education and Prevention* 14(2): 102–17.
Bayer, Ronald
    2000   "Privacy and the Public Health: Conflict and Change in the AIDS Epidemic." In *The Emergence of AIDS. The Impact of Immunology, Microbiology and Public Health.* Kenneth H. Mayer and H. F. Pizer, eds. Pp. 163–78. Washington, D.C.: American Public Health Association.

Bayer, Ronald, and Gerald M. Oppenheimer
   2000   *AIDS Doctors: Voices from the Epidemic*. New York: Oxford University Press.
BBC News UK Edition
   2004   *The Global Spread of HIV*. Electronic document, http://news.bbc.co.uk/1/shared/spl/hi/africa/03/aids_debate/html/default.stm, accessed September 24, 2005.
Becker, Jasper
   2003   "Beijing Wakes to Health Disaster Threat." *San Francisco Chronicle*, February 9: A14.
Beckett, Alison C.
   1997   "Ethical Dilemmas for Psychiatrists: Assisted Suicide in AIDS." In *Mental Health and HIV Infection: Psychological and Psychiatric Aspects*. Jose Catalan, ed. Pp. 223–33. London: UCL Press.
Becklerleg, Susan, Maggie Telfer, and Gillian Lewando Hundt
   2005   "The Rise of Injecting Drug Use in East Africa: A Case Study from Kenya." *Harm Reduction Journal* 2(1)(August): 1–9.
Beil, Laura
   1999   "(DMN) Tests trace HIV's origin to chimps: 'Missing link funding could boost research.'" *Dallas Morning News*, February 1. Electronic document, http://www.aegis.com/news/dam/1999/DN99020.html, accessed February 1, 2006.
Bennett, L., D. Miller, and M. Ross, eds.
   1995   *Health Workers and AIDS: Research, Intervention and Current Issues in Burnout and Response*. Chur: Harwood Academic.
Bennett, Rebecca
   1999   "Should We Routinely Test Pregnant Women for HIV?" In *HIV and AIDS: Testing, Screening and Confidentiality*. Rebecca Bennett and Charles A. Erin, eds. Pp. 228–39. New York: Oxford University Press.
Bennett, Rebecca, and Charles A. Erin, eds.
   1999   *HIV and AIDS: Testing, Screening and Confidentiality*. New York: Oxford University Press.
Beyrer, Chris
   1998   "War in the Blood: Sex, Politics and AIDS in Southeast Asia." New York: Zed Books.
Bhutani, L., and N. Khanna
   2001   *Sexually Transmitted Diseases: An Asian Perspective. A Common Wealth Response to a Global Health Challenge*. London: Common Wealth Secretariat.
Biehl, João, with Denise Coutinho and Ana Luzia Outeiro
   2001   "Technology and Affect: HIV/AIDS Testing in Brazil." *Culture, Medicine and Psychiatry* 25: 87–129.
Billowitz, Marissa
   2004   "Doing Gender the 'Rights' Way. Gender Roles: What Are We Really Teaching Young People?" *SIECUS Report* 32(3): 5–10.

Bingman, Cherilyn R., Gary Marks, and Nicole Crepaz
    2001   "Attributions about One's HIV Infection and Unsafe Sex in Seropositive Men Who Have Sex with Men." *AIDS and Behavior* 5(3): 283–90.

Blackwood, Evelyn, and Saskia E. Wieringa, eds.
    1999   *Female Desires: Same-Sex Relations and Transgender Practices.* New York: Columbia University Press.

Blankenship, Kim
    1997   "Social Context and HIV: Testing and Treatment Issues among Commercial Sex Workers." In *The Gender Politics of HIV/AIDS in Women: Perspectives on the Pandemic in the U.S.* Nancy Goldstein and Jennifer L. Manlowe, eds. Pp. 252–69. New York: New York University Press.

Bloem, Maurice, Enamul Hoque, Lusy Khanam, Trisna Selina Mahbub,Moshtaqua Salehin, and Shanaz Begum
    1999   "HIV/AIDS and Female Street-Based Sex Workers in Dhaka City, What About Their Clients?" In *Resistances to Behavioural Change to Reduce HIV/ AIDS Infection in Predominantly Heterosexual Epidemics in Third World Countries.* John C. Caldwell, Pat Caldwell, John Anarfi, Kofi Awusabo-Asare, James Ntozi, I. O. Orubuloye, Jeff Marck, Wendy Cosford, Rachel Colombo, and Elaine Hollings, eds. Pp. 197–210. Canberra: Health Transition Centre, National Centre for Epidemiology and Population Health, Australian National University.

Bloom, David E., and Ajay S. Mahal
    1997   "The AIDS Epidemic and Economic Policy Analysis." In *The Economics of HIV and AIDS: The Case of South and Southeast Asia.* David E. Bloom and Peter Godwin, eds. Pp. 9–21. New York: Oxford University Press.

Bloom, David, E., Ajay, S. Mahal, Lene Christiansen, Amala De Silva, Doma de Sylva, Malsiri Dias, Saroj Jayasinghe, Soma Mahawewa, Thana Sanmugam, and Gunatillake Tantrigana
    1997   "Socio-economic Dimensions of the HIV/AIDS Epidemic in Sri Lanka." In *The Economics of HIV and AIDS: The Case of South and Southeast Asia.* David E. Bloom and Peter Godwin, eds. Pp. 155–263. New York: Oxford University Press.

Blower, Sally, Katia Koelle, and John Mills
    2002   "Health Policy Modeling: Epidemic Control, HIV Vaccines and Risky Behavior." In *Quantitative Evaluation of HIV Prevention Programs.* Edward H. Kaplan and Ron Brookmeyer, eds. Pp. 260–89. New Haven: Yale University Press.

Bockting, Walter O., and Sheila Kirk, eds.
    2001   *Transgender and HIV.* Binghamton: Haworth Press.

Bockting, Walter O., B. R. Simon Rosser, and Eli Coleman
    2001   "Transgender HIV Prevention. Community Involvement and Empowerment." In *Transgender and HIV.* Walter O. Bockting and Sheila Kirk, eds. Pp. 119–44. Binghamton, N.Y.: Haworth Press.

Body AIDS and HIV Information Resources
    2003a "AIDS Forum." Electronic document, http://www.thebody.com/Forums/

AIDS/SideEffects/Archive/Information/Q12611.htm, accessed August 5, 2003.

2003b "HIV Testing. Names Reporting and Partner Notification." Electronic document, http://www.thebody.com/govt/reporting.html, accessed December 8, 2003.

Bodzin, Steven

2005   "Students Tap New Vein of Gay Issue: The FDA has Refused to End Its Ban on Donations of Blood from Men Who Have Had Sex With Men. Now, Campuses Take The Fight to the Red Cross." *Los Angeles Times.* July 10. http://www.aegis.com/news/lt/2005/ LT050704.html, accessed August 4, 2006.

Bolin, Anne, and Patricia Whelehan

1999   *Perspectives on Human Sexuality.* Albany: SUNY Press.

Bolton, Ralph

2000   "Real and Raw: Sexual Definitions & Motivations in Gay Barebacking." Paper Presented at the Society for Cross-Cultural Research, New Orleans, February 23–27.

1994   "Sex, Science and Social Responsibility: Cross-Cultural Research On Same-Sex Eroticism and Sexual Intolerance." *Cross-Cultural Research* 28(2): 134–90.

1992   "AIDS and Promiscuity: Muddles in the Models of HIV Prevention." *Medical Anthropology.* 14: 145–223.

Bolton, Ralph, John Vincke, Rudolf Mak, and Ellen Dennehy

1992   "Alcohol and Risky Sex. In Search of an Elusive Connection." *Medical Anthropology.* 14: 323–63.

Bonavida, Benjamin

2002   "Natural Killer Cells in HIV Infection and Role in the Pathogenesis of AIDS." In *Cellular Aspects of HIV Infection.* Andrea Cossarizza and David Kaplan, eds. Pp. 183–205. New York: Wiley-Liss.

Bond, Katherine C., David D. Delentianio, and Chayan Vaddhanaphuti

1996   "'I'm Not Afraid of Life or Death:' Women in Brothels in Northern Thailand." In *Women's Experiences with HIV/AIDS.* An International Perspective. Lynellen D. Long and E. Maxine Ankrah, eds. Pp. 123–49. New York: Columbia University Press.

Bond, Virginia

1997   "'Between a Rock and a Hard Place': Applied Anthropology and AIDS Research on a Commercial Farm in Zambia." *Health Transition Review.* 7 (Supplement 3): 69–83.

Bonivento, Cesare, Bishop of Vanimo

2001   "Do Condoms Stop or Spread AIDS?" Gorok: Family Life Apostolate. "AIDS and Condoms: The Teachings of the Church." Vanimo. Pastoral Letter. Foreword, pages 5–8. Vanimo Family Life Apostolate. Information from the Agencies Promoting Condoms as Protective from AIDS: 1–22.

Bradley, Joanne

1995   "Cultural Sensitivity." In *Primary Care of Women and Children with HIV*

Infection: A Multidisciplinary Approach. Patricia Kelly, Susan Holman, Rosalie Rothenberg, and Stephen P. Holzemer, eds. Pp. 189–93. Boston: Jones and Bartlett.

Bray-Preston, Deborah, Anthony R. D'Augelli, Cathy D. Kassab, and Michael T. Starks

    2007   "The Relationship of Stigma to the Sexual Risk Behavior of Rural Men Who Have Sex with Men." *AIDS Education and Prevention* 19(3)(June): 218–30.

Breitbart, William

    1996   "Pharmaco Therapy of Pain in AIDS." In *A Clinical Guide to HIV and AIDS.* Gary Wormser, ed. Pp. 359–78. Philadelphia: Lippincott-Raven.

Brenner, Bluma G., and Mark Wainberg

    2000   "The Role of Antiretrovirals and Drug Resistance in Vertical Transmission of HIV-1 Infection." *Prevention and Treatment of HIV Infection in Infants and Children* 918: 9–15.

Brimlow, Deborah L., and Michael W. Ross

    1998   "HIV-Related Communication and Power in Women Injection Drug Users." In *Women and AIDS. Negotiating Safer Practices, Care and Representation.* Nancy L. Roth and Linda K. Fuller, eds. Pp. 71–80. Binghamton, N.Y.: Haworth Press.

Brookmeyer, Ron

    2002   "Statistical Issues in HIV Prevention." In *Quantitative Evaluation of HIV Prevention Programs.* Edward H. Kaplan and Ron Brookmeyer, eds. Pp. 55–78. New Haven: Yale University Press.

Brooks, Ronald, Mary Jane Rotheram-Borus, and Eric G. Bing, eds.

    2003   "HIV Prevention for Men of Color Who Have Sex with Men (MSM) and Men of Color Who Have Sex with Men and Women (MSM/W)." A Special Supplement to *AIDS Education and Prevention* 15 (Supplement A, 1–6): 1–138.

Brown, J. E., O. B. Ayowa, and R. C. Brown

    1993   "Dry and Tight: Sexual Practices and Potential AIDS Risk in Zaire." *Social Science and Medicine* 37(8) (1993): 989–94.

Brown, Lisanne, K. MacIntyre, and Lea Trujillo

    2003   "Interventions to Reduce HIV/AIDS Stigma. What Have We Learned?" *AIDS Education and Prevention* 15(1): 49–69.

Bruce, Katherine E., and Lori J. Walker

    2001   "College Students' Attitudes about AIDS: 1986–2000." *AIDS Education and Prevention* 13(5): 428–37.

Buchanan, David, Susan Shaw, Amy Ford, and Merrill Singer

    2004   "Empirical Science Meets Moral Panic: An Analysis of the Politics of Needle Exchange." *Journal of Public Health Policy.* 24(3/4): 427–44.

Bucher, J. B., K. M. Thoma, D. Guzman, E. Riley, N. DelaCruz, and D. R. Bangsberg

    2007   Community-Based Rapid HIV Testing in Homeless and Marginally Housed Adults in San Francisco. Electronic Document, http:www.medscape.com/viewarticle/554783_1, accessed April 24, 2007

Bujra, Janet

    2000   "Risk and Trust: Unsafe Sex, Gender and AIDS in Tanzania." In *Risk Revisited.* Pat Caplan, ed. Pp. 59–84. London: Pluto Press.

Bulterys, Marc, Steven Nesheim, Elaine Abrams, J., Paul Palumbo, John Farley, Margaret Lampe, and Mary Glenn Fowler

    2000   "Lack of Evidence of Mitochondrial Dysfunction in the Offspring of HIV-Infected Women. Retrospective Review of Perinatal Exposure to Antiretroviral Drugs in the Perinatal AIDS Collaborative Transmission Study." *Prevention and Treatment of HIV Infection in Infants and Children* 918: 212–21.

Burhansstipanov, Linda, Carole laFavor, Shirley Hoskins, Gloria Bellymule, and Ronald M. Rowell

    1997   "Native Women Living Beyond HIV/AIDS Infection." In *The Gender Politics of HIV/AIDS in Women: Perspectives on the Pandemic in the U.S.* Pp. 337–56. Nancy Goldstein and Jennifer L. Manlowe, eds. New York: New York University Press.

Burke, Jean

    2004   "Infant HIV Infection: Acceptability of Prevention Strategies in Central Tanzania." *AIDS Education and Prevention* 16(5): 415–25.

Butt, Leslie, Jenny Munro, and Joanne Wong

    2004   "Border Testimonials: Patterns of AIDS Awareness Across the Island and New Guinea." *Papua New Guinea Medical Journal.* 47 (1–2) (March–June): 65–76.

Byrnes, Brian T.

    1996   "Building a Proud Gay Identity: Adult Responsibility for Ending the Expanding HIV Epidemic among Gay Male Youth." In *AIDS Education: Reaching Diverse Populations.* Melinda K. Moore and Martin L. Forst, eds. Pp. 27–40. Westport, Conn.: Praeger.

Cáceres, Carlos, K. Konda, M. Pecheny, A. Chatterjee, and R. Lyera

    2006   "Estimating the Number of Men Who Have Sex with Men in Low and Middle Income Countries." *Sexually Transmitted Infections.* 82 (Suppl 3): iii3–iii9.

Cameron, D. W., J. N. Simonsen, L. J. D'Costa, A. R. Ronald, G. M. Maitha, M. N.Gakinya, M. Cheang, J. O. Ndinya-Achola, P. Piot, and R. C. Brunham

    1989   "Female to Male Transmission of Human Immunodeficiency Virus Type 1: Risk Factors for Seroconversion in Men." *Lancet.* 2 (8660) (August 19): 403–7.

Campbell, Carole A.

    1999   *Women, Families and HIV/AIDS: A Sociological Perspective on the Epidemic in America.* New York: Cambridge University Press.

Canadian Aboriginal AIDS Network

    2000   Electronic Document, http://www.linkup-connection.ca/catalog/prod Images/02230201364147.pdf, accessed August 2, 2007.

Caplan, Patricia, ed.

    2000   *Risk Revisited.* London: Pluto Press.

Carballo-Dieguez, Alex

    1995   "The Sexual Identity and Behavior of Puerto Rican Men Who Have Sex with Men." *AIDS, Identity and Community. The HIV Epidemic and Lesbians and Gay Men* 2 (Psychological Perspectives on Lesbian and Gay Issues).

Carlson, Robert G., Harvey A. Siegel, Jichuan Wang, and Russel S. Falk
  1996   "Attitudes Toward Needle "Sharing" among Injection Drug Users: Combining Qualitative and Quantitative Research Methods." *Human Organization.* 55 (3) (Fall): 361–69.
Carovano, Kathryn, and Helen Schietings
  1996   "The Developing World: Caring for the Caregivers." In *Until the Cure: Caring for Women with HIV.* Ann Kurth, ed. Pp. 165–82. New Haven: Yale University Press.
Carrier, Joseph
  2001   "Some Reflections on Ethnographic Research on Latino and Southeast Asia Male Homosexuality and AIDS." *AIDS and Behavior* 5(2): 183–91.
Carrier, Joseph M., and Ralph Bolton
  1991   "Anthropological Perspectives on Sexuality and HIV Prevention." *Annual Review of Sex Research* 21: 49–74.
Cash, Kathleen
  1996   "Women Educating Women for HIV Prevention." In *Women's Experiences with HIV/AIDS: An International Perspective.* Lynellen D. Long and E. Maxine Ankrah, eds. Pp. 311–32. New York: Columbia University Press.
Catalan, Jose
  1999   "Psychological Problems in People with HIV." In *Mental Health and HIV Infection: Psychological and Psychiatric Aspects.* Jose Catalan, ed. Pp. 21–41. London: UCL Press.
Centers for Disease Control and Prevention (CDC)
  2005a   *CDC's Reproductive Health Information Source. "ART 2002 Report."* Electronic document, 2005a, http://apps.nccd.cdc.gov/ ART2002/clinlist02.asp?State=IL, accessed March 25, 2005.
  2005b   "HIV Test Counseling Protocols-CDC Standard and Rapid." Electronic document, http://www.cdc.gov/hiv/projects/respect-2/counseling.htm, accessed December 26, 2005.
  2003a   "Advancing HIV Prevention: New Strategies for a Changing Epidemic— United States, 2003." *Morbidity and Mortality Weekly Report* (MMWR) 52: 329–32.
  2003b   "Condoms Fact Sheet." Electronic document, http://www.cdc.gov/hiv/pubs/facts/condoms.htm, accessed August 5, 2005.
  2002   "Surveillance of Health Care Personnel with HIV/AIDS, as of December 2002." Electronic document, http://www.cdc.gov/ncidod/hip/BLOOD/hivpersonnel.htm, accessed April 30, 2004.
  2001a   "HIV/AIDS among African-Americans. Key Facts." Electronic document, http://www.cdc.gov/hiv/pubs/facts/afam/pdf, accessed May 19, 2003.
  2001b   "HIV and AIDS—United States, 1981–2001." *Morbidity and Mortality Weekly Report 2001* 50 (2001): 430–34.
  2000   XIIIth International AIDS Conference 2000. Electronic document, http://www.cdc.gov/nchstp/od/Durban/default.htm, accessed December 15, 2004.
  1999   "Youth Risk Behavior Surveillance—United States, 1999." *Morbidity and Mortality Surveillance Summary* 49: 1–96.

Center for Disease Control/Health and Human Services (HHS)

1999   Electronic document, http://www.cdc.gov/hiv/stats/addendum.htm, accessed December 15, 2004.

Center for Health and Gender Equity (CHANGE)

2004a "Bush's Global AIDS Plan: Long on Rhetoric, Short on Science and Solutions. 'Smoke and Mirrors Strategy' Fails to Meet Needs of Women and Girls." Electronic document, http://www.genderhealth.org/globalAIDSstrategy.php , accessed March 9, 2005.

2004b *Debunking the Myths in the U.S. Global AIDS Strategy: An Evidence Based Analysis.* Takoma Park.

Chapkis, Wendy

1997   *Live Sex Acts. Women Performing Erotic Labor.* New York: Routledge.

Chase, Marilyn

2006   Plans to Expand AIDS Testing Alarm Activists. Electronic document, http://www.ph.ucla.edu/epi/seaids/plansexpandtesting.html, accessed April 24, 2007.

Cheever, Laura W.

2001   "Adherence to HIV Therapies."'" In *A Clinical Guide to the Care of Women with HIV.* Jean Anderson, ed. Pp. 139–48. Rockville: Womencare.

Cherry, Michael

2000a "Are AIDS Dissidents Advising South Africa?" *Nature* 404(6775): 216.

2000b "Mbeki Agrees to Step Back from AIDS Debate." *Nature* 407(6806): 822.

Child and Adolescent Health and Development

2003   *Consultation to discuss revisions of HIV and Infant Feeding Guidelines.* Electronic document, http://www.who.int/child-adolescent.health/NEWS/news_16.html, accessed March 13, 2006.

CHIRON

2003   Electronic document, http://www.chiron.com, accessed June 12, 2006.

Chng, Chwee Lye, Frank Y. Wong, Royce J. Park, Mark C. Edberg, and David S. Lai

2003   "A Model for Understanding Sexual Health among Asian American/Pacific Islander Men Who Have Sex with Men (MSM) in the United States. HIV Prevention for Men of Color Who Have Sex with Men (MS) and Men of Color Who Have Sex with Men and Women (MSM/W)." A Special Supplement to *AIDS Education and Prevention* 15 (Supplement A, 1–6): 21–38.

Choi, Kyung-Hee, Chong-suk Han, Esther Sid Hudes, and Susan Kegeles

2002   "Unprotected Sex and Associated Risk Factors among Young Asian and Pacific Islander Men Who Have Sex with Men." *AIDS Education and Prevention* 14(6): 472–81.

Choi, Kyung-Hee, N. Salazaar, S. Lew, and Thomas J. Coates

1995   "AIDS Risk, Dual Identity and Community Response among Gay Asian Islander Men in San Francisco." *AIDS, Identity and Community. The HIV Epidemic and Lesbians and Gay Men 2* (Psychological Perspectives on Lesbian and Gay Issues): 115–34.

Choi, Kyung-Hee, Zheng Xiwen, Qu Shuquan, Kevin Yiee, and Jeffrey Mandell

2000   "HIV Risk among Patients attending Sexually Transmitted Disease Clinics in China." *AIDS and Behavior* 4(1): 111–19.

Chu, S. Y., T. A. Hammett, and J. W. Buehler
  1992   "Update: Epidemiology of reported cases of AIDS in women who report sex only with women, United States, 1981–1991." *AIDS* 6(5): 518–19.

Clatts, Michael C.
  1999   "Integrating Ethnography and Virology in the Study of Transmission of Blood-borne Pathogens among IDUs." Paper presented at the Annual Meeting of the Society for Applied Anthropology, April, Tucson, Arizona.

Clatts, Michael C., and Jo L. Sotheran
  2000   "Challenges in Research on Drug and Sexual Risk Practices of Men Who Have Sex with Men: Applications of Ethnography in HIV Epidemiology and Prevention." *AIDS and Behavior* 4(2): 169–79.

Clay, S. B.
  2002   "Villains or Victims?" *HIV Plus* 5(7): 28–31.

Cleland, John G., with Benoit Ferry and M. Carael
  1995   "Summary and Conclusions." In *Sexual Behavior and AIDS in the Developing World*. J.G. Cleland and Benoit Ferry, eds. Pp. 208–31. Bristol, U.K.: Taylor and Francis.

Clements-Noelle, K., W. Wilkinson, K. Kitano, and R. Marx
  2001   "HIV Prevention and Health Service Needs of the Transgender-Community in San Francisco." In *Transgender and HIV*. Walter O. Bockting and Sheila Kirk, eds. Pp. 69–89. Binghamton: Haworth Press.

CNN Live
  2004   *AIDS Orphans*. CNN, July 13.

Cocina, Elizabeth R., and Cassandra R. Thomas
  1996   "HIV Education and the Sexual Assault Survivor." In *AIDS Education: Reaching Diverse Populations*. Melinda K. Moore and Martin L. Forst, eds. Pp. 163–71. Westport, Conn.: Praeger.

Cohen, Jon
  2004a   "HIV/AIDS in China: Poised for Takeoff." *Science* 304: 1430–32.
  2004b   "HIV/AIDS in China: Vaccine Development with a Distinctly Chinese Flavor." *Science* 304: 1437.

Cohen, Judith B.
  1999   "Sexual Transmission of HIV in Prostitutes." In *The AIDS Knowledge Base: A Textbook on HIV Disease from the University of California, San Francisco School of Medicine and San Francisco General Hospital*. Philip T. Cohen, Merle A. Sande, and Paul Volberding, eds. Pp. 1.15-1–1.15-9. Philadelphia: Lippincott Williams and Wilkins.

Cohen, Madge H., and Patricia Kelly
  1995   "HIV Disease in the Primary Care Setting. Primary Care of Women and Children with HIV Infection: A Multidisciplinary Approach." Patricia Kelly, Susan Holman, Rosalie Rothenberg and Stephen Holzemer, eds. Pp. 9–18. Boston: Jones and Bartlett.

Cohen, Philip T., Merle A. Sande and Paul Volberding, eds., D. Osmond (associated)
  1999   *The AIDS Knowledge Base: A Text book on HIV Disease from the University of California, San Francisco, School of Medicine and San Francisco General Hospital*. Philadelphia: Lippincott Williams and Wilkins.

Cold, C. J., and J. R. Taylor
  1999 "The Prepuce." *British Journal of Urology.* 83. (Suppl. 1) (January): 34–44.
Colón, Héctor M., H. Ann Finlinson, Martin Fishbein, Rafaela R. Robles, Mayra Soto-
  López, and Héctor Marcano
  2005 "Elicitation of Salient Beliefs Related to Drug Preparation Practices among
        Injection Drug Users in Puerto Rico." *AIDS and Behavior.* 9 (3)(September):
        363–75.
Commentary
  2000 "The Durban Declaration." Conference: 15th Annual International AIDS
        Conference. *Nature* 406(6791): 15–16.
Coodvadia, Hoosen M.
  2000 "Access to Voluntary Counseling and Testing for HIV in Developing Coun-
        tries." In *Prevention and Treatment of HIV Infection in Infants and Children*
        918: 57–63. Arthur J. Ammann and Ayre Rubenstein, eds. New York: New
        York Academy of Sciences.
Corea, Gena
  1992 *The Invisible Epidemic: The Story of Women and AIDS.* New York: Harper-
        Collins.
Cummings, Gayle, Robins Battle, Judith C. Barker, and Flora M. Krasnovsky
  1999 "Are African-American Women Worried about Getting AIDS? A Qualita-
        tive Analysis." *AIDS Education and Prevention: An Interdisciplinary Journal*
        11(4): 331–42.
d'Adesky, Anne-Christine
  2002a "India's Generics Play a High Stakes Game." *The AmFar Treatment Insider
         in HIV Plus* 5(4): 1–6.
  2002b "Mexico's Rural HIV Fighters Forced to Improvise Amid Official Neglect."
         The AmFar Treatment Insider 3(6): 4–7.
  2002c "Uganda Confronts Limits to Preventing Mother-to-Child Transmission."
         HIV Plus 5(1): 6–7.
Daley, C. L.
  1999 "HIV Disease in Africa." In *The AIDS Knowledge Base: A Textbook on HIV
        Disease from the University of California, San Francisco School of Medicine
        and San Francisco General Hospital.* Philip T. Cohen, Merle A. Sande and
        Paul Volberding, eds. Pp. 1.6-1–1.6-21. Philadelphia: Lippincott Williams
        and Wilkins.
Daniels, Norman
  1995 *Seeking Fair Treatment: From the AIDS Epidemic to National Healthcare
        Reform.* New York: Oxford University Press.
Dawson, Alvin G., Michael W. Ross, Doug Henry, and Anne Freeman
  2005 "Deliberate or Indifferent to HIV Transmission? Evidence of Barebacking
        Risk Levels from an Internet Site." *Journal of Gay and Lesbian Psychothera-
        py.* 9 (3/4): 73–83.
Day, S.
  2000 "The Politics of Risk among London Prostitutes." In *Risk Revisited.* Patricia
        Caplan, ed. Pp. 29–58. London: Pluto Press.

Dean, Laura

 1995 "Psychosocial Stressors in a Panel of New York City Gay Men During the AIDS Epidemic, 1985–1991." In *AIDS, Identity and Community. The HIV Epidemic and Lesbians and Gay Men 2* (Psychological Perspectives on Lesbian and Gay Issues): 135–49.

De Graaf, Ron, Gertjan van Zessen, Ine Vanwesenbeeck, Cees J. Straver, and Jan H. Visser

 1997 "Condom Use by Dutchmen with Commercial Heterosexual Contacts: Determinants and Considerations." *AIDS Education and Prevention. An Interdisciplinary Journal* 9(5): 411–23.

Delacoste, Frederique, and Priscilla Alexander, eds.

 1987 *Sex Work, Writings by Women in the Sex Industry.* Pittsburgh: Cleis Press.

de la Gorgendière, Louise

 2005 "Rights and Wrongs. HIV/AIDS Research in Africa." *Human Organization.* 64(2)(Summer): 166–78.

Desclaux, Alice, Mounirou Ciss, Bernard Taverne, Papa S. Sow, Marc Egrot, Mame A. Faye, Isabelle Lancièce, Omar Sylla, EricDelaporte, and Ibrahima Ndoye

 2003 "Access to Antiretroviral Drugs and AIDS Management in Senegal." *AIDS.* 17 (Supplement 3): 595–S101.

Desgrees du Lou, Annabel

 1999 "Reproductive Health and AIDS in Sub-Saharan Africa. Problems and Prospects." *An English Selection.* 11: 61–87.

DesJarlais, Don C., Katchit Choopanya, Peggy Millson, PatriciaFriedmann, and Samuel R. Friedman

 1998 "The Structure of Stable Seroprevalence HIV-1 Epidemics among Injecting Drug Users." In *Drug Injecting and HIV Infection. Global Dimensions and Local Responses.* Gerry Stimson, Don DesJarlais, and Andrew Ball, eds. Pp. 91–100. Bristol, U.K.: UCL Press.

de Vincenzi, Isabelle, and Thierry Mertens

 1994 "Male Circumcision: A Role in HIV Prevention?" *AIDS.* 8. (2): 153–60.

Diaz, F. J., J. A. Vega, P. J. Patino, G. Bedoya, J. Nagles, C.Villegas, R. Vesga, and M. T. Rugeles

 2000 "Frequency of CCR5 Delta 32 Mutation in Human Immunodeficiency Virus (HIV)-seropositive and HIV-exposed seronegative Individuals and in General Population of Medellin, Colombia." *MemInst Oswaldo Cruz* 95(2): 237–42.

Diaz, Rafael

 2000 "Cultural Regulation, Self-Regulation and Sexuality." In *Framing the Sexual Object: The Politics of Gender, Sexuality and Power.* Richard Parker, R. Barbosa and Peter Aggleton, eds. Pp. 191–215. Berkeley: University of California Press.

 1998 *Latino Gay Men and HIV: Culture, Sexuality and Risk Behavior.* New York: Routledge.

Dickson, David

 2000 "Tests Fail to Support Claims for Origin." *Nature* 407(6801): 117.

DiClemente, Ralph J., Katherine A. Forrest, Susan Mickler, and Prinicipal Site Investigators
  1990   "College Students Knowledge and Attitudes About AIDS and Changes in HIV-Preventive Behaviors." *AIDS Education and Prevention* 2(3): 201–12.
Dilger, Hanjorg
  2007   "Healing the Wound of Modernity: Salvations, Community and Care in a Neo-Pentecostal Church in Dar Es Salaam, Tanzania." *Journal of Religion in Africa* 37(1)(February): 59–83.
Ditmore, Melissa
  2005   "New U.S. Funding Policies on Trafficking Affect Sex Work and HIV-Prevention Efforts WorldWide." *SIECUS Report.* 33(2)(Spring): 26–29.
Dolcini, Margaret, and Joseph A. Catania
  2000   "Psycho social Profiles of Women with Risky Sexual Partners: The Natural AIDS Behavioral Survey." *AIDS and Behavior* 4(3): 297–308.
Doll, Linda S., John Peterson, J. Raul Magana, and Joe M. Carrier
  1991   "Male Bisexuality and AIDS in the United States." In *Bisexuality and HIV/AIDS: A Global Perspective.* Rob Tielman, Manuel Carballo and Aart Hendriks, eds. Pp. 27–39. Buffalo, N.Y.: Prometheus.
Doran, Terence I., Howard Lune, and Rachel Davis
  2002   "Immigrants and Migrant Families." In *Invisible Caregivers: Older Adults Raising Children in the Wake of HIV/AIDS.* Daphne Joslin, ed. Pp. 228–47. New York: Columbia University Press.
Dowsett, Gary
  1999   "Understanding Cultures and Sexuality: Lessons Learned from HIV/AIDS Education and Behaviour Change among Gay Men in Australia." In *Resistances to Behavioural Change to Reduce HIV/AIDS Infection in Predominantly Heterosexual Epidemics in Third World Countries.* John Caldwell, Pat Caldwell, John Anarfi, Kofi Awusabo-Asare, James Ntozi, I. O. Orubuloye, Jeff Marck, Wendy Cosford, Rachel Colombo, and Elaine Hollings, eds. Pp. 223–31. Canberra: Health Transition Centre, National Centre for Epidermiology and Population Health, Australian National University.
Dowsett, Gary W., Jeffrey W. Grierson, and Stephen P. McNally
  2006   "A Review of Knowledge about the Sexual Networks and Behaviours of Men Who Have Sex with Men in Asia: Annotated Bibliography-Bangladesh." Australian Research Centre in Sex, Health and Society. La Trobe University, Melbourne, Australia. Monograph Series Number 59.
Duesberg, Peter
  1996   *Inventing the AIDS Virus.* Washington, D.C.: Regnery.
Dugan, Anne B.
  1988   "Compadrazgo as a Protective Mechanism in Depression." In *Women and Health. Cross-Cultural Perspectives.* Patricia Whelehan, ed. Pp. 143–52. Granby, Conn.: Bergin and Garvey.
Editorial
  2003   "Bush Steps Up on AIDS." *San Francisco Chronicle,* February 9: Insight.
  2004   "Leadership Needed on AIDS." *New York Times,* May 29: A14.

Edwards, Michael, W. E.

2005   "In Your Face." *HIVPlus*. December: 4–7.

Ehrardt, Anke A.

1996   "Sexual Behavior among Heterosexuals." In *AIDS in the World II. Global Dimensions, Social Roots and Responses*. Jonathan M. Mann and Daniel J. M. Tarantola, eds. Pp. 259–63. New York: Oxford University Press.

Ehrenreich, Barbara

2002   *Nickel and Dimed. On (Not) Getting By in America*. Bellingham: Owl Books.

Elders, Jocelyn

1994   Address to the World AIDS Day Conference at the United Nations. New York.

Eldred, Lois, and Richard Chiasson

1996   "The Clinical Course of HIV Infection in Women." In *HIV, AIDS and Childbearing. Public Policy, Private Lives*. Ruth R. Faden and Nancy E. Kass, eds. Pp. 15–30. New York: Oxford University Press.

Elias, Christopher J., and Lori L. Heise

1996   "Challenge for the Development of Female-Controlled Vaginal Microbicides." In *Women's Experiences with HIV/AIDS: An International Perspective*. Lynellen Long and E. Maxine Ankrah, eds. Pp. 351–69. New York: Columbia University Press.

Epstein, Steven

1996   *Impure Science: AIDS, Activism and the Politics of Knowledge*. Berkeley: University of California Press.

Erikson, Erik

1963   *Childhood and Society*. 2nd edition. New York: W. W. Norton.

Erni, John N.

1998   "Redressing Sanuk: 'ASIAN AIDS' and the Practices of Women's Resistance." In *Women and AIDS: Negotiating Safer Practices, Care and Representation*. Nancy Roth and Linda K. Fuller, eds. Pp, 231–56. Binghamton, N.Y.: Harrington Park Press.

Faden, Ruth R., Gail Geller, and Madison Powers, eds.

1991   *AIDS, Women and the Next Generation: Towards a Morally Acceptable Public Policy for HIV Testing of Pregnant Women and Newborns*. New York: Oxford University Press.

Faden, Ruth R., and Nancy E. Kass, eds.

1996   *HIV, AIDS and Childbearing. Public Policy, Private Lives*. New York: Oxford University Press.

Faden, Ruth R., Nancy E. Kass, Katherine Acuff, Anita Allen, Jean Anderson, Taunya L. Banks, M. Gregg Bloche, Richard Chiasson, Sylvia Cohn, Nancy Hutton, Patricia A. King, Marsha Lillie-Blanton, Mary E. McCaul, Madison Powers, Karen H. Rothenberg, Alfred Saah, Liza Solomon, and Lawrence Wissow

1996   "HIV-Infection and Childbearing: A Proposal for Public Policy and Clinical Practice." In *HIV, AIDS, and Childbearing. Public Policy, Private Lives*. Ruth R. Faden and Nancy E. Kass, eds. Pp. 447–61. New York: Oxford University Press.

Fan, Hung Y., Ross F. Conner, and Luis P. Villarreal
  2004 *AIDS—Science and Society*. 4th edition. Sudbury: Jones and Bartlett.
Farber, Celia
  2006 "Out of Control. AIDS and the Corruption of Medical Science." *Harper's Magazine*. 312(1870) (March 2006): 37–52.
Farmer, Paul
  1999 *Infections and Inequalities: The Modern Plagues*. Berkeley: University of California Press.
  1992 "AIDS and Accusation. Haiti and the Geography of Blame." *Comparative Studies of Health Systems and Medical Care* 33.
Farmer, Paul, Margaret Connors, and Janie Simmons, eds.
  1996 *Women, Poverty and AIDS: Sex, Drugs and Structural Violence*. Monroe, Maine: Common Courage Press.
Farmer, Paul, David A. Walton, and Jennifer J. Furin
  2000 "The Changing Face of AIDS: Implications for Policy and Practice." In *The Emergence of AIDS. The Impact of Immunology, Microbiology and Public Health*. Kenneth H. Mayer and H. F Pizer, eds. Pp. 139–61. Washington, D.C.: American Association of Public Health.
Farook, Norman
  2007 "HIV Risk Associated with Different Types of Sexual Activity." Electronic document, http://74.125.47.132/search?q=cache:YYZq27BOpkMJ:www.pnac.net.pk/Reports/RC-Emails/June-28-HIVRisk-Associated-with-Different-Types-of-SexualActivity.pdf+HIV+risks+associated+with+different+types+of+sexual+activity&hl=en&ct=clnk&cd=1&gl=us, accessed December 6, 2008.
Fawzi, Wafaie
  2000 "Nutritional Factors and Vertical Transmission of HIV-1. Epidemiology and Potential Mechanisms." *Prevention and Treatment of HIV Infection in Infants and Children* 918: 99–114.
Feldman, Douglas
  2003a "Reassessing AIDS Priorities and Strategies for Africa: ABCvsACCDG-LMT." *AIDS & Anthropology Bulletin*. The Newsletter of the AIDS and Anthropology Research Group 15(2): 5–8.
  2003b "Problems with the Uganda Model for HIV/AIDS Prevention." *Anthropology News*. October: 6, 2003.
Feldman, Jaime
  1995 *Plague Doctors: Responding to the AIDS Epidemic in France and America*. Westport, Conn.: Bergin and Garvey.
Ferry, Benoit
  1995 "Risk Factors Related to HIV Transmission: Sexually Transmitted Disease, Alcohol Consumption and Medically Related Injuries." In *Sexual Behavior and AIDS in the Developing World*. John Cleland and Benoit Ferry, eds. Pp. 193–207. Bristol, U.K.: Taylor and Francis.
Fethers, Katherine, Caron Marks, Adrian Mindel, and Claudia S. Estcourt
  2000 "Sexually Transmitted Infections and Risk Behaviours in Women Who Have Sex with Women." *Sexually Transmitted Infections*. 76: 345–49.

Feuer, Cindra

    2006   "Rectal Microbicides. Investments & Advocacy." International Rectal Mi-
           crobicides Working Group (IRMWG). April.: 1–28. Electronic Document,
           http://www.aidschicago.org/pdf/2006/adv_rectalreport.pdf, accessed April
           29, 2006.

    2004a "Can PEPFAR Save the Most Vulnerable?" amfAR GLOBAL LINK *HIV/*
           AIDS TREATMENT INSIDER 5(4): 1–3, 7.

    2004b "HIV Drugs Trickle into Uganda." amfAR GLOBAL LINK *HIV/AIDS*
           TREATMENT INSIDER 5(4): 6.

Fletcher, John C., M. Meyer, and Brian Wispelwey

    1999   "AIDS and Ethics: Clinical, Social and Global." In *Textbook of AIDS Medi-*
           cine. 2nd edition. Thomas C. Merigan, John G. Bartlett and Dani Bolognesi,
           eds. Pp. 951–78. Baltimore: Williams and Wilkers.

Forbes, Anna

    2006   "Moving Toward Assured Access to Treatment in Microbicide Trials." *PLoS.*
           3 (7) (July): e153.

Forst, Martin L., and Melinda K. Moore

    1996   "Effective Program Evaluation." In *AIDS Education: Reaching Diverse Popu-*
           lations. Melinda K. Moore and Martin L. Forst, eds. Pp. 201–20. Westport,
           Conn.: Praeger.

Fowke, Keith R., Nico J. D. Nagelkerke, Joshua Kimani, J. NeilSimonsen, Aggrey
    O.Anzala, Job J. Bwayo, Kelly S. MacDonald, Elizabeth N. Ngugi, and Fran-
    cis A. Plummer.

    1996   "Resistance to HIV-1 Infection among Persistently Seronegative Prostitutes
           in Nairobi, Kenya." *Lancet* 348(9038): 1347–51.

Fowler, Mary G.

    2000   "Prevention of Perinatal HIV Infection. What Do We Know? Where Should
           Future Research Go?" *Prevention and Treatment of HIV Infection in Infants*
           and Children 918: 45–52.

Francis, Henry L., and Victoria A. Cargill

    2001   "Substance Abuse." In *A Guide to the Clinical Care of Women with HIV.*
           2001 edition. Jean Anderson, ed. Pp. 313–33. Rockville: Womencare.

Friedman, Samuel R., Richard Curtis, Alan Neaigus, Benny Jose,and Don C. DesJarlais

    1999   *Social Networks, Drug Injectors' Lives and HIV/AIDS.* New York: Kluwer
           Academic.

Furlonge, Colin, Steven E. Gregorich, Samuel Kalibala, Olga A. Grinstead, Thomas A.
    Coates, and Kevin R. O'Reilly

    2000   "HIV-Related Risk Factors in a Population-Based Probability Sample of
           North and Central Trinidad: The Voluntary HIV-Counseling and Testing
           Efficacy Study." *AIDS and Behavior* 4(1) (2000): 49–62.

FXB Foundation

    2004   Electronic document, http://www.fxbfoundation.org/mann.htm, accessed
           August 6, 2005.

Gallo, Robert, Nathan Geffen, Gregg Gonsalves, Richard Jeffreys, Daniel Kuritzes,
    Bruce Mirken, John P. Moore, and Jeffrey T. Safrit

    2006   "Errors in Celia Farber's March 2006 article in *Harper's Magazine.*" Draft for *Harper's Magazine* and public distribution: 4 March (version 2). Electronic document, http://www.tac.org.za/, accessed March 17, 2006.

Gamella, Juan F.
    1994   "The Spread of Intravenous Drug Use and AIDS in a Neighborhood in Spain." *Medical Anthropology Quarterly.* New Series. 8(2)(June): 131–60.

Garcia, Maria de Lourdes, Jose Valdespino, Jose Izazola, Manuel Palacios, and Jaime Sepulveda
    1991   "Bisexuality in Mexico: Current Perspectives." In *Bisexuality and HIV/ AIDS: A Global Perspective.* Rob Tielman, Manuel Carballo, and Aart Hendriks, eds. Pp. 41–58. Buffalo, N.Y.: Prometheus.

Garrett, Laurie
    1994   *The Coming Plague.* Toronto: HarperCollins Canada.

Gay Men's Health Crisis (GMHC)
    2003   Electronic document, http://www.gmhc.org, accessed December 15, 2004.

Gayle, Helene
    2003   "International Conference on Women and AIDS." CBS News Report, March 8.

Gee, Royal
    2006   "Primary Care Health Issues among Men Who Have Sex with Men." *Journal of the American Academy of Nurse Practitioners.* 18: 144–53.

Geller, Gail, and Nancy Kass
    1991   "Informed Consent in the Context of Prenatal HIV Testing." In *AIDS, Women and the Next Generation: Towards a Morally Acceptable Public Policy for HIV Testing of Pregnant Women and Newborns.* Ruth R. Faden, Gail Geller, and Madison Powers, eds. Pp. 288–307. New York: Oxford University Press.

Gender-AIDSeForum
    2003   Electronic document, af-aids@eforums.healthdev.org, accessed December 15, 2005.
    2004   Electronic document, gender_aids@healthdev.net, accessed December 15, 2004.

Gerbert, Barbara, Barbara Brown, Paul Volberding, Molly Cooke, Nona Caspers, Candace Love, and Amy Bonstone
    1999   Physicians Transmission Prevention Assessment and Counseling Practices with Their HIV Positive Patients." *AIDS Education and Prevention* 11(4): 307–20.

Gielen Andrea C., Linda A. Fogarty, Kay Armstrong, Brian M. Green, Rebecca Cabral, Bobby Milstein, Christine Galavotti, and
Charles, M. Heilig
    2001   "Promoting Condom Use with Main Partners: A Behavioral Intervention Trial for Women." *AIDS and Behavior* 5(3): 193–204.

Gifford, S., N. Suanching, J. Tusing, N. Lian, B. Langkham, an V. Muana
    1999   "The Social Context of Risk and Protection amongst Young People and Women in Churachandpur, India." In *Resistances to Behavioural Change to Reduce HIV/AIDS Infection in Predominantly Heterosexual Epidemics in Third World Countries.* John Caldwell, Pat Caldwell, John Anarfi, Kofi

Awusabo-Asare, James Ntozi, I. O. Orubuloye, Jeff Marck, Wendy Cosford, Rachel Colombo, and Elaine Hollings, eds. Pp. 171–84. Canberra: Health Transition Centre, National Centre for Epidermiology and Population Health, Australian National University.

Gillett, James, Dorothy Pawluch, and Roy Cain
   2005   "Complementary Approaches to Health Care: Diverse Perspectives among People Living with HIV/AIDS." *AIDS& Public Policy Journal.* 16 (1–2): 16–27.

Girard, Francoise
   2004   "Global Implications of U.S. Domestic and International Policies on Sexuality." The Center for Gender, Sexuality and Health. Columbia University. Mailman School of Public Health: 1–30. Electronic document, http:ww. www.mailman.hs.columbia.edu/cgsh/cgsh.html, accessed June 30, 2006.

Global Fund to Fight AIDS, Tuberculosis, and Malaria
   2004   Electronic document, http://www.theglobalfund.org, accessed July 9, 2004.

Global Health Council
   2005   "HIV/AIDS." Electronic document, http://globalhealth.org/view_top. php3?id=227, accessed March 3, 2006.

Goden, Gaston, Helene Gagnon, Michel Alary, Lina Noel, and Michel P. Morissette
   2001   "Correctional Officers' Intention of Accepting or Refusing to Make HIV Preventive Tools Accessible to Inmates." *AIDS Education and Prevention* 13(5): 462–73.

Gogna, Monica, and Silvina Ramos
   2000   "Gender Stereotypes and Power Relations. Unacknowledged Risks for STDs in Argentina." In *Framing the Sexual Object: The Politics of Gender, Sexuality and Power.* Robert Parker, Regina Maria Barbosa, and Peter Aggleton, eds. Pp. 117–40. Berkeley: University of California Press.

Goldstein, Nancy
   1997   "Lesbians and the Medical Profession: HIV/AIDS and the Pursuit of Visibility." In *The Gender Politics of HIV/AIDS in Women: Perspectives on the Pandemic in the U.S.* Nancy Goldstein and Jennifer L. Manlowe, eds. Pp. 86–110. New York: New York University Press.

Golin, Carol, Frederick Isasi, Jean Breny Bontempi, and Eugenia Eng
   2002   "Secret Pills: HIV Positive Patients' Experiences taking Antiretroviral Therapy in North Carolina." *AIDS Education and Prevention* 14(4): 318–29.

Gomez, Cynthia A.
   1995   "Lesbians at Risk for HIV. The Unresolved Debate." *AIDS, Identity and Community. The HIV Epidemic and Lesbians and Gay Men 2* (Psychological Perspectives on Lesbian and Gay Issues): 19–31.

Goode, Erica
   2003   "AIDS Researchers get Warning: Federal Health Officials Advise Them to Avoid Controversial Topics." *San Francisco Chronicle*, February 18.

Goodman, Billy
   1995   "A Controversy That Will Not Die: The Role of HIV in Causing AIDS." *The Scientist* 9(6): 1.

Gostlin, Lawrence O., and Zita Lazzarini
  1997 *Human Rights and Public Health in the AIDS Pandemic.* New York: Oxford University Press.
Grady, Christine
  1995 *The Search for an AIDS Vaccine: Ethical Issues in the Development and Testing of a Preventive HIV Vaccine.* Bloomington: Indiana University Press.
Grandi, Joa Luiz, Samuel Goihman, Mirtes Ueda, and George W. Rutherford
  2000 "HIV Infection, Syphilis and Behavioral Risks in Brazilian Male Sex Workers." *AIDS and Behavior* 4(1): 129–35.
Gray, Peter B.
  2003 "HIV and Islam: Is HIV Prevalence Lower among Muslims?" *Social Science and Medicine.* 58: 1751–56.
Green, Edward, C.
  2003 *Rethinking AIDS Prevention: Learning from Successes in Developing Countries.* Portsmouth, N.H.: Greenwood.
Green, Gill, and Elisa Sobo
  2000 *The Endangered Self: Managing the Social Risks of HIV.* London: Routledge.
Greenblatt, Ruth M., and Nancy A. Hessol
  2001 "Epidemiology and Natural History of HIV Infection in Women." In *A Guide to the Clinical Care of Women with HIV.* Jean Anderson, ed. 2001 ed. Pp. 1–33. Rockville: Womencare.
Gupta, Geeta R.
  2000 "The Best of Times and the Worst of Times: Implications of Scientific Advances in HIV Prevention for Women in the Developing World." In *Prevention and Treatment of HIV Infection in Infants and Children* 918: 16–26. Arthur J. Ammann and Ayre Rubenstein, eds. New York: New York Academy of Sciences.
Gupta, Geeta R., Ellen Weiss, and Purnima Mane
  1996 "Talking about Sex: A Prerequisite for AIDS Prevention." In *Women's Experiences with HIV/AIDS: An International Perspective.* Lynellen Long and E. Maxine Ankrah, eds. Pp. 333–50. New York: Columbia University Press.
Gupta, Geeta R., Ellen Weiss, and Daniel J. Whelan
  1996 "Women and AIDS: building a new HIV Prevention Strategy." In *AIDS in the World II. Global Dimensions, Social Roots and Responses.* Jonathan M. Mann and Daniel J.M. Tarantola, eds. Pp. 215–28. New York: Oxford University Press.
Guydish, Joseph, Clare Brown, Renee Edgington, Heather Edney, and Delia Garcia
  2000 "What Are the Impacts of Needle Exchange on Young Injectors?" *AIDS and Behavior* 4(2): 137–46.
Hahn, Beatrice H., George M. Shaw, Kevin M. DeCock, and Paul Sharp M.
  2000 "AIDS as a Zoonosis: Scientific and Public Health Implications." *Science* 287(5453): 607–14.
Hahn, Robert A.
  1995 *Sickness and Healing: An Anthropological Perspective.* New Haven: Yale University Press.

Halkitis, Perry N.

    2003   "Gay Culture in the Third Decade of AIDS: The Emergence of Barebacking." *CHIP Brown Bag Lecture Series 03–04*. University of Connecticut. September 25.

Halperin, Daniel

    2000   "Is Poverty the Root Cause of African AIDS?" *AIDS Analysis in Africa* 11: 1, 3, 15.

    1999   "Heterosexual Anal Intercourse: Prevalence, Cultural Factors and HIV Infection and Other Health Risks, Part I." *AIDS Patient Care and STDs* 13(12): 717–30.

    1998   "HIV, STS, anal sex and AIDS prevention policy in a Northeastern Brazilian City." *International Journal of STD and AIDS* 9: 294–98.

Halperin, Daniel, and Robert C. Bailey

    1999   "Male Circumcision and HIV Infection. 10 Years and Counting." *Lancet* 354(9190): 1813–15.

Halperin, Daniel, T., Marcus J. Steiner, Michael M. Cassell, Edward C. Green, Norman Hearst, Douglas Kirby, Helene D. Gayle, and Willard Cates

    2004   "Comment. The Time Has Come for Common ground on Preventing Sexual Transmission of HIV." *Lancet*. 364 (November 27): 1913–14.Halperin, Daniel T., and Brian Williams

    2001   "This Is No Way to Fight AIDS in Africa." Electronic document, Washingtonpost.com, August 26: B01, accessed September 24, 2003.

Hammar, Lawrence

    2004   "Editorial. Sexual Health, Sexual Networking and AIDS in Papua New Guinea and West Papua." *Papua New Guinea Medical Journal*. 47 (1–2) (March-June): 1–12.

Harder, Ben

    2005   "Striking a Better Bargain with HIV: New Interventions Needed to Save Infants and to Spare Mothers." *Science News*. June 18.

Heald, Suzette

    2006   "Abstain or Die: The Development of HIV/AIDS Policy in Botswana." *Journal BioSoc Science*. 38: 29041.

Hedge, Barbara

    1999   "The Impact of HIV Infection on Partners and Relatives." In *Mental Health and HIV Infection: Psychological and Psychiatric Aspects*. Jose Catalan, ed. Pp. 66–89. London: UCL Press.

Heitman, Elizabeth, and Michael Ross

    1999   "Ethical Issues in the Use of New Treatments for HIV." In *Psychosocial and Public Health Impacts of New HIV Therapies*. David G. Ostrow and Seth C. Kalichman, eds. Pp. 113–35. New York: Kluver Academic.

Helfferich, Cornelia

    2000   "The Meaning of HIV Prevention in the Context of Heterosexual Relationships. What Are Women Protecting Themselves From?" In *Partnership and Pragmatism: Germany's Response to AIDS Prevention and Care*. Rolf Rosenbrock and Michael T. Wright, eds. Pp. 171–81. New York: Routledge.

Henry J. Kaiser Family Foundation

 2005 "HIV Testing in the United States." HIV/AIDS Policy Fact Sheet. Electronic document, http://www.kff.org/hivaids/upload/ 6094–05.pdf, accessed June 28, 2006.

Hepeng, Jia

 2004 "China Approves Traditional Medicine for AIDS Patients." SciDevNet, accessed April 26, 2006.

Herdt, Gil

 2001 "Stigma and the Ethnographic Study of HIV: Problems and Prospects." *AIDS and Behavior* 5(2): 141–49.

Herdt, Gil, and Robert Stoller

 1990 *Intimate Communications: Erotics and the Study of Culture.* New York: Columbia University Press.

Herdt, Gilbert, Francis Paine Conant, E. Michael Gorman, Stephanie Kane, Norris Lang, William Leap, Michael D. Quam, Ernest Quimby, Brooke Grundfest Schoepf, and Martha C. Ward

 1990 "AIDS on the Planet: The Plural Voices of Anthropology." *Anthropology Today.* 6(3)(June): 10–15.

Herek, Gregory M., and Eric K. Glunt

 1995 "Identity and Community among Gay and Bisexual Men in the AIDS Era. Preliminary Findings from the Sacramento Men's Health Study." *AIDS, Identity and Community. The HIV Epidemic and Lesbians and Gay Men 2* (Psychological Perspectives on Lesbian and Gay Issues): 55–84.

 1991 "AIDS Related Attitudes in the United States: A Preliminary Conceptualization." *The Journal of Sex Research* 28(1): 99–125.

Herek, Gregory M., and Beverly Greene, eds.

 1995 "AIDS, Identity and Community." *AIDS, Identity and Community. The HIV Epidemic and Lesbians and Gay Men 2* (Psychological Perspectives on Lesbian and Gay Issues).

Herrell, Richard, K.

 1991 "Research and the Social Sciences." *Current Anthropology.* 32(2)(April): 199–203.

Herrn, Rainer

 2000 "Western-Style Prevention for Eastern Gay Men? AIDS Prevention in the Former East Germany." In *Partnership and Pragmatism: Germany's Response to AIDS Prevention and Care.* Rolf Rosenbrock and Michael T. Wright, eds. Pp. 143–59. New York: Routledge.

Hingson, Ralph W., Lee Strunin, Timothy Heeren, and Beth M. Berlin

 1990 "Beliefs about AIDS, Use of Alcohol and Drugs, and Unprotected Sex among Massachusetts Adolescents." *American Journal of Public Health* 80(3): 295–99.

HIV Education and Training Programs

 2000 "HIV Reporting and Partner Notification: Assisting Persons Living with HIV/AIDS." *Participant Manual April 2000.* Albany: NYSDOH AIDS Institute.

HIV-Prevent.com

　　2003　Electronic document, http://www.prevent- hiv.com/Pages/preventing. html, accessed May 7, 2006.

Hogan, Katie

　　2001　*Women Take Care: Gender, Race, and the Culture of AIDS.* Ithaca, N.Y.: Cornell University Press.

　　1998　"Sentimentality, Race and Boys on the Side." In *Women and AIDS: Negotiating Safer Practices, Care and Representation.* Nancy Roth and Linda K. Fuller, eds. Pp. 293–317. Binghamton, N.Y.: Harrington Park Press.

Hogle, Janice, A., Edward C. Green, Vinand Nantulya, Rand Stoneburner, and John Stover

　　2002　"What Happened in Uganda? Declining HIV Prevalence, Behavior Change and National Response." Washington, D.C. The Synergy Project.

Hojer, B.

　　1999　"The Community-Health Services Interface: The Critical Issue for AIDS Prevention." In *Resistances to Behavioural Change to Reduce HIV/AIDS Infection in Predominantly Heterosexual Epidemics in Third World Countries.* J. Caldwell, et al., eds. Pp. 59–80. Canberra: Health Transition Centre, National Centre for Epidermiology and Population Health, Australian National University.

Holmes, King, and William C. Miller

　　2007　*Circumcision Status Does Not Affect Women's STI Risk.* Paper Presented at the 17th Meeting of the International Society for Sexually Transmitted Diseases Research. Abstract 449. Presented July 30.

Holtgrave, David, R.

　　2007　"Costs and Consequences of the U.S. Centers for Disease Control and Prevention's Recommendations for Opt-Out HIV Testing." *PLoS Med* 4(6): e194. Electronic Document, http://medicine.plosjournals.org/perlserv/?request=get-document&doi=10.1371/journal.pmed.0040194, accessed June 12, 2007.

　　1998　*Handbook of Economic Evaluation of HIV Prevention Programs.* New York: Plenum Press.

Howell, Amy

　　2007　"UC Studies HIV Patients. Religious Support, Alienation Scrutinized." *The Enquirer.* Friday, August 10.

Hudis, Jan, and Jerome Brown

　　2002　"Custody and Permanency Planning." In *Invisible Caregivers: Older Adults Raising Children in the Wake of HIV/AIDS.* Daphne Joslin, ed. Pp. 170–86. New York: Columbia University Press.

Hughes, Jenny

　　2004　"Sexually Transmitted Infections: A Medical Anthropological Study from the Tari Research Unit, 1990–1991." *Papua New Guinea (PNG) Medical Journal.* 45 (1–2) (March–June): 128–33.

Human Rights Watch

　　2004　"A Test of Inequality: Discrimination against Women Living with HIV in the Dominican Republic." Electronic document, http://www.hrw.org/re-ports/2004/dr0704/, accessed August 3, 2006.

Hunter, Joyce, and Priscilla Alexander

1996   "Women Who Sleep with Women." In *Women's Experiences with HIV/ AIDS: An International Perspective.* Lynellen Long and E. Maxine Ankrah, eds. Pp. 43–55. New York: Columbia University Press.

Hutchinson, Janis Faye

2001   "The Biology and Evolution of HIV/AIDS." *Annual Review of Anthropology.* 30: 108–32.

Hutchison, Margaret, and Maureen Shannon

1993   "Reproductive Health and Counseling." In *Until the Cure: Caring for Women with HIV.* Ann Kurth, ed. Pp. 47–65. New Haven: Yale University Press.

Hutton, Nancy

1996   "Health Prospects for Children Born to HIV Infected Women." In *HIV, AIDS and Childbearing. Public Policy, Private Lives.* Ruth R. Faden and Nancy Kass, eds. Pp. 63–77. New York: Oxford University Press.

Hutton, Nancy, and Lawrence Wissow

1991   "Material and Newborn HIV Screening, Implications for Children and Families." In *AIDS, Women and the Next Generation: Towards a Morally Acceptable Public Policy for HIV Testing of Pregnant Women and Newborns.* Ruth R. Faden, Gail Geller, and Maxine Powers, eds. Pp. 105–18. New York: Oxford University Press.

Im-em, Wassana

2000   "Changing Partner Relations in the Era of AIDS in Upper-North Thailand." In *Resistances to Behavioural Change to Reduce HIV/AIDS Infection in Predominantly Heterosexual Epidemics in Third World Countries.* John Caldwell, Pat Caldwell, John Anarfi, Kofi Awusabo-Asare, James Ntozi, I.O. Orubuloye, Jeff Marck, Wendy Cosford, Rachel Colombo, and Elaine Hollings, eds. Pp. 157–70. Canberra: Health Transition Centre, National Centre for Epidermiology and Population Health, Australian National University.

Im-em, Wassana, Mark VanLandingham, John Knodel and Chanpen Saengtienchai

2002   "AIDS-Related Knowledge and Attitudes: A Comparison of Older Persons and Young Adults in Thailand." *AIDS Education and Prevention* 14(3): 246–62.

Inciardi, James A., Hilary L.Surratt, Paolo R.Telles, and Bin H. Pok

2001   "Sex, Drugs and the Culture of Travestismo in Rio de Janeiro." In *Transgender and HIV.* Walter O. Bockting and Sheil Kirk, eds. Pp. 1–12. Binghamton, N.Y.: Haworth Press.

Infectious Disease News

2004   Electronic document, http://www.infectiousdiseasenews.com, accessed April 30, 2005.

Innocenti, Nicol D., and Pilling, David

2001   "A Crack in the Resolve of an Industry: South Africa and the Drug Companies Have Changed Forever." *London Financial Times*, April 19.

Institute of Medicine
  2001   *No Time to Lose: Getting More from HIV Prevention.* Washington, D.C.: National Academy of Sciences.
International Center for Research on Women (ICRW)
  2005   "Common at Its Core: HIV-Related Stigma Across Contexts." (Jessica Ogden and Laura Nyblade). Electronic document, http://www.icrw.org/docs/2005_report_stigma_synthesis.pdf.: 1–45, accessed April 14, 2005.
International Committee for Prostitutes' Rights (ICPR)
  1987   "World Charter and World Whores' Congress Statements." In *Sex Work, Writings by Women in the Sex Industry.* F. Delacoste and P. Alexander, eds. Pp. 305–21. Pittsburgh: Cleis Press.
Inungu, Joseph, Eileen Malone Beach, and Jeffrey Betts
  2005   "Male Circumcision and the Risk of HIV Infection." *AIDS Read.* 15 (3): 130–35.
IOM/HDN Project Team
  2005   "The Brain Drain of Health Care Professionals from Southern Africa." AF-AIDSeForum 2005, accessed June 24, 2005.
IOM-UNAIDS Reports on Mobile Populations and HIV/AIDS 2006
  2006   "A Review of Risks and Programmes among Truckers in West Africa." Electronic document, http://www.iom.int/DOCUMENTS/PUBLICATION/EN/MIL6010070.pdf, accessed February 20, 2006.
Irvine, Mary K.
  1996   "Targeting Education for Women Who Have Sex with Women." In *AIDS Education: Reaching Diverse Populations.* Melinda K. Moore and Martin L. Forst, eds. Pp. 41–69. Westport, Conn.: Praeger.
Jacobs, Sue-Ellen, Sabine Lang, and Wesley Thomas, eds.
  1997   *Two Spirit People: Native American Gender Identity, Sexuality, and Spirituality.* Chicago/Urbana: University of Illinois Press.
Jang, Michael
  1996   "HIV/AIDS Education and Prevention in the Asian American and Pacific Islander Communities." In *AIDS Education: Reaching Diverse Populations.* Melinda K. Moore, and Martin L. Forst, eds. Pp. 83–96. Westport, Conn.: Praeger.
Jemmott, Loretta Sweet, and Suellen Miller
  1996   "Women's Reproductive Decisions in the Context of HIV Infection." In *Women and AIDS: Coping and Care.* Anne O'Leary and Loretta Sweet Jemmott, eds. Pp. 167–84. New York: Plenum Press.
Jenkins, Carol
  1999   "Resistance to Condom Use in a Bangladesh Brothel." In *Resistances to Behavioural Change to Reduce HIV/AIDS Infection in Predominantly Heterosexual Epidemics in Third World Countries.* John Caldwell, Pat Caldwell, John Anarfi, Kofi Awusabo-Asare, James Ntozi, I. O. Orubuloye, Jeff Marck, Wendy Cosford, Rachel Colombo, and Elaine Hollings, eds. Pp. 211–22. Canberra: Health Transition Centre, National Centre for Epidermiology and Population Health, Australian National University.

Jenkins, Carol, Habibur Rahman, Tobi Saidel, Jana Smarajit, and A. M. Zakir Hussain
    2002   "Rapidly Changing Conditions in the Brothels of Bangladesh: Impact on HIV/STD." *AIDS Education and Prevention* 14: 97–106.
    2001   "Measuring the Impact of Needle Exchange Programs among Injecting Drug Users through the National Behavior Surveillance in Bangladesh." *AIDS Education and Prevention* 13(5): 452–61.

Jiraphongsa, Chuleeporn, Wanna Danmoensawat, Sander Greenland, Ralph Frerichs, Taweesap Siraprapasiri, Deborah C. Glik, and
Roger Detels
    2002   "Acceptance of HIV testing and Counseling among Unmarried Young Adults in Northern Thailand." *AIDS Education and Prevention. An Interdisciplinary Journal* 14(2): 89–101.

Johnston, William I.
    1995   *HIV-Negative: How the Uninfected Are Affected by AIDS*. New York: Plenum Press.

Jooma, Miriam Bibi
    2006   "Southern Africa Assessment. Food Security and HIV/AIDS." *Africa Watch*. (14) (1): 1–8. Electronic document, http://www.iss.co.za/pubs/ASR/14No1/jooma.pdf, accessed March 17, 2006.

Joralemon, Donald
    2006   *Exploring Medical Anthropology*. 2nd ed. Boston: Pearson, Allyn, and Bacon.

Joslin, Daphne, ed.
    2002   *Invisible Caregivers: Older Adults Raising Children in the Wake of HIV/AIDS*. New York: Columbia University Press.

Kahn, James G., Elliott Marseille, and Joseph Saba
    2002   "Feeding Strategies for Children of HIV-Infected Mothers: Modeling the Trade-Off Between HIV Infection and Non-HIV Mortality." In *Quantitative Evaluation of HIV Prevention Programs*. Edward H. Kaplan and Ron Brookmeyer, eds. Pp. 202–19. New Haven: Yale University Press.

Kaiser, Shari M., Harmit S. Malik, and Michael Emerman
    2007   "Restriction of an Extinct Retrovirus by the Human TRIM5a Antiviral Protein. *Science* 316 (5832) June 22: 1756–58.

Kaiser Daily HIV/AIDS Report
    2006a   "Global Challenges. Shortage of Health Workers in Developing Countries Impeding Fight against HIV/AIDS, TB, Malaria, WHO Report Says." Electronic document, http://www.kaisernetwork.org/ daily_reports/rep_index. cfm?DR_ID=36483, accessed April 7, 2006.
    2006b   "Primate Expert to Urge U.S. Wildlife Agency to Reject HIV/AIDS Experiments on Monkeys." Electronic document, http://www.kaisernetwork. org/daily_reports/rep_index.cfm?DR_ID=38089, accessed June 23, 2006.
    2006c   "Oraquick HIV Test Accurate Despite False Positives." Electronic document, http://www.kaisernetwork.org/daily_reports/rep_index. cfm?DR_ID=34775, accessed July 15, 2006.

2006d "AP/CNN.com Examines Botswana's Routine HIV Testing Policy." Electronic document, http://www.kaisernetwork.org/daily_reports /rep_index. cfm?DR_ID=34651, accessed January 9, 2006.

2006e "IRIN News/All Africa.com Examines Debate over Focus on Abstinence in Uganda's Fight against HIV/AIDS," April 7. Electronic document, http:// www.kaisernetwork.org/daily_reports/rep_index.cfm. ?DR-ID=36482, accessed July 6, 2006.

2006f "Number of New HIV Cases in Uganda Increasing, AIDS Commission Official Says,'" May 22. Electronic document, http://www.kaisernetwork.org/ daily_reports/rep_index.cfm? DR_ID=37396, accessed May 22, 2006.

2006g "Politics and Policy: New CDC HIV Testing Recommendations Could Compromise Patients' Civil Rights, ACLU Statement Says." Electronic document, http://us.f368.mail.yahoo.com/ym/ShowLetter?MsgId=6588_1 4599298_255756_3028_12326_0_50053_46776_3770719451&Idx= 6&Y Y=49236&inc=25&order=down&sort=date&pos=0&view=a&head=b&b ox=Inbox, accessed September 25, 2006.

2006h "Reuters Examines How Some New York City Public Bathhouses Serve as Venues for Awareness of Safer Sex." Electronic document, http://www. kaisernetwork.org/daily_reports/rep_index.cfm? DR_ID=39765, accessed September 13, 2006.

2005   "Lesotho's Health Minister to Announce Plan for Universal Testing in Country." Electronic document, http://www.kaisernetwork.org/daily_ reports/rep_index.cfm?DR_ID=33296, accessed, October 25, 2005.

Kaiser Daily Women's Health Policy
2007   Lack of Sex Education in U.S. Increases Vulnerability to Sexual Assault, STIS, Former Surgeon General Elders Says. Electronic Document, http:// www.Kaisernetwork.org/daily_reports/rep_index.cfm?DR_ID=46943, accessed August 17, 2007.

Kaiser Family Foundation
2005   "Women and HIV/AIDS in the United States: Setting an Agenda for the Future." Electronic document, http://www.kff.org/hivaids/hiv102303 package. cfm., accessed March 3, 2006.

2004   The Global HIV/AIDS Epidemic: A Timeline of Key Milestones. Electronic document, http://www.kff.org/hivaids/timeline, accessed November 19, 2005.

Kaiser Family statehealthfacts.org
2006a "HIV/AIDS," Electronic document, http://www.statehealthfacts.org/cgi-bin/ healthfacts.cgi?action=compare&welcome=1&category=HIV/AIDS, accessed June 30, 2006.

2006b "New HIV/AIDS Funding Data." Electronic document, http://www.state-healthfacts. org/ linking.html, accessed September 15, 2006.

Kaiser, Jocelyn
2003   "NIH Roiled by Inquiries Over Grants Hit List." *Science.* 32(5646)(October 31): 758.

Kaisernetwork

2004a "Briefing: Survey of African Americans and Latinos on HIV/AIDS." Electronic document, http://www.kaisernetwork.org/health_cast/uploaded_files/080404_kff_aids.pdf, accessed August 6, 2005.

2004b CNN vs. ABC. Electronic document. http://www.Kaisernetwork.org/health_cast/uploaded_files/071204_ias_cnn.pdf, accessed August 11, 2005.

Kaisernetwork.org Daily Reports. National Politics and Policy

2004 "Prominent Scientists Criticize Bush Administration for Suppressing, Distorting Science, Including Abortion, Condom Data." Electronic document, http://www.kaisernetwork.org/dailyreports/rep.index.cfm?DRID=22269, accessed February 24, 2004.

Kaiser Public Opinion Spotlight

2006 "The Public's Experiences with and Attitudes about HIV Testing." Electronic document, http://www.kff.org/spotlight/hivtest/ index.cfm, accessed September 15, 2006.

Kammerer, Nina, Theresa Mason, Margaret Connors, and Rebecca Durkee

2001 "Transgenders, HIV/AIDS and Substance Abuse: From Risk Groups to Group Prevention." In *Transgender and HIV*. Walter O. Bockting and Sheila Kirk, eds. Pp. 13–38. Binghamton, N.Y.: Haworth Press.

Kane, Stephanie

1998 *AIDS Alibis: Sex, Drugs and Crime in the Americas*. Philadelphia: Temple University Press.

Kane, Stephanie, and Theresa Mason

2001 "AIDS and Criminal Justice." *Annual Review of Anthropology* 30: 457–79.

Kanuha, Vallikalei

2000 "Impact of Sexuality and Race/Ethnicity on HIV/AIDS Risk among Asian and Pacific Island American (A/PIA) Gay and Bisexual Men in Hawaii." *AIDS Education and Prevention* 12(6): 505–18.

Kaplan, Edward H. and Ron Bookmeyer, eds.

2002 *Quantitative Evaluation of HIV Prevention Programs*. New Haven: Yale University Press.

Karim, Quarraisha A.

2000 "Global Strategies for the Prevention of HIV Transmission from Mothers to Infants." *Prevention and Treatment of HIV Infection in Infants and Children* 918: 36–44.

Kaschak, Ellyn, and Leonore Tiefer, eds.

2002 *A New View of Women's Sexual Problems*. Binghamton, N.Y.: Haworth Press.

Kass, Nancy, and Ruth R.Faden

1996a "In Women's Words, The Values and Lived Experiences of HIV-Infected Women." In *HIV, AIDS and Childbearing. Public Policy, Private Lives*. Ruth R. Faden and Nancy Kass, eds. Pp. 426–43. New York: Oxford University Press,

1996b "Practices and Opinions of Health-care Providers serving HIV-Infected Women." In *HIV, AIDS and Childbearing. Public Policy, Private Lives*. Ruth R. Faden and Nancy Kass, eds. Pp. 411–25. New York: Oxford University Press.

Kates, Jennifer

    2006 "The HIV/AIDS Epidemic in the United States." Kaiser Family Foundation. February. Electronic document, http://www.kaiseredu.org/tutorials_index. asp#domestichiv., accessed February 27, 2006.

Keele, Brandon, F., Fran Van Heuveswyn, Yingying Li, Elizabeth Bailes, Jun Take-hisa, Mario L. Santiago, Frederic Bibollet-Ruche, Yalu Chen, Louise V. Wain, Florian Liegeois, Severin Loul, Eitel Mpoudi Ngole, Yanga Bienvenue, Eric Delaporte, John F. Y. Brookfield, Paul M. Sharp, George M. Shaw, Martine Peeters, and Beatrice H. Hahn

    2006 "Chimpanzee Reservoirs of Pandemic and Nonpandemic HIV-1." *Science Express*. Electronic document, www.scienceexpress.org/25May2006/ Page1/10. 1126/science.1126531, accessed May 26, 2006.

Keersmaekers, K., and A. Meheus

    1998 "Epidemiology of Sexually Transmitted Infections and AIDS in Developing Countries." In *Sexually Transmitted Infections and AIDS in the Tropics*. O. Arya and C. Hart, eds. Pp. 3–30. New York: CABI.

Kegeles, Susan M., and Joseph Catania

    1991 "Understanding Bisexual Men's AIDS Risk Behavior: The AIDS Risk-Re-duction Model." In *Bisexuality and HIV/AIDS: A Global Perspective*. Rob Tielman, Manuel Carballo, and Aart Hendriks, eds. Pp. 139–47. Buffalo, N.Y.: Prometheus.

Keinin, T.

    2002 "Governments Need to Provide Sexual Health Services to Their Clients." *Siecus Report* 30(5): 5–6.

Keller, M.

    1993 Why Don't Young Adults Protect Themselves against Sexual Transmission of HIV? Possible Answers to a Complex Question." *AIDS Education and Prevention* 5(3): 220–34.

Kelly, J.

    1995 *Changing HIV Risk Behaviors. Practical Strategies*. New York: Guilford Press.

Kempadoo, Kamala, and Jo Doezema, eds.

    1998 *Global Sex Workers. Rights, Resistance and Redefinition*. New York: Rout-ledge.

Kendall, Carl

    1996 "The Ethics of Social and Behavioral Research on Women and AIDS." In *Women's Experiences with HIV/AIDS: An International Perspective*. Lynel-len Long and E. Maxine Ankrah, eds. Pp. 370–87. New York: Columbia University Press.

Kennedy, Edward, and Henry Waxman

    2006 "Press Release: Sen. Kennedy and Rep. Waxman Call for Investigation of U.S. Trade Agreements and International Health." October 13, 2006. GenderAIDSeforum. http://www.healthdev.org/eforum, accessed October 18, 2006.

Khoshnood, Kaveh, and P. Clay Stephens

1997   "Can Needle Exchange Better Serve Women?" In *The Gender Politics of HIV/AIDS in Women: Perspectives on the Pandemic in the U.S.* Nancy Goldstein and Jennifer L. Manlowe, eds. Pp. 357–72. New York: New York University Press.

Kimoto, Diane M.

1998   "Affirming the Role of Women as Carers: The Social Construction of AIDS Through the Eyes of Mother, Friend, and Nurse." In *Women and AIDS: Negotiating Safer Practices, Care and Representation.* Nancy Roth and Linda K. Fuller, eds. Pp. 155–79. Binghamton, N.Y.: Harrington Park Press.

Kirkland, Michael

1998   "Court: HIV Covered by Federal Law." United Press International (UPI), June 25. Electronic document, http://www.aegis.com/news/upi/1998/UP980608.html, accessed May 7, 2003.

Kirshenbaum, Sheri B., and Jeffrey S. Nevid

2000   "The Specificity of Maternal Disclosure of HIV/AIDS in Relation to Children's Adjustment." *AIDS Education and Prevention* 14(1) (2000): 1–16.

Klasse, Per Johan, Robin J. Shattuck, and John P. Moore

2006   "Which Topical Microbicides for Blocking HIV-1 Transmission Will Work in the Real World?" *PLoS* 3 (9) (August).

Klein, Daniel, Leo B. Hurley, Deanna Merrill, and Charles P. Quesenberry Jr. for Consortium for HIV/AIDS Interregional Research (CHAIR)

2003   "Review of Medical Encounters in the 5 Years Before a Diagnosis of HIV-1 Infection: Implications for Early Detection." *Journal of Acquired Immune Deficiency Syndromes* 32(2): 143–52.

Klein-Alonso, Luiza

1993   "Women's Social Representation of Sex, Sexuality and AIDS in Brazil." In *Until the Cure: Caring for Women with HIV.* Ann Kurth, ed. Pp. 150–59. New Haven: Yale University Press.

Kleinman, Arthur

2000   *Writing at the Margin: Discourse Between Anthropology and Medicine.* Berkeley: University of California Press.

Koenig, Serena, Jennifer Furin, and Paul Farmer

2004   "Scaling-up Antiretroviral Therapy in Resource-limited Settings." Business Briefing: *Clinical Virology and Infectious Disease.*: 1–5.

Koo, Helen P., Cynthia Woodsong, Barbara T. Dalberth, Pheera Viswanathan, and Ashley Simons-Rudolph

2005   "Context of Acceptability of Topical Microbicides: Sexual Relationships." *Journal of Social Diseases.* 61 (1): 67–93.

Korvick, Joyce A.

1993   "Trends in Federally Sponsored Clinical Trials." In *Until the Cure: Caring for Women with HIV.* Ann Kurth, ed. Pp. 96–103. New Haven: Yale University Press.

Kottak, Conrad

   2000   *Cultural Anthropology*. New York: McGraw-Hill.

Kropp, Rhonda Y., Clea C. Samquist, Elizabeth T. Montgomery, Juan D. Ruiz, and
      Yvonne A. Maldonado

   2006   "A Comparison of Preinatal HIV Prevention Opportunities for Hispanic
           and Non-Hispanic Women in California." *AIDS Education and Prevention*.
           18 (5): 430–43.

Kruger, Jill M., and L. M. Richter

   2003   "South African Street Children at Risk for AIDS." *Children, Youth and En-
           vironments*. 13(1)(Spring): 1–15.

Kumar, Bushan

   1991   "Patterns of Bisexuality in India." In *Bisexuality and HIV/AIDS: A Global
           Perspective*. Rob Tielman, Manuel Carballo, and Aart Hendriks, eds. Pp.
           91–96. Buffalo, N.Y.: Prometheus.

Kurth, Ann

   1993   "Introduction." In *Until the Cure: Caring for Women with HIV*. Ann Kurth,
           ed. Pp. 1–18. New Haven: Yale University Press.

Kwakwa, Helena, and M. W. Ghobrial

   2003   "Female-to-Female Transmission of Human Immunodeficiency Virus."
           Clinical Infectious Diseases. 36(1 February): e40–41.

   1996   "Orphans of the HIV/AIDS Epidemic." In *AIDS in the World II. Global Di-
           mensions, Social Roots and Responses*. Jonathan M. Mann and Daniel J. M.
           Tarantola, eds. Pp. 278–86. New York: Oxford University Press.

Kwiatkowski, Carol F., and Robert E. Booth

   2000   "Differences in HIV Risk Behavior among Women who Exchange Sex for
           Drugs, Money, or Both Drugs and Money." *AIDS and Behavior* 4(3): 233–
           40.

LaBrie, Joseph, Mitch Earlywine, Jason Schiffman, Eric Pedersen, and Charles Marriot

   2005   "Effects of Alcohol, Expectancies, and Partner Type on Condom Use in
           College Males: Event-Level Analyses." *Journal of Sex Research*. 42(3)(Au-
           gust): 259–366.

Lahey, Timothy, P.

   2004   "Controversy over Vaccine Trial." AIDS Clinical Care. March 1. Elec-
           tronic document, http://www.aids-clinical-care.jwatch.org/cgi/content /
           full/2004/0301/1, accessed June 29, 2006.

Larsen, Janet

   2003   Iran: A Model for Family Planning?" Electronic document, http://www.
           theglobalist.com/DBWeb/StoryID.aspx?StoryID=2269, accessed May 3,
           2006.

Lather, Patricia Ann, and Chris Smitheres

   1997   *Troubling the Angels: Women Living with HIV/AIDS*. Boulder, Colo.: West-
           view Press.

Lau, Joseph T. F, P. C. Siah, and H. Y. Tsui

   2002   "Behavioral Surveillance and Factors Associated with Condom Use and
           STD Instances among the Male Commercial Sex Client Population in Hong

Kong-Results of Two Surveys." *AIDS Education and Prevention* 14(4): 306–17.

Lau, Joseph T. F., and H. Y. Tsui

2002 "Surveillance of HIV/AIDS-Related Attitudes and Perceptions among the General Public in Hong Kong from 1994–2000." *AIDS Education and Prevention* 14(5)(October): 419–31.

Lauter, D.

1997 "Man Infects 9 with AIDS Virus in Semi-rural NY. Health: He Reportedly Traded Drugs for Sex, Even After Diagnosed. Youngest Victim Is 13. Number Could Multiply." *Los Angeles Times*, October 28: A1.

LeClerc-Madlala, Suzanne

2005 "Popular Responses to HIV/AIDS and Policy." *Journal of Southern African Studies*. 31 (4) (December): 845–56.

2001 "Virginity Testing: Managing Sexuality in a Maturing HIV/AIDS Epidemic." *Medical Anthropology Quarterly*. 15(4): 533–52.

Leveton, Lauren B., Harold C. Sox Jr., and Michael A. Soto, eds.

1995 "HIV and the Blood Supply. An Analysis of Crisis Decision-Making." *Committee to Study HIV Transmission Through Blood and Blood Products*. Division of Health Promotion and Disease Prevention. Institute of Medicine. Washington, D.C.: National Academy Press.

LeVine, Carol

1993 "Ethical Issues." In *Until the Cure: Caring for Women with HIV*. Ann Kurth, ed. Pp. 112–24. New Haven: Yale University Press.

Levine, Martin P., Peter M. Nardi, and John H. Gagnon, eds.

1997 *Changing Times. Gay Men and Lesbians Encounter HIV/AIDS*. Chicago: University of Chicago Press.

LeVine, Robert J.

2000 "Some Recent Developments in the International Guidelines on the Ethics of Research Involving Human Subjects." *Prevention and Treatment of HIV Infection in Infants and Children* 918: 170–78.

Lhotska, Ludmilla, and Helen Armstrong

2000 "Future Directions Reinforces Previous Statement in Previous Article." In *Prevention and Treatment of HIV Infection in Infants and Children* 918: 145–55. Arthur J. Ammann and Ayre Rubenstein, eds. New York: New York Academy of Sciences.

Lightfoot-Klein, Hanny

1989 *Prisoners of Ritual: An Odyssey into Female Genital Circumcision in Africa*. New York: Harrington Park Press.

Lindegren, Mary Lou, Philip Rhodes, Laura Gordon, Patricia Fleming, State and Local Health Department HIV/AIDS Surveillance Programs, and the Perinatal Safety Review Working Group

2000 "Affirms Results of Previous Listed Study and Also Calls for Long Term Studies of Effects on Children Exposed to Antivirals Invitero, at Birth, Post Partum." *Prevention and Treatment of HIV Infection in Infants and Children* 918: 222–35.

Liu, Juliana

 2003 "HIV Positive Couple Make History in China." Reuters, August 4. Electronic document, http://story/news.yahoo.com/news?tmpl=story&cid=56 4&ncid=564&e=10&u=/nm/200–30804/+s_nm/health_china_aids_dc-2, accessed August 5, 2004.

Lochhead, Carolyn

 2003 "Gay Rights Affirmed in Historic Ruling 6–3 Decision: Supreme Court Throws Out Sodomy Law." *San Francisco Chronicle*, June 27: A1.

Long, Iris L.

 1996 "An Advocate's View of Clinical Research." In *Until the Cure: Caring for Women with HIV*. Ann Kurth, ed. Pp. 110–11. New Haven: Yale University Press.

Long, Lynellen, and E. Maxine Ankrah, eds.

 1996 *Women's Experiences with HIV/AIDS: An International Perspective*. New York: Columbia University Press.

Loue, Sana

 1999 *Gender, Ethnicity and Health Research*. New York: Klewer Academic/Plenum Press.

 1995 *Legal and Ethical Aspects of HIV-Related Research*. New York: Plenum Press.

Love, James

 2003 "Oxfam, TWN, MSF, and CPTech Press Conference Notes on Doha Exports Issue." Electronic document, http://lists.essential.org/pipermail/ip-health/2002–June/003183.html, accessed June 24, 2004.

Lovgren, Stefan

 2003 "HIV Originated with Monkeys, Not Chimps, Study Finds." *National Geographic News*, June 12. Electronic document, http://news.nationalgeographic.com, accessed June 26, 2003.

Low-Beer, Daniel, and Rand L. Stoneburner

 2003 "Behavioural and Communication Change in Reducing HIV: Is Uganda Unique?" *African Journal of AIDS Research*. 2 (1): 9–21.

Luna, Cajetan

 1997 *Youths Living with HIV: Self Evident Truths*. New York: Haworth Press.

Lyttleton, Chris

 2004 "Fleeing the Fire: Transformation and Gendered Belonging in Thai HIV/AIDS Support Groups." *Medical Anthropology*. 23: 1–40.

 2000 *Endangered Relations: Negotiating Sex and AIDS in Thailand*. Amsterdam: Harwood Academic.

Machekano, Rhoderick, William McFarland, Esther S.Hudes, Mary T.Bassett, Michael T. Mbizvo, and D. Katzenstein

 2000 "Correlates of HIV Test Results Seeking and Utilization of Partner Counseling Services in a Cohort of Male Factory Workers in Zimbabwe." *AIDS and Behavior* 4(1): 63–70.

Madhok, R., C. Forbes, and B. Evatteds

 1994 *Blood, Blood Products, and HIV*. 2nd edition. London: Chapman and Hall Medical.

Magana, J. R.
    1991   "Sex, Drugs, and HIV. An Ethnographic Approach." *Social Science and Medicine* 33: 5–9.

Malungo, Jacob R. S.
    2001   "Sexual Cleansing (Kusalazya) and Levirate Marriage (Kunjiliamung'anda) in the Era of AIDS: Changes in Perceptions and Practices in Zambia." *Social Science and Medicine* 53(3): 371–82.

    1999   "Challenges to Sexual Behavioural Changes in the Era of AIDS: Sexual Cleaning [Kusalazya] and Levirate Marriage in Zambia." In *Resistances to Behavioural Change to Reduce HIV/AIDS Infection in Predominantly Heterosexual Epidemics in Third World Countries.* John Caldwell, Pat Caldwell, John Anarfi, Kofi Awusabo-Asare, James Ntozi, I. O. Orubuloye, Jeff Marck, Wendy Cosford, Rachel Colombo, and Elaine Hollings, eds. Pp. 44–57. Canberra: Health Transition Centre, National Centre for Epidermiology and Population Health, Australian National University.

Manlowe, Jennifer, L.
    1997   "Gender, Freedom and Safety: Does the U.S. Have Anything to Learn from Cuban AIDS Policy." In *The Gender Politics of HIV/AIDS in Women: Perspectives on the Pandemic in the U.S.* Nancy Goldstein and Jennifer L. Manlowe, eds. Pp. 385–400. New York: New York University Press.

Marck, Jeff
    1999   "Long Distance Truck Drivers' Sexual Cultures and Attempts to Reduce HIV Risk Behavior amongst Them: A Review of The African and Asian Literature." In *Resistances to Behavioural Change to Reduce HIV/AIDS Infection in Predominantly Heterosexual Epidemics in Third World Countries.* John Caldwell, Pat Caldwell, John Anarfi, Kofi Awusabo-Asare, James Ntozi, I. O. Orubuloye, Jeff Marck, Wendy Cosford, Rachel Colombo, and Elaine Hollings, eds. Pp. 91–100. Canberra: Health Transition Centre, National Centre for Epidermiology and Population Health, Australian National University.

Margillo, Gina, and Todd Imahori
    1998   "Understanding Safer Sex Negotiation in a Group of Low-Income African American Women." In *Women and AIDS: Negotiating Safer Practices, Care and Representation.* Nancy Roth and Linda K. Fuller, eds. Pp. 43–69. Binghamton, N.Y.: Harrington Park Press.

Mariano, Esmeralda
    2005   "Clients' Perceptions of HIV/AIDS Voluntary Counseling and Testing (VCT) in Mozambique." Training in Sexual Health Research, Geneva 2005. WHO Scholarship: 1–6. Electronic document, http://www.gfmer.ch/Medical_education_En/PGC_SH_2005/csh_lectureplan2005.htm, accessed April 8, 2006.

Marins, Jose R., Kimberly Page-Shafer, Bertide de Azevedo, Barros Marlisa, Esther Hudes, Sanny Chen, and Norman Hearst
    2000   "Sero Prevalence and Risk Factors for HIV Infection among Incarcerated Men in Sorocaba, Brazil." *AIDS and Behavior* 4(1): 121–28.

Marks, Gary, Gordon Mansergh, Nicole Crepaz, Sheila Murphy, Lynn C. Miller, and Paul R. Appleby

    2000   "Future HIV Prevention Options for Men Who Have Sex with Men: Intention to Use a Potential Microbicide During Anal Intercourse." *AIDS and Behavior* 4(3): 279–87.

Marseille, Elliot, James G. Kahn, Francis M. Miro, Laura Guay, Philippa Musoke, Mary G. Fowler, and J. Brooks Jackson

    2000   "The Cost Effectiveness of a Single-Dose Nevirapine Regimen to Mother and Infant to Reduce Vertical HIV-1 Transmission in Sub-Sahara Africa." *Prevention and Treatment of HIV Infection in Infants and Children* 918: 53–56.

Marte, Carola, and Theresa McGovern

    2000   "Gender Equity in HIV/AIDS Clinical Trials." In *The Emergence of AIDS. The Impact on Immunology, Microbiology and Public Health.* Kenneth H. Mayer and H. F. Pizer, eds. Pp. 99–116. Washington, D.C.: American Public Health Association.

Martindale, Linda

    2007a   "Being HIV-Negative." Pamphlet, Elon University, Elon, N.C.

    2007b   "Being HIV-Positive." Pamphlet, Elon University,Elon, N.C.

    2007c   "Why Should I Worry About HIV?" Pamphlet, ElonUniversity, Elon, N.C.

Masenior, Nicole Franck, and Chris Beyrer

    2007   "The U.S. Anti-Prostitution Pledge: First Amendment Challenges and Public Health Priorities." PLoSMed 4(7):e207. Electronic document, http://medicine.plosjournals.org/perlserv/?request=get-documents&doi=10.1371/journal.pmed.0040207, accessed July 24, 2007.

Mayer, Kenneth H., and H. F Pizer, eds.

    2000   *The Emergence of AIDS: The Impact on Immunology, Microbiology and Public Health.* Washington, D.C.: American Public Health Association.

McBride, W. J., and D. Bradford

    2004   "Antiretroviral Therapy for HIV-Infected People in Papua New Guinea: Challenges and Opportunities." *Papua New Guinea Medical Journal.* 47(1–2) (March–June): 22–30.

McCaul, Mary E., Marsha Lillie-Blanton, and Dace S. Svikus

    1996   "Drug Use, HIV Stakes and Reproduction." In *HIV, AIDS and Childbearing. Public Policy, Private Lives.* Ruth R. Faden and Nancy Kass, eds. Pp. 110–39. New York: Oxford University Press.

McFarland, Willi, Sanny Chen, Darlene Weide, Robert Kohn, and Jeffrey Klausner

    2004   "Gay Asian Men in San Francisco Follow the International Trend: Increases in Rates of Unprotected Anal Intercourse and Sexually Transmitted Diseases, 1999–2002." *AIDS Education and Prevention* 16(1): 13–18.

McGrath, Janet W., David Mafigiri, Moses Kamya, Kathleen George, Richard Senvewo, Grace Svilar, Michael Kabugo, and Emmanual Mugisha

    2001   "Developing AIDS Vaccine Trials. Educational Programs in Uganda." *JAIDS. Journal of Acquired Immune Deficiency Syndromes.* 26: 176–81.

McGrath, Janet W., Charles B. Rwabukwali, Debra A. Schumann, Jonnie Pearson-

Marks, Sylvia Nakayiwa, Barbara Namande, Lucy Nakyobe, and Rebecca Mukasa

1993   "Anthropology and AIDS: The Cultural Context of Sexual Risk Behavior among Urban Baganda Women in Kampala, Uganda." *Social Science and Medicine*. 36(4): 429–39.

McGuire, Jean

2000   "Inclusion, Representation and Parity: The Making of a Public Health Response to HIV." In *The Emergence of AIDS. The Impact of Immunology, Microbiology and Public Health*. Kenneth H. Mayer and H. F. Pizer, eds. Pp.181–205. Washington, D.C.: American Public Health Association.

McIlvenna, Ted, and Clark Taylor, eds.

1999   *The Complete Guide to Safer Sex. The Institute for the Advanced Study of Human Sexuality*. 2nd edition. Ft. Lee, N.J.: Barricade Books.

McKeganey, Neil, Samuel R.Friedman, and Fabio Mesquita

1998   "The Social Context of Injectors' Risk Behavior." In *Drug Injecting and HIV Infection. Global Dimensions and Local Responses*. Gary Stimson, Don Des-Jarlais, and Andrew L. Ball, eds. Pp. 22–41. Bristol, U.K.: UCL Press.

MEDSCAPE

2004   "Combivir Added to Nevirapine May Reduce HIV Transmission." Electronic document, http://www.medscape.com/viewarticle/483512?src=mp, accessed August 3, 2005.

Melendez, Rita M., Theresa A. Exner, Anke A. Ehrhardt, Brian Dodge, Robert H. Reimen, Mary-Jane Rotheram-Borus, Marguerita Lightfoot, Daniel Hong, and the National Institute of Mental Health and Healthy Living Project Team

2006   "Health and Health Care among Male-to-Female Transgender Persons Who Are HIV-Positive." *American Journal of Public Health*. 96 (6): 1034–37.

Mellins, Claude A., Anke A. Ehrhardt, Lucille Newman, and MichaelConard

1996   "Selective Kin: Defining the Caregivers and Families of Children with HIV disease." In *Women and AIDS: Coping and Care*. Ann O'Leary and Loretta Sweet Jemmott, eds. Pp. 123–49. New York: Plenum Press.

Merson, Michael H., and Julia M. Dayton

2002   "Overview of HIV Prevention Programs in Developing Countries." In *Quantitative Evaluation of HIV Prevention Programs*. Edward H. Kaplan and Ron Brookmeyer, eds. Pp. 13–31. New Haven: Yale University Press.

Metsch, Lisa R., Clyde B.McCoy, Judy Wingerd, and Christine C. Miles

2001   "Alternative Strategies for Sexual Risk Reduction Used by Active Drug Users." *AIDS and Behavior* 5(1): 75–84.

Meursing, Karla

1999   "Barriers to Sexual Behavior Change After an HIV Diagnosis in Sub-Sahara Africa." In *Resistances to Behavioural Change to Reduce HIV/AIDS Infection in Predominantly Heterosexual Epidemics in Third World Countries*. John Caldwell, Pat Caldwell, John Anarfi, Kofi Awusabo-Asare, James Ntozi, I. O. Orubuloye, Jeff Marck, Wendy Cosford, Rachel Colombo, and Elaine Hollings, eds. Pp. 35–39. Canberra: Health Transition Centre, National Centre for Epidermiology and Population Health, Australian National University.

Meyer-Bahlburg, H.F.L, Theresa M. Exner, G. Lorenz, R. S. Gruen, J. M. Gorman, and
    Anke A. Ehrhardt
    1991   "Sexual Risk Behavior, Sexual Functioning and HIV-Disease Progression in
           Gay Men." *The Journal of Sex Research* 28(1): 3–29.
Miguez-Burbano, Maria Jose, Ricardo Navas, Mario German Forero, Ximena Bur-
bano, Noaris Rodriquez, and Gail Shor-Posner
    2002   "Evaluation of HIV Prevention and Counseling Practices of Obstetrician/Gy-
           necologist in Bogota, Colombia: Impacts on Women's Knowledge and Risk
           Practices." *AIDS Education and Prevention* 14 (Supplement A): 72–80.
Mills, Edward J., Jean B. Nachega, Ian Buchan, James Orbinski, Amir Attaran, Sonal
Singh, Beth Rachlis, Ping Wu, Curtis Cooper, Lehana Thabane, Kumahari Wilson, Gor-
don H. Guyatt, and David R. Bangsberg
    2006   "Adherence to Antiretroviral Therapy in Sub-Saharan Africa and North
           America." *Journal of the American Medical Association.* 296 (6) (August):
           679–90.
Mirochnick, Mark
    2000   "Antiretroviral Pharmacology in Pregnant Women and Their Newborns."
           Prevention and Treatment of HIV Infection in Infants and Children 918:
           287–97.
Mitchell, Carole
    1999   "Suicidal Behavior and HIV Infection." In *Mental Health and HIV Infection:
           Psychological and Psychiatric Aspects.* Jose Catalan, ed. Pp. 14–131. Lon-
           don: UCL Press.
Mitchell, Christina M., Carol E. Kaufman, and the Pathways of Choice and Healthy
    Ways Project Team
    2002   "Structure of HIV Knowledge, Attitudes and Behaviors among American
           Indian Young Adults." *AIDS Education and Prevention* 14(5): 401–18.
Mitchell, Janet L., Ilene Fennoy, John Tucker, Patricia O. Loftman, and Sterling B. Wil-
    liams
    1993   "Obstetrical Management." In *Until the Cure: Caring for Women with HIV.*
           Ann Kurth., ed. Pp. 66–80. New Haven: Yale University Press.
MMWR (Mortality and Morbidity Weekly Report)
    2006a "The Global HIV/AIDS Pandemic, 2006. August. 55 (31): 841–44. Elec-
           tronic   document,   http://www.cdc.gov/mmwr/preview/mmwrhtml   /
           mm5531a1.htm., accessed August 11, 2006.
    2006b "Revised Recommendations for HIV Testing of Adults, Adolescents and
           Pregnant Women in Health Care Settings." Prepared by Bernard M. Branson,
           M.D., H. Hunter Hansfield, M.D., Margaret A. Lampe, MPH, Robert S. Jans-
           sen, M.D., Allan W. Taylor, M.D., Sheryl B. Lyss, M.D., Jill E. Clark, MPH.
           Electronic   document,   http://www.cdc.gov/mmwr/preview/mmwrhtml/
           rr5514a1.htm, Accessed September 22, 2006.
    2003   "Advancing HIV Prevention: New Strategies for a Changing Epidemic—in
           the United States, 2003." *MMWR* 53(15): 329–32.
Moatti, Jean-Paul, and Bruno Spire
    2000   "Living with HIV/AIDS and Adherence to Antiretroviral Treatments." In

AIDS in Europe: New Challenges for the Social Sciences. Jean-Paul Moatti, Yves Souteyrand, Annick Prieur, Theo Sandfort, and Peter Aggleton, eds. Pp. 57–73. New York: Routledge.

Monti-Catania, Diane
   1997   "Women, Violence and HIV/AIDS." In *The Gender Politics of HIV/AIDS in Women: Perspectives on the Pandemic in the U.S.* Nancy Goldstein and Jennifer L. Manlowe, eds. Pp. 242–51. New York: New York University Press.

Moore, Ami, Mark Vosvick, and Foster K. Amey
   2006   "Stress, Social Support, and Derpression in Informal Caregivers to People with HIV/AIDS in Lomé, Togo." *International Journal of Sociology and Social Policy.* 26. (1/2): 63–73.

Moore, Jan, Merle E. Hamburger, David Vlahov, Ellie E. Schoenbaum, Paula Schuman, and Kenneth Mayer
   2001   "Longitudinal Study of Condom Use Patterns among Women with or at Risk for HIV." *AIDS and Behavior* 5(3): 263–73.

Morof, Diane, Asibo Wahasoka, Hannah Nivia, Tony Lupiwa, and Charles Mgone
   2004   "Sex Workers' Sexual Health and Peer Education Project in Goroka, Eastern Highlands Province, Papua, New Guinea." *Papua New Guinea Medical Journal.* 47(1–2) (March–June): 50–64.

Moynihan, Ray, and Ala Cassels
   2005   *Selling Sickness.* New York: Nation Books.

Mufune, Pemplani
   2003   "Changing Patterns of Sexuality in Northern Namibia: Implications for the Transmission of HIV/AIDS." *Culture, Health, and Sexuality* 5(5)(September):425–38.

Murphy, Laura L., Paul Harvey, and Eva Silvestre
   2005   "How Do We Know What We Know about the Impact of AIDS on Food and Livelihood in Society? A Review of Empircial Research from Rural Sub-Saharan Africa." *Human Organization.* 64(3): 265–75.

Murrain, Michelle
   1997   "Caught in the Crossfire: Women and the Search for the Magic Bullet." In *The Gender Politics of HIV/AIDS in Women: Perspectives on the Pandemic in the U.S.* Nancy Goldstein and Jennifer L. Manlowe, eds. Pp. 63–73. New York: New York University Press.

Musher, Daniel M., and Robert E. Baughn
   1999   "Syphillis." In *Textbook of AIDS Medicine.* 2nd edition. Thomas C. Merigan, John G. Bartlett, and Dani Bolognesi, eds. Pp. 297–302. Baltimore: Williams and Wilkers.

Namaste, Vivian K.
   2001   "HIV/AIDS and Female to Male Transsexuals and Transvestites: Results from a Needs Assessment." In *Transgender and HIV.* Walter O. Bockting and S. Kirk, eds. Pp. 91–99. Binghamton, N.Y.: Haworth Press.

Nanda, Serena
   2000   *Gender Diversity. Crosscultural Variations.* Prospect Heights: Waveland Press.

NASTAD (National Alliance of State and Territorial AIDS Directories)

2007   "The ADAP Watch, August 16, 2007." Electronic document, http://www.
nastad.org/Docs/Public/InFocus/2007816   NASTAD%20ADAP%20
Watch%20–%208%2016%2007%FINAL.pdf,accessed August 17, 2007.

The Nation

2004   "HIV and AIDS." Electronic document, http://www/thenation.com/direc-
tor/view.html?t=OB0301, accessed July 11, 2004.

National Institute of Allergy and Infectious Diseases (NIAID)

2002   "HIV/AIDS News. Study Shows Why Some Immune Systems Control HIV."
AIDS Community Resources Newsletter, December 14.

National Institutes of Health (NIH)

2002   "HIV/AIDS Statistics February 2002. Fact Sheet. Office of Communications and Public Liaison." National Institute of Allergy and Infectious Disease. Electronic document, http://www.niaid.nih.gov/Factsheets/aidsstaat.
htm, accessed May 27, 2002.

National Women's Health Report

2006   "Women and HIV." National Women's Health Resource Center. Electronic
document,   http://www.healthywomen.org/Documents/NationalWomen-
sHealthReport.June2006.pdf, accessed June 26, 2006.

Nedeljkovic, Srdjan

2002   "Pain Syndromes and Their Causes in HIV Infection." In *Pain Management
of HIV/AIDS Patients*. Srdjan Nedeljkovic, ed. Pp. 85–106. Boston: Butterworth-Heinemann.

Needle, R. H., S. Coyle, H. Cessari, R. Trotter, M. Clatts, S. Koester, L. Price, E. McLel-
lan, A. Finlinson, R. Bluthenthal, T. Pierece, J. Johnson, S. Jones, S., and M.
Williams

1998   "HIV Risk Behaviors Associated with the Injection Process: Multiperson
Use Drug Injection Equipment and Paraphernalia in IDU Networks." *Substance Use and Misuse*. 33: 2403–23.

Newman, Peter A.

2004   "The Sonagachi Project: A Sustainable Community Intervention Program."
AIDS Education and Prevention 16(5): 405–14.

News Feature

2003   "AIDS Vaccines: Back to Plan "A." *Nature* 423: 912–14.

Newsweek

2006   "AIDS at 25. "A Global Menace." (Global Incidence and Prevalence Map).
CXLV11 (20) (May 15): 52–53.

New York State Department of Education

1990   "Commissioner's Regulations. Subchapter G. Part 135. Health, Physical
Education, and Recreation. Section 135. 1. Health Education. (b). Health
Education in the Elementary School 2. (c) Health Education in the Secondary schools. (2)(i)(ii)." Electronic document, http://www.emso.nysed.gov/
rscs/chaps/Law-Regs/135%20Regulations.html, accessed April 27, 2004.

IXth International Conference on AIDS in Affiliation with the IVth STD World Congress

1993   Programme. Berlin: International AIDS Society, WHO, Berline Medizinis,

Che. Gesellschaft, International Union against the Venereal Diseases and Treponematoses.

Noar, Seth, Patricia J. Morokoff, and Colleen A.Redding

2002   "Sexual Assertiveness in Heterosexual Man: A Test of Three Samples." *AIDS Education and Prevention* 14(4): 330–42.

Nokes, Kathleen M.

1996   *HIV/AIDS and the Older Adult.* Washington, D.C.: Taylor and Francis.

Northridge, Mary E., and Richard Mack

2002   "Integrating Ethnomedicine into Public Health." *American Journal of Public Health* 92(10): 1561.

Nyblade, Laura, Rohini Pande, Sanyukta Mathur, Kerry MacQuarrie, Ross Kidd, Hailom Banteyerga, Akiliu Kidanu, Gad Kilonzo, Jessie Mbwambo, and Virgina Bond (ICRW)

2003   "Disentangling HIV and AIDS Stigma in Ethiopia, Tanzania and Zambia." Electronic document, http://www.icrw.org/docs/stigmareport093003.pdf, accessed March 5, 2004.

Obermeyer, Carla Makhlouf

2003   "Health Consequences of Female Circumcision: Science, Advocacy and Standards of Evidence." *Medical Anthropology Quarterly.* 17 (3): 394–412.

Odets, Walt

1995   *In the Shadow of the Epidemic: Being HIV-Negative in the Age of AIDS.* Durham, N.C.: Duke University Press.

O'Donnell, Lydia, Gail Agronick, Alexi SanDoval, Richard Duran, Athi Myint-u and Ann Stueve

2002   "Ethnic and Gay Community Attachments and Sexual Risk Behaviors among Urban Latino Young Men Who Have Sex with Men." *AIDS Education and Prevention* 14(6): 457–71.

Oetomo, Dede

2000   "Masculinity in Indonesia. Genders, Sexualities, and Identities in a Changing Society." In *Framing the Sexual Object: The Politics of Gender, Sexuality, and Power.* Robet Parker, Regina Maria Barbosa, and Peter Aggleton, eds. Pp. 46–57. Berkeley: University of California Press.

1991   "Patterns of Bisexuality in Indonesia." In *Bisexuality and HIV/AIDS: A Global Perspective.* Rob Tielman, Manuel Carballo and Aart Hendriks, eds. Pp. 119–26. Buffalo, N.Y.: Prometheus.

Office of the Medical Director

2000   "HIV Reporting and Partner Notification: Assisting Persons Living with HIV/AIDS." *Participant Manual April 2000.* Albany, N.Y.: HIV Education and Training Programs. NYSDOH AIDS Institute.

Office of the Surgeon General

2001   *The Surgeon General's Call to Action to Promote Sexual Health and Responsible Sexual Behavior 2001.* Rockville: Office of the Surgeon General.

O'Gara, Chloe, and Anna C. Martin

1993   "HIV and Breast Feeding: Informed Choice in the Face of Medical Ambiguity." In *Until the Cure: Caring for Women with HIV.* Ann Kurth, ed. Pp. 220–35. New Haven: Yale University Press.

Okie, Susan

    2006   "Fighting HIV-Lessons from Brazil." *The New England Journal of Medicine.*
           354 (19) (May 11): 1977–81.

O'Leary, Ann, and Loretta Sweet Jemmott, eds.

    1996   *Women and AIDS: Coping and Care.* New York: Plenum Press.

O'Leary, Ann, May Kennedy, Katina A. Pappas-DeLuca, Marlene Nkete, Vicki Beck,
      and Christine Galavotti

    2007   Association Between Exposure to an HIV Storyline in the "Bold and the
           Beautiful" and HIV-Related Stigma in Botswana. *AIDS Education and Pre-*
           vention (19) (3) (June): 209–17.

Omohundro, John T.

    2000   *Careers in Anthropology.* 2nd edition. New York: McGraw-Hill.

Orubuloye, I. O, John C. Caldwell, and Pat Caldwell

    1994   "Sexual Networking in the Ekti District of Nigeria." In *Sexual Network-*
           ing and AIDS in Sub-Saharan Africa: Behavioural Research and the Social
           Context. I. O. Orubuloye, John C. Caldwell, Pat Caldwell, and Gigi Santow,
           eds. Pp. 13–32. Canberra: Health Transition Centre, Australian National
           University.

Orubuloye, I. O., John C. Caldwell, Pat Caldwell, and Gigi Santow, eds.

    1994   *Sexual Networking and AIDS in Sub-Saharan Africa: Behavioural Research*
           and the Social Context. Canberra: Health Transition Centre, Australian Na-
           tional University.

Orubuloye, I. O., and Folakemi Orguntimehin

    1999   "Death Is Preordained, It Will Come When It Is Due: Attitudes of Men to
           Death in the Presence of AIDS in Nigeria." In *Resistances to Behavioural*
           Change to Reduce HIV/AIDS Infection in Predominantly Heterosexual Epi-
           demics in Third World Countries. John Caldwell, Pat Caldwell, John Anarfi,
           Kofi Awusabo-Asare, James Ntozi, I. O. Orubuloye, Jeff Marck, Wendy
           Cosford, Rachel Colombo, and Elaine Hollings, eds. Pp. 101–11. Canberra:
           Health Transition Centre, National Centre for Epidermiology and Popula-
           tion Health, Australian National University.

Osmond, Dennis H., and Nancy Padian

    1999   "Sexual Transmission of HIV." In *The AIDS Knowledge Base: A Textbook on*
           HIV Disease from the University of California, San Francisco School of Med-
           icine and San Francisco General Hospital. Philip T. Cohen, Merle A. Sande,
           and Paul Volberding, eds. Pp. 1.9–17. Philadelphia: Williams and Wilkins.

Ostrow, David G.

    2000   "Sex and Drugs and the Virus." In *The Emergence of AIDS. The Impact on*
           Immunology, Microbiology, and Public Health. Kenneth H. Mayer and H. F.
           Pizer, eds. Pp. 63–76. Washington, D.C.: American Public Health Associa-
           tion.

O'Sullivan, Sue, and Pratibha Parmer

    1992   *Lesbians Talk (Safer) Sex.* London: Scarlett Press.

Outwater, Anne

    1996   "The Socioeconomic Impact of AIDS on Women in Tanzania." In *Women's*
           Experiences with HIV/AIDS: An International Perspective. Lynellen Long

and E. Maxine Ankrah, eds. Pp. 112–22. New York: Columbia University Press.

Owens, Douglas K.

1998   "Economic Evaluations of HIV Screening Interventions." In *Handbook of Economic Evaluation of HIV Prevention Programs*. David R. Holtgrave, ed. Pp. 81–101. New York: Plenum Press.

Owens, Douglas K., D. M. Edwards, and Ross Schacter

2002   "Costs and Benefits of Imperfect HIV Vaccines: Implications for Vaccine Development and Use." In *Quantitative Evaluation of HIV Prevention Programs*. Edward H. Kaplan and Ron Brookmeyer, eds. Pp. 143–71. New Haven: Yale University Press.

Padian, Nancy

1998   "Prostitute Women and AIDS: Epidemiology." *AIDSCare* 2(6): 413–19.

Padian, Nancy S., Stephen C. Shiboski, and Nicholas P. Jewell

1991   "Female to Male Transmission of Human Immunodeficiency Virus." *Journal of the American Medical Association* 266(12): 1664–67.

PAEG (SUNY Potsdam AIDS Education Group)

2002   Electronic document, http://www2.potsdam.edu/clubs/aeg/index.html, accessed April 3, 2003.

Palmedo, M.

2002   "EU, U.S. Accused of Backing Out of AIDS Drug Pledge." Reuters, June 25.

Pankhurst, Alula

2006   "Conceptions of and Responses to HIV/AIDS: Views from Twenty Ethiopian Rural Villages." *ESRC Research Group on Wellbeing in Developing Countries*. WeD Ethiopia. Electronic document, http://www.wed-ethiopia.org/working.htm, accessed March 1.

Papua New Guinea Medical Journal

2004   "Focus Issue on Sexual Health." 47(1–2)(March–June).

Parameswaran, Gowri

2004   "The Cuban Response to the AIDS Crisis. Human Rights Violation or Just Plain Effective?" *Dialectica Anthropology*. 28: 289–305.

Parker, Barbara, and David W. Patterson

1996   "Sexually Transmitted Diseases as Catalysts of HIV/AIDS in Women." In *Women's Experiences with HIV/AIDS. An International Perspective*. Lynellen Long and E. Maxine Ankrah, eds. Pp. 205–19. New York: Columbia University Press.

Parker, Richard G.

2001   "Sexuality, Culture, and Power in HIV/AIDS research." *Annual Review of Anthropology* 30: 163–79.

1994   "Sexual Cultures, HIV Transmission, and AIDS Prevention." *AIDS* 8:S309–S314.

Parker, Richard G., and Peter Aggleton, eds.

1999   *Culture, Society and Sexuality. A Reader*. London: UCL Press.

Parker, Richard G., Regina Maria Barbosa, and Peter Aggleton, eds.

2000   *Framing the Sexual Subject: The Politics of Gender, Sexuality and Power*. Berkeley: University of California Press.

Parker, Richard G., Delia Easton, and Charles Klein
    2000   "Structural Barriers and Facilitators in HIV Prevention: A Review of International Research." *AIDS* 14 (Supplement 1): S22–S32.

Parker, Richard G., and Anke A. Ehrhardt
    2001   "Through an Ethnographic Lens: Ethnographic Methods, Comparative Analysis and HIV/AIDS Research." *AIDS and Behavior* 5(2): 105–14.

Parker, Richard G., Gil Herdt, and Manuel Carallo
    1991   "Sexual Culture, HIV Transmission, and AIDS Research." *The Journal of Sex Research* 28(1): 77–98.

Parker, Robert, and Peter Aggleton
    2003   "HIV and AIDS-Related Stigman and Discrimination: A Conceptual Framework and Implication for Action." *Social Science and Medicine* 57 (1) (July): 13–24.

Parsons, Jeffrey T., Perry N. Halkitis, Richard J. Wolkowitz, Cynthia A. Gómez, and the Seropositive Urban Men's Study Team
    2003   "Correlates of Sexual Risk Behaviors among HIV Positive Men Who Have Sex with Men." *AIDS Education and Prevention* 15(5): 383–400.

Pastore, Doris R., Pamela J. Murray, and Linda Juszczak
    2001   "Position Paper. School-Based Health Center. Position Paper of the Society for Adolescent Medicine." *Journal of Adolescent Health*. 29: 448–50.

Patton, Cindy
    1994   *Last Served?: Gendering the HIV Epidemic*. Bristol, U.K.: Taylor and Francis.

PBS (Public Broadcasting System)
    2004   "AIDS Warriors." PBS, August 15.

PEPFARWATCH
    2006   Electronic document, http://www.pepfarwatch.org/, accessed September 15, 2006.

Perrone, Bobette, H. Henrietta Stockel, and Victoria Krueger
    1989   *Medicine Women, Curanderas, and Women Doctors*. Norman: University of Oklahoma Press.

Peterson, John L.
    1995   "AIDS-Related Risk and Same-Sex Behaviors among African-American Men." *AIDS, Identity and Community. The HIV Epidemic and Lesbians and Gay Men 2* (on Lesbian and Gay Issues):85–104.

Peterson, John L., Susan Folkman, and Roger Bakeman
    1996   Stress, Coping, HIV Status, Psycho-social Resources, and Depressive Mood in African-American Gay, Bisexual, and Heterosexual Men. *American Journal of Community Psychology* 24(4):461–87.

Pfeiffer, James
    2004   Condom Social Marketing, Pentecostalism, and Structural Adjustment in Mozambique: A Clash of AIDS Prevention Messages. *Medical Anthropology Quarterly* 18(1): 77–103.

Phanuphak, P., and D. Serwadda
    1998   "HIV Infection and AIDS." In *Sexually Transmitted Infections and AIDS in the Tropics*. O. Arya and C. Hart, eds. Pp. 67–98. New York: CABI.

Pilkington, Constance J., Whitney Kern, and David Indest
    1994   "Is Safer Sex Necessary with a 'Safe' Partner? Condom Use and Romantic
            Feelings." *The Journal of Sex Research* 31: 203–11.
Pitayanon, Sumalee, Sukontha Kongsin, and Wattana Janjareon
    1997   "The Economic Impact of HIV/AIDS Mortality on Households in Thai-
            land." In *The Economics of HIV and AIDS: The Case of South and Southeast
            Asia*. David Bloom and Peter Godwin, eds. Pp. 53–101. New York: Oxford
            University Press.
Planned Parenthood Federation of America
    2004   *Fact Sheets, Reports and White Papers*. Electronic document, http://www.
            plannedparenthood.org/library/factsheets.htm, accessed April 9, 2005.
Podolefsky, Aaron, and Peter J. Brown, eds.
    2002   *Applying Anthropology: An Introductory Reader*. 7th edition. New York:
            McGraw-Hill.
Pointdexter, Cynthia C.
    2002   "Stigma, Isolation, and Support for HIV-Affected Elder Parental Surro-
            gates." In *Invisible Caregivers: Older Adults Raising Children in the Wake of
            HIV/AIDS*. Daphne Joslin, ed. Pp. 42–63. New York: Columbia University
            Press.
Policy Watch
    2003a   *September 2003 Policy Watch*. San Francisco: SFAF.
    2003b   *October 2003 Policy Watch*. San Francisco: SFAF.
Population Resource Center 2001
    2001   "Executive Summary: Child and Infant Health and Mortality." Electronic
            document, http://www.prcdc.org/summaries/childinfant/childinfant.html,
            accessed December 15, 2003.
Pott, Elisabeth
    2000   "AIDS Prevention Campaigns for the General Public. The Work of the Fed-
            eral Centre for Health Education." In *Partnership and Pragmatism: Germa-
            ny's Response to AIDS Prevention and Care*. Rolf Rosenbrock and Michael
            T. Wright, eds. Pp. 61–72. New York: Routledge.
Powers, Madison
    1991   "Legal Protections of Confidential Medical Information and the Need for
            Antidiscrimination Laws." In *AIDS, Women and the Next Generation: To-
            wards a Morally Acceptable Public Policy for HIV Testing of Pregnant Wom-
            en and Newborns*. Ruth R. Faden, Gail Geller, and Madison Powers, eds. Pp.
            221–55. New York: Oxford University Press.
Preidt, Robert
    2005   "Placental Leak Drives Mom-to-Baby HIV Transmission." University of
            North Carolina at Chapel Hill, News Release, November 21.
Preston-Whyte, Eleanor
    1999   "Reproductive Health and the Condom Dilemma: Identifying Situational
            Barriers to HIV Protection in South Africa." In *Resistances to Behavioural
            Change to Reduce HIV/AIDS Infection in Predominantly Heterosexual Epi-
            demics in Third World Countries*. John Caldwell, Pat Caldwell, John Anarfi,
            Kofi Awusabo-Asare, James Ntozi, I. O. Orubuloye, Jeff Marck, Wendy

Cosford, Rachel Colombo, and Elaine Hollings, eds. Pp. 139–55. Canberra: Health Transition Centre, National Centre for Epidermiology and Population Health, Australian National University.

Preston-Whyte, Eleanor, Christine Varga, Herman Oosthuizen, Rachel Roberts, and Frederick Blasé

2000   "Survival Sex and HIV/AIDS in an African City." In *Framing the Sexual Object: The Politics of Gender, Sexuality and Power.* Richard G. Parker, Regina Maria Barbosa, and Peter Aggleton, eds. Pp. 165–90. Berkeley: University of California Press.

Quinn, Andrew

2004   "S. Africa to Limit Use of AIDS Drug Nevirapene." Electronic document, http://www.alertnet.org/thenews/newsdesk/L1335224.2.htm, accessed July 14, 2004.

Quist-Arcton, Ofeibea

2001   "Kenya: Powell Hears Demand for More U.S. Action on AIDS." Electronic document, http://allafrica.com/stories/200105270001.html, accessed September 15, 2006.

Raffaelli, Marcela, and Mariana Suarez-Al-Adam

1998   "Reconsidering the HIV/AIDS Prevention Needs of Latino Women in the United States." In *Women and AIDS: Negotiating Safer Practices, Care, and Representation.* Nancy Roth and Linda K. Fuller, eds. Pp. 9–41. Binghamton, N.Y.: Harrington Park Press.

Rambaut, Andrew, David L. Robertson, Oliver G. Pybus, Martine Peeters and Edward C. Holmes

2001   "Human Immunodeficiency virus: Phylogeny and the origin of HIV-1." *Nature* 410: 1047–48.

Ramirez, Juan R., William D. Crano, Ryan Quist, Michael Burgoon, Eusebio M.Alvaro and Joseph Grandpere

2002   "Effects of Fatalism and Family Communication on HIV/AIDS Awareness Variations in Native American and Anglo Parents and Children." *AIDS Education and Prevention. An Interdisciplinary Journal* 14(1): 29–40.

Ramos, Laura J.

1997   "Si Tenemos Sexo con Mujeres, pero no somos Marimachas." In *The Gender Politics of HIV/AIDS in Women: Perspectives on the Pandemic in the U.S.* Nancy Goldstein and Jennifer L. Manlowe, eds. Pp. 127–54. New York: New York University Press.

Rasing, Thera

2003   "HIV/AIDS and Sex Education among the Yough in Zambia: Towards Behavioural Change." Electronic Document, http://www.ascleiden.nL/pdf/paper09102003.pdf, accessed July 31, 2007.

Reaney, Patricia

2004   "AIDS Robs 15 Million Children of Parents—U.N. Report." Electronic document, http://www.reuters.com/newsArticle.jhtml?type=topNews&storyID=6560892, accessed July 14, 2005.

Reback, Cathy J., and Emilia L. Lombardi

2001   "HIV Risk Behaviors of Male-to-Female Transgenders in a Community-

Based Harm Reduction Program." In *Transgender and HIV. Risks, Prevention and Care.* Walter O. Bockting and Sheila Kirk, eds. Pp. 59–68. Binghamton, N.Y.: Haworth Press.

Reilly, Thom, and Grace Woo
  2001   "Predictors of High-Risk Sexual Behavior among People Living with HIV/
          AIDS." *AIDS and Behavior* 5(3): 205–17.

ReligiousTolerance.org
  2007   "Prohibiting Same-Sex Marriages in the U.S.: Federal and State DOMA." De-
          cember 22. Electronic document, http://www.religioustolerance.org/hom_
          Mar6.htm, accessed April 15, 2008.

Renaud, Michelle Lewis
  1997   *Women at the Crossroads. A Prostitute Community's Response to AIDS in
          Urban Senegal.* Netherlands: Gordon and Breach.

Repke, J., and T. Johnson
  1991   "HIV Infection and Obstetric Care." In *AIDS, Women and the Next Genera-
          tion: Towards a Morally Acceptable Public Policy for HIV Testing of Preg-
          nant Women and Newborns.* R. Faden, G. Geller, and M. Powers, eds. Pp.
          94–104. New York: Oxford University Press.

Rhodes, Tim, and Alan Quirk
  1998   "Drug Users' Sexual Relationships and the Social Organization of Risk." *So-
          cial Science and Medicine.* 46 (2): 157–69.

Roberts, Leslie, and Jon Cohen
  2006   "Special Online Collection: HIV/AIDS-Latin America & Caribbean." *Sci-
          ence.* 313 (5786) (July 28): 467–89.

Robertson, Jennifer, ed.
  2005   *Same-Sex Cultures and Sexualities. An Anthropological Reader.* Malden,
          Mass.: Blackwell.

Robinson, Beatrice "Bean" E., Gary Uhl, Michael Miner, Walter O. Bockting, Karen E.
Schletema, B. R. Simon Rosser, and Bonita Westover
  2002   "Evaluation of a Sexual Health Approach to Prevent HIV among Low-In-
          come Urban Primarily African-American Women: Results of a Random-
          ized Control Trial." *AIDS Education and Prevention* 14 (Supplement A):
          81–96.

Rochman, Sue
  2002a "A Woman's Needs." *HIV Plus* 5(3): 23–26.
  2002b "Parental Rites." *HIV Plus* 5(1): 16–20.
  2001a "A Tropical Timebomb." *HIV Plus* 4(5): 28–32.
  2001b "Conscience or a Con of Science." *HIV Plus* 4(5): 16–20.

Rogers, Lesley
  2001   *Sexing the Brain.* New York: Columbia University Press.

Rogers, Susan J., Liu Ying, Xin Yan Tao, Kee Fung, and Joan Kaufman
  2002   "Reaching and Identifying the STD/HIV Risk of Sex Workers in Beijing."
          AIDS Education and Prevention 14(3): 217–27.

Rom, Mark C.
  1997   *Fatal Extraction: The Story Behind the Florida Dentist Accused of Infecting*

His Patients with HIV and Poisoning Public Health. 1st edition. San Francisco: Jossey-Bass.

Roscoe, Will
   1998   *Changing Ones. Third and Fourth Genders in Native North America.* New York: St. Martin's Press.

Roscoe, Will, ed.
   1988   *Living the Spirit—Gay Indians Tell Their Own Stories: A Gay American Indian Anthology.* New York: St. Martin's Press.

Rosenbrock, Rolf, and Michael T. Wright, eds.
   2000   *Partnership and Pragmatism: Germany's Response to AIDS Prevention and Care.* New York: Routledge.

Ross, Michael W., B. R. Simon Rosser, Greta R. Bauer, Walter O. Bockting, Beatrice "Bean" E. Robinson, Deborah L. Rugg, and Eli Coleman
   2001   "Drug Use, Unsafe Sexual Behavior and Internalized Homonegativity in Men Who Have Sex with Men." *AIDS and Behavior* 5(1): 97–103.

Roth, Nancy
   1995   "Structuring Burnout: Interactions among HIV/AIDS Health Workers, Their Clients, Organizations, and Society." In *Health Workers and AIDS: Research, Intervention and Current Issues in Burnout and Response.* Lydia Bennett, David Miller, and Michael Ross, eds. Pp. 73–91. Chur: Harwood Academic.

Roth, Nancy, Myra S. Nelson, C. Collins, P. Emmons, M. Alderson,Frank Hatcher, Barbara Nabrit-Stephens and Mary Ann South
   1998   "Enacting Care: Successful Recruitment, Retention and Compliance of Women in HIV/AIDS Medical Research." In *Women and AIDS: Negotiating Safer Practices, Care and Representation.* N. Roth and L. Fuller, eds. Pp. 181–207. Binghamton, N.Y.: Harrington Park Press.

Roth, Nancy L., and Fuller, L. K., eds.
   1998   *Women and AIDS. Negotiating Safer Practices, Care and Representation.* Binghamton, N.Y.: Harrington Park Press.

Rothenberg, Karen H.
   1996   "Reproductive Choice and Reality: An Assessment of Tort Liability for Health-Care Providers and Women with AIDS." In *HIV, AIDS and Childbearing. Public Policy, Private Lives.* Ruth R. Faden and Nancy Kass, eds. Pp. 178–213. New York: Oxford University Press.

Rotheram-Borus, Mary Jane, Joyce Hunter, and Margaret Rosario
   1995   "Coming Out as Lesbian or Gay in the Era of AIDS." *AIDS, Identity and Community. The HIV Epidemic and Lesbians and Gay Men* 2 (Psychological Perspectives on Lesbian and Gay Issues).

Rotheram-Borus, Mary Jane, Mark Kuklinski, and Kathyrn Mattes
   2001   "Providers' Awareness of HIV Testing Policies and Perceived Testing Practices." *AIDS and Behavior* 4(4): 411–13.

Rowland, Laura Joh
   1994   *Shinju.* New York: HarperCollins.

Ruan, Fang Fu
  1991   *Sex in China: Studies in Sexology in Chinese Culture*. New York: Plenum
         Press.
Rubin, Gayle S.
  1997   "Elegy for the Valley of Kings: AIDS and the Leather Community in San
         Francisco, 1981–1996." In *In Changing Times. Gay Men and Lesbians En-
         counter HIV/AIDS*. Martin P. Levine, Peter M. Nardi, and John H. Gagnon,
         eds. Chicago: University of Chicago Press: 101–44.
Rubin, Lillian
  1983   *Intimate Strangers: Men and Women Together*. Scranton, Pa.: HarperCol-
         lins.
Russell, Sabin
  2004   "AIDS in India. First of a Five-Part Series. South Asia's Smoldering Threat."
         San Francisco Chronicle, July 4: A1.
Rust, Paula C., ed.
  2000   *Bisexuality in the United States. A Social Science Reader*. New York: Co-
         lumbia University Press.
Saah, Alfred
  1996   "The Epidemiology of HIV and AIDS in Women." In *HIV, AIDS and Child-
         bearing. Public Policy, Private Lives*. Ruth R. Faden and Nancy Kass, eds. Pp.
         3–14. New York: Oxford University Press.
San Francisco AIDS Foundation
  2004   Electronic document, http://www.sfaf.org, accessed November 19, 2004.
Sanguiwa, M. Gloria, Olga A. Grinstead, Margaret Hogan, Davis Mwakagile, Japhet
Z. L. Killewo, Steven E. Gregorich, M. Claudes Kamenga, Michael D. Sweat, Kevin R.
O'Reilly, Samuel Kalibala, Eric van Praag, and Thomas J. Coates
  2000   "Characteristics of Individuals and Couples Seeking HIV-1 Prevention Ser-
         vices in Dar Es Salaam, Tanzania: The Voluntary HIV-1 Counseling and
         Testing Efficacy Study." *AIDS and Behavior* 4(1): 25–33.
Sarche, Jennifer
  2003   "The Quest for an HIV Vaccine." *San Francisco Chronicle*, May 18: D5.
Sargeant, Carolyn F., and Caroline B. Bretell, eds.
  1996   *Gender and Health. An International Perspective*. Upper Saddle River, N.J.:
         Prentice Hall.
Satcher, David
  2001   *The Surgeon General's Call to Action to Promote Sexual Health and Re-
         sponsible Sexual Behavior*. Washington, D.C.: United States Department of
         Health and Human Services, June 28.
Saul, Janet, Fran H. Norris, Kelly K. Bartholow, Denise Dixon, Mike Peters, and Jan
     Moore
  2000   "Heterosexual Risk for HIV among Puerto Rican Women." *AIDS and Be-
         havior* 4(4): 361–71.
Scheper-Hughes, Nancy
  1994   "AIDS, Public Health and Human Rights in Cuba." *Anthropology Newsletter*
         34(7): 48, 46.

1993   "AIDS, Public Health and Human Rights in Cuba." *Lancet*. 342 (8877) (October):965–67.

Schneider, Beth E., and Nancy E. Stoller, eds.

1995   *Women Resisting AIDS. Feminist Struggles of Empowerment*. Philadelphia: Temple University Press.

Schoepf, Brooke

2004   "Review of African Political Economy. Briefing. #3(No.100): 372–76. Filed in Book as ROAPE UGA 04.

2003a   "What Happened in Uganda?" *AIDS and Anthropology Bulletin*. The Newsletter of the AIDS and Anthropology Research Group 15(2): 8–13.

2003b   "Uganda: Lessons for AIDS Control in Africa." *Review of African Political Economy*. #30(No.98): 553–72.

2001   "International AIDS Research in Anthropology: Taking a Critical Perspective on the Crisis." *Annual Review of Anthropology* 30: 335–61.

1993   "AIDS Action Research with Women in Kinshasa, Zaire." *Social Science and Medicine* 33(11): 1401–13.

Schoofs, Mark

1999   "AIDS: The Agony of Africa: Part 1: The Virus Creates a Generation of Orphans." *The Village Voice*, November 3–9. Electronic document, http://www.villagevoice.com/specials/africa/, accessed March 23, 2003.

Schooley, Robert T.

1996   "Antiretroviral Chemotherapy." In *A Clinical Guide to HIV and AIDS*. Gary Wormser, ed. Pp. 273–95. Philadelphia: Lippincott-Raven.

SciDev.Net

2003   Electronic document, http://www.scidev.net/, accessed December 13, 2005.

Seabrook, Jeremy

2001   *Travels in the Skin Trade. Tourism and the Sex Industry*. 2nd edition. Sterling, U.K.: Pluto Press.

Semba, Richard D.

2000   "Mastitis and Transmission of Human Immunodeficiency Virus Through Breast Milk." *Prevention and Treatment of HIV Infection in Infants and Children* 918: 156–62.

Setel, Philip

1999   *A Plague of Paradoxes: AIDS, Culture and Demography in Northern Tanzania*. Chicago: University of Chicago Press.

Sex Information and Education Council of the United States (SIECUS)

2002   "Sexuality Education in the United States. A Decade of Controversy: Special Edition" 31(6): 1–47.

2000   "Current Issues Relating to Pregnancy and Parenting" 30(3): 1–29.

Sex Toys

2006   "Using Toys. Cleaning and Caring for Your Sex Toy." Electronic document, http://www.sextoys.co.uk/buyers-guide/lifetime.asp, accessed July 26, 2006.

Sherman, Mark

    2003 "NIH Questions Researchers on AIDS Grants." Electronic document, http://www.newsday.com/news/nationworld/nation/sns-ap-nih-sex-aids,0,392560.story?coll=ny-news-navigation, accessed December 15, 2004.

Shernoff, Michael, ed.

    1999 *AIDS and Mental Health Practice: Clinical and Policy Issues.* Binghamton, N.Y.: Haworth Press.

Sherr, Lorraine

    1999 "HIV Disease and Its Impact on the Mental Health of Children." In *Mental Health and HIV Infection: Psychological and Psychiatric Aspects.* Jose Catalan, ed. Pp. 42–65. London: UCL Press.

Shilts, Randy

    1987 *And the Band Played On: Politics, People, and the AIDS Epidemic.* New York: St. Martin's Press.

SIECUS Report

    2006 "Revamped Federal Abstinence-Only-Until-Marriage Programs Go Extreme." Electronic document, http://www.siecus.org/media/press/press 0124.html, accessed February 18, 2006.

    2005 "Sex Workers: Perspectives in Public Health and Human Rights." 33(2) (Spring).

    2003 "Sexuality and Education in the United States. A Decade of Controversy." Special Edition. 31 (6): 1–47.

    2001 "Current Issues Related to Pregnancy and Parenting." 30 (3): 1–29.

Simoni, Jane M., Penelope Demas, Hyacinth R. C. Mason, Jill, A. Drossman, and Michelle Davis

    2000 "HIV Disclosure among Women of African Descent: Associations with Coping, Social Support and Psychological Adaptation." *AIDS and Behavior* 4(2): 147–58.

Simpson, B. Joyce, and Ann Williams

    1993 "Caregiving: A Matriarchal Tradition Continues." In *Until the Cure: Caring for Women with HIV.* Ann Kurth, ed. Pp. 210–11. New Haven: Yale University Press.

Singer, Merrill

    2005 *Something Dangerous. Emergent and Changing Illicit Drug Use and Community Health.* Long Grove, Ill.: Waveland Press.

    2003a "As Goes the Drug Trade, So Goes the Drug-Related AIDS Epidemic. Breaking the Link." *AIDS and Anthropology Bulletin.* The Newsletter of The AIDS and Anthropology Research Group 15(2): 3–4.

    2003b "Stigma Still: HIV Stigmatization as Social Terrorism." *AIDS & Anthropology Bulletin* 15(1): 1–2.

Singer, Merrill, Elsa Huertas, and Glenn Scott

    2000 "Am I My Brother's Keeper?: A Case Study of the Responsibilities of Research." *Human Organization.* 59(4)(Winter): 389–400.

Singer, Merrill, Tom Stopka, Susan Shaw, Claudia Santelices, David Buchanan, Wei Tang, Karen Khooshnood, and Robert Heyner
>   2005   "Lessons from the Field: The Fight against AIDS among Injection Drug Users in Three New England Cities." *Human Organization*. 64(2): 179–91.

Sittitrai, Wiresit, Tim Brown and Sirapone Virulrak
>   1991   "Patterns of Bisexuality in Thailand." In *Bisexuality and HIV/AIDS: A Global Perspective*. Rob Tielman, Manuel Carballo and Aart Hendriks, eds. Pp. 97–117. Buffalo, N.Y.: Prometheus.

Sobo, Elisa
>   1995   *Choosing Unsafe Sex: AIDS—Risk Denial among Disadvantaged Women*. Philadelphia: University of Pennsylvania Press.

Solomon, Suniti, Aylur Ganesh, Maria Ekstrand, John Barclay, Narayan Kumarasamy, Jeffrey Mandel and Christina Lindan
>   2000   "High HIV Seropositivity at an Anonymous Testing Site in Chennai, India: Client Profile and Trends over Time." *AIDS and Behavior* 4(1): 71–81.

Somlai, Anton M., Jeffrey A. Kelly, Eric Benotsch, Cheryl Gore-Felton, Dmitri Ostrovski, Timothy McAuliffe, and Andrei P. Zozlov
>   2002   "Characteristics and Predictors of HIV Risk Behaviors among Injection-Drug-Using Men and Women in St. Petersburg, Russia." *AIDS Education and Prevention* 14(4): 295–305.

Sontag, Susan
>   1995   *Illness as Metaphor and AIDS and Its Metaphors*. London: Peter Smith.

Sottile, A., S. Nedeljkovic, and C. Warfield
>   2002   "Postoperative Pain Management for the HIV-Infected Patient." In *Pain Management of HIV/AIDS Patients*. Srdjan Nedeljkovic, ed. Pp. 107–18. Boston: Butterworth-Heinemann.

South African Development Commission (SADC)
>   2006   "Expert Think Tank Meeting on HIV Prevention in High- Prevalence Countries in Southern Africa." REPORT. Maseru, Lesotho. 10–12 May. Electronic document, http://www.sadc.int/attachments/news/ SADCPrev Report. pdf, accessed August 17, 2006.

Spira, Rosemary, Emmanuel Lagarde, Jean Bouyea, Karim Seck, Catherine Enel, Ndeye Toure Kane, Jean-Pierre Piau, Ibrahima Ndoye, Souleymayne Mboup and Gilles Pison, for the MECORA Group
>   2000   "Preventive Attitudes Toward the Treatment of AIDS: Process and Determinants in Rural Senegal." *AIDS Education and Prevention. An Interdisciplinary Journal* 12(6): 544–56.

Stall, Ron, and David W. Purcell
>   2000   "Intertwining Epidemics: A Review of Research on Substance Use Among." *AIDS and Behavior* 4(2): 181–92.

Stanley, Laura D.
>   1999   "Transforming AIDS. The Moral Management of Stigmatized Identity." *Anthropology and Medicine* 6(1)(April): 103–20.

Stanmeyer, Anastasia
>   2003   "New freedom for Gays in China. A challenge for an activist." *San Francisco Chronicle*, February 9: A14.

Steffan, Elfriede, and Michael Kraus

2000   "The Umbrella Network. AIDS, STD Prevention and Prostitution on the Eastern Border of Germany." In *Partnership and Pragmatism: Germany's Response to AIDS Prevention and Care.* Rolf Rosenbrock and Michael T. Wright, eds. Pp. 182–92. New York: Routledge.

Stimson, Gerry V., and Katchit Choopanya

1998   "Global Perspectives on Drug Injecting." In *Drug Injecting and HIV Infection. Global Dimensions and Local Responses.* Gerry V. Stimson, Don C. DesJarlais and Andrew Ball, eds. Pp. 1–21. Bristol, U.K.: UCL Press.

Stimson, Gerry V., Don C. DesJarlais and Andrew Ball, eds.

1998   *Drug Injecting and HIV Infection.* Global Dimensions and Local Responses. Bristol, U.K.: UCL Press.

Stine, Gerald

1997   *Acquired Immune deficiency Syndrome. Biological, Medical, Social and Legal Issues.* 3rd edition. Upper Saddle River: Prentice Hall.

Stoller, Nancy, E.

1998   *Lessons from the Damned: Queers, Whores and Junkies Respond to AIDS.* New York: Routledge.

Stoto, Michael A., Donna A. Almario and Marie C. McCormick, eds., Committee on Perinatal Transmission of HIV, Division of Health Promotion and Disease Prevention, Institute of Medicine and Board on Children, Youth and Families, Commission on Behavioral and Social Sciences and Education, National Research Council, Institute of Medicine

1999   *Reducing the Odds. Preventing Perinatal Tranmission of HIV in the U.S.* Washington, D.C.: National Academy Press.

Strauss, Sheila M., and Gregory P. Falkin

2001   "HIV-Negative Women's Communication of Their HIV Status to Their Intimate Partners." *AIDS Education and Prevention. An Interdisciplinary Journal* 13(5): 403–12.

Stryker, Jeff, and Thomas J. Coates

1997   "Home Sccess HIV Testing. What Took So Long?" (editorial comment). *Archives of Internal Medicine* 157 (3): 261–62.

Stumpf, Terrill Lee

1996   "Hospice Care for Persons with AIDS in the United States." Ph.D. dissertation, School of Nursing, University of California, San Francisco.

SUNY Potsdam AIDS Education Group (SUNY-PAEG)

2003   Electronic document, http://www2.potsdam.edu/clubs/aeg/index.html, accessed April 30, 2003. State University of New York (SUNY).

Susser, Ida

2001   "Sexual Negotiations in Relation to Political Mobilization: The Prevention of HIV in a Comparative Context." *AIDS and Behavior* 5(2): 163–72.

Svenson, G., K. Johnson, and B. Hanson

1999   "Utilising Peer Education and Target Group Empowerment to Induce Behaviour Change on a University Campus." In *Mental Health and HIV Infection: Psychological and Psychiatric Aspects.* J. Catalan, ed. Pp. 43–50. London: UCL Press.

Svensson, Jonas

2007   HIV/AIDS and Islamic Religious Education in Kisumu, Kenya. *International Journal of Qualitative Studies on Health and Well Being* 2(3):179–92.

Synergy Project

2003   "Women's Experiences with HIV Serodisclosure in Africa: Implications for VCT and PMTCT." Washington, D.C.: USAID Office of HIV/AIDS. Electronic document, http://www.synergyaids.com/documents/VCTDisclosureReport.pdf, accessed March 18, 2004.

TAC (Treatment Action Campaign)

2004a "Invest in Health, Not War." Electronic document, http://www.tac.org.za/HealthNotWar.htm, accessed June 14, 2004.

2004b Electronic document, http://www.tac.org.za, accessed June 14, 2004.

Tavris, Carol

1992   *The Mismeasure of Woman. Why Women Are Not the Better Sex, the Inferior Sex, or the Opposite Sex.* London: Touchstone Press.

Taylor, Clark L., and David Lourea

1992   "HIV Prevention: A Dramaturgical Analysis and Practical Guide to Creating Safer Sex Interventions." *Medical Anthropology* 14 (2–4) (May): 243–84.

Teunis, Niels

2001   "Same-Sex Sexuality in Africa: A Case Study from Senegal." *AIDS and Behavior* 5(2): 173–82.

Thomas, Lewis

1984   *The Lives of a Cell. Notes of a Biology Watcher.* New York: Bantam.

Thomas, Patricia

2001   *Big Shot. Passion, Politics, and the Struggle for an AIDS Vaccine.* New York: Public Affairs Press.

Thornton, Robert

2002   *Traditional Healers, Medical Doctors, and HIV/AIDS in Gauteng and Mpumalanga Provinces, South Africa.* Report to the Margaret Sanger Institute and Medical Care Development International Center. October 16.

Thuy, Nguyen Thi Than, Christina P. Landan, Nguyen Xuan Hoan, John Barclay and Ha Ba Khiem

2000   "Sexual Risk Behavior of Women in Entertainment Services, Vietnam." *AIDS and Behavior* 4(1): 93–101.

Tielman, Rob

1991   "Conclusions." In *Bisexuality and HIV/AIDS: A Global Perspective.* Rob Tielman, Manuel Carballo and Aart Hendriks, eds. Pp. 211–20. Buffalo, N.Y.: Prometheus.

Tielman, Rob, Manuel Carballo and Aart Hendriks, eds.

1991   *Bisexuality and HIV/AIDS. A Global Perspective.* Buffalo, N.Y.: Prometheus.

Tokars, Jerome I., and William J. Martone

1996   "Infection Control Considerations in HIV Infection." In *A Clinical Guide to HIV and AIDS.* Gary Wormser, ed. Pp. 253–71. Philadelphia: Lippincott-Raven.

Torres, M. I., S. Tuthill, S. Lyon-callo, C. M. Hernandez, and P. Epkind
    1999   Focused Female Condom Education and Trial: Comparison of Young Af-
            rican-American and Puerto Rican Women's Assessments. *International
            Quarterly of Community Health Education* 18(1):49–68.
Tortu, Stephanie, James McMahon, Rahul Hamid, and Alan Neaigus
    2000   "Drug-Using Women's Sexual Risk: An Event Analysis." *AIDS and Behavior*
            4(4): 329–40.
Traditional Medicine and HIV/AIDS Workshop
    2006   (April 18 and 19) Anthropology Department SOAS. Centre for African
            Studies and Support from UNESCO Culture and HIV/AIDS Programme
            and the British Academy.
Treichler, Paula
    1999   "The Burdens of History: Gender and Representation in AIDS Discourse,
            1981–1988." In *How to Have Theory in an Epidemic: Cultural Chronicles of
            AIDS*. Paula Treichler, ed. Durham, N.C.: Duke University Press: 42–98.
Tross, Susan
    2001   "Women at Heterosexual Risk for HIV in Inner-City New York: Reaching
            the Hard Reach." *AIDS and Behavior* 5(2): 131–39.
Trotter II, Robert T., Anne M. Bowen, and James M. Potter
    1995   "Network Models for HIV Outreach and Prevention Programs for Drug
            Users." *NIDA Monograph Series*. Washington, D.C. National Institute on
            Drug Abuse NIDA Monograph Series No. 151: 144–80.
Ulin, Priscilla R., Michel Cayemittes, and Robert Gringle
    1996   "Bargaining for Life: Women and the AIDS Epidemic in Haiti." In *Women's
            Experiences with HIV/AIDS: An International Perspective*. Lynellen Long
            and E. Maxine Ankrah, eds. Pp. 90–111. New York: Columbia University
            Press.
UNAIDS
    2007   "2007 AIDS Epidemic Update." Electronic document, http://www.unaids.
            org/en/knowledgecentre/HIV/Data/EipUpdate/EpiUpdArchive/2007, ac-
            cessed April 11, 2008.
    2006   "Report on the Global Epidemic." Electronic document, http://www.unaids.
            org/en/HIV_data/2006GlobalReport/default.a sp, accessed July 6, 2006.
    2004   "UNAIDS 2004 Report on the Global AIDS Epidemic 2004." Electronic
            document, http://www.unaids.org/bangkok2004/report_pdf.html, ac-
            cessed July 12, 2004.
    2002   "Report on the Global HIV/AIDS Epidemic." Geneva, Switzerland: UN-
            AIDS. Electronic document, www.unaids.org, accessed December 15,
            2004.
UNAIDS/UNFPA/UNIFEM
    2004   "Woman and AIDS: Confronting the Crisis." Electronic document, http://
            www.unaids.org/NetTools/Misc/DocInfo.aspx?href=http:/lgra_doc_ow/
            WEBcontent1Documents/pub/Publications/External_D   ocuments/UN-
            FPA_UNAIDS_UNIFEM_womenAIDS_en.pdf, accessed December 15,
            2004.

Underhill, Kristen, Paul Montgomery, and Don Operario
    2007   Sexual Abstinence-Only programmes in High-Income Countries: A System-
            atic Review. *British Medical Journal* (BMJ). Published July 26, 2007. Elec-
            tronicdocument,http://www.bjm.com/cgi/content/full/bmj39245.446586.
            BEv1, accessed August 14, 2007.

UNFPA
    2007a   Gender Responsive Budgeting and Women's Reproductive Rights: A Re-
            source Pack. Electronic document, http://www.unfpa.org/upload/lib_pub_
            file/686_filename_gender_eng.pdf, accessed August 16,2007.
    2007b   Culture in the Context of UNFPA Programming. ICPD+10 Survey Results
            on Culture and Religion. Electronic document, http://www.unfpa.org/up-
            load/lib_pub_file/528_filename_culture_religion.pdf, accessed August 16,
            2007.

United Nations Events and Observances. World AIDS Day
    2003   "Live and . . . Let Live!" Secretary-General Kofi Annan's message on the
            occasion of World AIDS Day, observed 1 December, 2003. Electronic doc-
            ument, http://www.un.org/events/aids/worldaidsday2003.html, accessed
            April 25, 2008.

United Nations Special Session on HIV/AIDS
    2001   "Declaration of Commitment on HIV/AIDS." Electronic document, http://
            www.unaids.org/whatsnew/others/un_specialdeclaration02081_en.htm, ac-
            cessed August 22, 2006.

Upton, Rebecca, L.
    2003   "Women Have No Tribe." Connecting Carework, Gender and Migration in
            an Era of HIV/AIDS in Botswana." *Gender and Society.* 17(2)(April): 314–
            22.

USAID/AIDSMark
    2003   "Male Circumcision: Current Epidemiological and Field Experience. Pro-
            gram and Policy Implications for HIV Prevention and Reproductive Health."
            Conference Report May: 1–34. Washington, D.C.: USAID.

U.S. Department of Health and Human Services (HHS)
    2003   "HHS Extends Use of Rapid HIV Test to New Sites Nationwide." Electronic
            document, http://www.hhs.gov/news/press/2003pres/20030131b.html, ac-
            cessed February 4, 2006.

U.S. Philanthropic Commitments for HIV/AIDS
    2006   "Funders Concerned About AIDS." Electronic document, http://
            www.fcaaids.org/   documents/FCAA_2006_ResourceTracking_comp.
            pdf#search= %22MAC%20Cosmetics%20Supports%20HIV%2FAIDS%20
            Interventions%22, accessed September 22, 2006.

Valdiserri, Ronald O.
    2004   "Mapping the Roots of HIV/AIDS Complacency: Implications for Program
            and Policy Development." *AIDS Education and Prevention* 16(5): 426–39.

van den Boom, Frans, Fabrizio Starace and Erik Hochheimer
    1999   "Euthansia, Physician-Assisted Suicide and AIDS." In *Mental Health and
            HIV Infection: Psychological and Psychiatric Aspects.* Jose Catalan, ed. Pp.
            132–50. London: UCL Press.

Van de Perre, Philippe
  2000 "Breast Milk Transmission of HIV-1. Laboratory and Clinical Studies." In *Prevention and Treatment of HIV Infection in Infants and Children* 918: 122–27. Arthur J. Ammann and Ayre Rubenstein, eds. New York: New York Academy of Sciences.

Van Der Straten, A., K.A. Vernon, K. R. Knight, C. A. Gomez, and Nancy S. Padian
  1998 "Managing HIV among Sero-Discordant Couples: Serostatus, Stigma, and Sex." *AIDS Care* 10(5)(October): 533–48.

Van Hollen, Cecilia
  2007 "Navigating HIV, Pregnancy, and Childbearing in South India: Pragmatics and Restraints in Women's Decision-Making." *Medical Anthropology* 26(1): 7–52.

Varga, Christina A.
  1999 "South African Young People's Sexual Dynamics: Implications for Behavioural Responses to HIV/AIDS." In *Resistances to Behavioural Change to Reduce HIV/AIDS Infection in Predominantly Heterosexual Epidemics in Third World Countries*. John Caldwell, Pat Caldwell, John Anarfi, Kofi Awusabo-Asare, James Ntozi, I. O. Orubuloye, Jeff Marck, Wendy Cosford, Rachel Colombo and Elaine Hollings, eds. Pp. 13–34. Canberra: Health Transition Centre, National Centre for Epidermiology and Population Health, Australian National University.

Vernon, Irene S.
  2001 *Killing Us Quietly*. Lincoln: University of Nebraska Press.

Viaud, Loune, Paul Farmer, and Guitele Nicoleau
  1997 "Haitian Teens Confront Aids: A Partners in Health Program on Social Justice and AIDS Prevention." In *The Gender Politics of HIV/AIDS in Women: Perspectives on the Pandemic in the U.S.* Nancy Goldstein and Jennifer L. Manlowe, eds. Pp. 302–36. New York: New York University Press.

Vincke, John, and Ralph Bolton
  2002 "Therapy Adherence and Highly Active Antiretroviral Therapy: Comparison of Three Sources of Information." *AIDS Patient Care and STDs*. 16(10): 487–95.

VitaminShoppe
  2003 Electronic document, http:www//vitaminshoppe.com, accessed December 15, 2004.

Volberding, Paul, Judith A. Aberg, and Philip P. Cohen, eds.
  1999 *The San Francisco General Hospital Handbook of HIV Management: The Practical Management of HIV-Infected Patients*. New York: Parthenon Publication Group.

Volk, Jonathan E., and Cheryl Koopman
  2001 "Factors Associated with Condom Use in Kenya: A Test of the Health Belief Model." *AIDS Education and Prevention*. An Interdisciplinary Journal 13(6): 495–508.

Vollmer, Tim
  2000 Editorial. "When Cultures Clash Over AIDS." *San Francisco Chronicle*, July.

VSO-RAISA

    2003   "Men, HIV and AIDS Regional Conference 2003 Report back." Electronic document, http://www.kubatana.net/docs/hivaid/vso_men_aids_2003.pdf, accessed December 15, 2004.

Walters, Karina L., and Jane M. Simoni

    2005   Trauma and HIV Risk among Urban Gay/Bisexual/Two Spirit American Indian Men: Research Findings and Decolonizing Practics Strategies. *National HIV Prevention Conference.*June 12–15. (Abstract # M2–D 1402): 1–2.

    2004   HIV Prevention Issues among American Indian and Alaska Native "Two Spirits." *The Linkage. Newsletter of the Behavioral and Social Science Volunteer Program* (Summer):1, 3.

Wang, Quanyi, and Michael W. Ross

    2002   "Differences Between Chat Room and E-Mail Sampling Approaches in Chinese Men Who Have Sex with Men." *AIDS Education and Prevention* 14(5): 361–66.

Waterston, Alisse

    1997   "Anthropological Research and the Politics of HIV Prevention: Towards a Critique of Policy and Priorities in the Age of AIDS." *Social Science and Medicine.* 44(9): 1381–91.

Watkins, Sherri A.

    2002   "Demographic Shifts Change National Face of HIV/AIDS." *SIECUS REPORT* 31(1): 10–12.

Waxman, Henry A.

    2006   "Waxman Response to New Federal Abstinence Programs." Electronic document, http://www.democrats.reform.house.gov/Documents/200602161212 50–30800.pdf, accessed February 23, 2006.

Weeks, Margaret R., Katie Mosack, Maryann Abbott, Laurie Novick Sylla, Barbara Valdes, and Mary Prince

    2004   "Microbicide Acceptability among High-Risk Urban U.S. Women: Experiences and Perceptions of Sexually Transmitted HIV Prevention." *Sexually Transmitted Diseases* 31 (11):682–90.

Weil, Andrew

    2004   *Health and Healing.* Boston: Houghton-Mifflin.

    1998   *Health and Healing.* Boston: Houghton-Mifflin.

Weiss, Helen A., Maria A. Quigley, and Richard J. Hayes

    2000   "Male Circumcision and Risk of HIV Infection in Sub-Saharan Africa: A Systematic Review and Meta-analysis." *AIDS* 14: 2361–70.

Westerhaus, Michael, and Arachu Castro

    2006   "How Do Intellectual Property Law and International Trade Agreements Affect Access to Antiretroviral Therapy?" *PLoS.* 3 (8) (August).

Whelehan, Patricia

    2001a   *An Anthropological Perspective on Prostitution.* Mellen Studies in Anthropology vol. 4. Lewiston: Edwin Mellen Press.

    2001b   "Cross-Cultural Sexual Practices." In *The Encyclopedia of Women and Gender.* J. Worell, ed. Pp. 291–302. San Diego: Academic Press.

White, Edith
    1999   *Breastfeeding and HIV/AIDS. The Research, the Politics, the Women's Responses*. Jefferson: McFarland.

White, Luise
    1990   *The Comforts of Home: Prostitution in Colonial Nairobi*. Chicago: University of Chicago Press.

Whitehead, Tony
    1997   Urban Low-Income African-American Men, HIV/AIDS, and Gender Identity. *Medical Anthropology Quarterly*. New Series 11(4)(December):411–47.

Wilkinson, Willy
    1997   "HIV/AIDS and Asian Pacific Islander Wome. In *The Gender Politics of HIV/ AIDS in Women: Perspectives on the Pandemic in the U.S.* Nancy Goldstein and Jennifer L. Mnlowe, eds. PP. 168–77. New York: New York University Press.

Williams, Brian G., James O. Lloyd-Smith, Eleanor Gouws, Catherine Hankins, Wayne M. Getz, John Hargrove, Isabelle de Zoysa, Christopher Dye, and Bertran Auvert
    2006   "The Potential Impact of Male Circumcision on HIV in Sub-Saharan Africa." *PloS Med*. 3 (7) (July): e 262, accessed July 11, 2006.

Williams, Mark, H. Virginia McCoy, Anne Bowen, Lori Saunders, Robert Freeman, and Danyang Chen
    2001   "An Evaluation of a Brief HIV Risk Reduction Intervention Using Empirically Derived Drug Use and Sexual Risk Indices." *AIDS and Behavior* 5(1): 31–44.

Wilson, Bianca D. M., and Robin L. Miller
    2003   "Examining Strategies for Culturally Grounded HIV Prevention: A Review." *AIDS Education and Prevention* 15(2):184–202.

Wissow, Lawrence, Nancy Hutton, and Deven C. McGraw
    1996   "Psycho Social Issues for Children Born to HIV-Infected Mothers." In *HIV, AIDS and Childbearing. Public Policy, Private Lives*. Ruth R. Faden and Nancy Kass, eds. PP. 78–95. New York: Oxford University Press.

Wolffers, Ivan, and Mascha Bevers
    1997   *Sex Work, Mobility and AIDS in Kuala Lumpur, Malaysia*. Amsterdam: Caram-Asia and the Free University of Amsterdam.

Wolffers, Ivan, and Fernandez I. Josie, eds.
    1999   *Health Compromised. Two Preliminary Studies of Bangladeshi Female Migrant Workers. One in Malaysia and One in Bangladesh*. Kuala Lumpur: CARAM Asia.

Women's Bulletin
    2003   "Hot Topic: HIV/AIDS: A Women's Human Rights Crisis." *Women's Human Rights Online Bulletin January*. Electronic document, http://www.amnestyusa.org/women, accessed June 4, 2004.

World Health Organization (WHO)
    2007   "WHO and UNAIDS Announce Recommendations from Expert Consultations on Male Circumcision for HIV Prevention." Electronic document, http://www.who/inthiv/mediacentre/news68/en/index.htm, accessed April 12, 2007.

2004a Electronic document, http://www.who.int/en/, accessed June 11, 2004.

2004b "XVth International AIDS Conference, Bangkok 2004." Electronic document, http://www.who.int/3by5/bangkok/en/, accessed July 13, 2004.

1946/1948 "1946/1948 Preamble to the Constitution of the World Health Organization as adopted by the International Health Conference New York, 19–22 June 1946. Signed on 22 July 1946 by the representatives of 61 States (Official Records of the World Health Organization, No.2, p 100) and entered into force on 7 April 1948." Electronic document, http://www.who.int/about/definition/enl, accessed February 18, 2003.

World Health Organization/CDC

2004 "Prevention of Mother-to-Child Transmission of HIV. Generic Training Package Participant Manual." Geneva, Switzerland: World Health Organization. Electronic document, http://womenchildrenhiv.org/pdf/p03–pi/pi-60/IntroOverview_PM.pdf, accessed October 1, 2004.

World Health Organization

2007 WHO and UNAIDS announce recommendations from expert consultation on male circumcision for HIV prevention. Electronic Document, http://www.who.int/hiv/mediacentre/news68/en/index.html, accessed April 2, 2007.

Working Groups on Girls

2004 "Empowering Girls to Beat HIV/AIDS." Electronic document, http://www.girlsrights.org/factsheets/Empower%20Girls%20web%20version.pdf, accessed May 14, 2004.

Wormser, Gary P., and Harold W. Horowitz

1996 "Care of the Adult Patient with HIV Infection." In *A Clinical Guide to HIV and AIDS*. Gary Wormser, ed. Pp. 21–68. Philadelphia: Lippincott-Raven.

Wu, Zunyou, Roger Detels, Guoping Ji, Chen Xu, Keming Rou, Huancheng Ding, and Virginia Li

2002 "Diffusion of HIV/AIDS Knowledge, Positive Attitudes and Behaviors ThroughTraining of Health Professionals in China." *AIDS Education and Prevention* 14(5): 379–90.

Wu, Zunyou, Guoming Qi, Yi Zeng, and Roger Detels

1999 "Knowledge of HIV/AIDS among Health Care Workers in China." *AIDS Education and Prevention. An Interdisciplinary Journal* 11(4): 353–64.

XIIIth International AIDS Conference

2000 Electronic document, http://www.cdc.gov/nchstp/od/Durban/default.htm, accessed December 15, 2004.

XVth International AIDS Conference (IAC)

2004 Electronic document, http://www.aids2004.org, accessed December 15, 2004.

Yanushka-Bunn, Janice, Sondra E. Solomon, Carol Miller, and Rex Forehand

2007 Management of Stigma in People with HIV: Re-examination of the HIV-Stigma Scale. *AIDS Education and Prevention* 19 (3)(June): 198–208.

Yee, Daniel

2003a "AIDS Spread Due to Complacency." *Lincoln Journal Star*, August 3: 3A.

2003b "CDC Has New Way to Track HIV cases." *Lincoln Journal Star*, July 27: 4A.

Yep, Gust A.

   1998   "Safer Sex Negotiation in Cross-Cultural Romantic Dyads: An Extension of Ting-Toomey's Face Negotiation Theory." In *Women and AIDS: Negotiating Safer Practices, Care and Representation*. N. Roth and L. Fuller, eds. Pp. 81–100. Binghamton, N.Y.: Harrington Park Press.

Zavos, Michael

   1993   "Legal Considerations." In *Until the Cure: Caring for Women with HIV*. Ann Kurth, ed. Pp. 126–43. New Haven: Yale University Press.

Zierler, Sally, and Nancy Krieger

   2000   "Social Inequality and HIV Infection in Women." In *The Emergence of AIDS. The Impact of Immunology, Microbiology and Public Health*. Kenneth H. Mayer and H. F. Pizer, eds. Pp. 77–97. Washington, D.C.: American Public Health Association.

Index

Patricia E. Whelehan, Ph.D., is professor of anthropology and AIDS Education Coordinator at the State University of New York, Potsdam. She is the editor of *Women and Health: Cross-Cultural Perspectives* (1988), coauthor of *Perspectives on Human Sexuality* with Anne Bolin (1999) and *Interdisciplinary Perspectives on Human Sexuality: Biological, Psychological, and Cultural Perspectives* (2009), and author of *An Anthropological Perspective on Prostitution: The World's Oldest Profession* (2001). In 2007, she received the President's Award for Excellence in Service. In 1999 and 2008, she received the Phi Eta Sigma award for Outstanding Teacher of the Year, and in 2008 she was inducted into Phi Kappa Phi, a national honor society that recognizes scholarly distinction.

Thomas Budd, Ph.D., is professor of biology at St. Lawrence University, Canton, N.Y., and has taught a seminar on the subject of AIDS/HIV for many years. His areas of scholarship include immunology, cell/molecular biology, and ultrastructural pathology, with the results of his research appearing in 50 peer-reviewed publications.

CPSIA information can be obtained
at www.ICGtesting.com
Printed in the USA
LVOW01s1922291015
460351LV00004B/6/P